BMA

IMMUNOLOGY
FOR MEDICAL STUDENTS

IMMUNOLOGY
FOR MEDICAL STUDENTS
THIRD EDITION

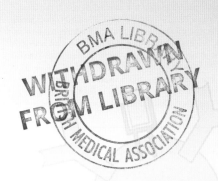

MATTHEW HELBERT, MBChB, FRCP, FRCPath, PhD
Consultant Immunologist
Yorkshire, United Kingdom

ELSEVIER

ELSEVIER

1600 John F. Kennedy Blvd.
Ste 1800
Philadelphia, PA 19103-2899

IMMUNOLOGY FOR MEDICAL STUDENTS, THIRD EDITION ISBN: 978-0-7020-6801-0

Notices

Knowledge and best practice in this field are constantly changing. As new research and experience broaden our understanding, changes in research methods, professional practices, or medical treatment may become necessary.

Practitioners and researchers must always rely on their own experience and knowledge in evaluating and using any information, methods, compounds, or experiments described herein. In using such information or methods they should be mindful of their own safety and the safety of others, including parties for whom they have a professional responsibility.

With respect to any drug or pharmaceutical products identified, readers are advised to check the most current information provided (i) on procedures featured or (ii) by the manufacturer of each product to be administered, to verify the recommended dose or formula, the method and duration of administration, and contraindications. It is the responsibility of practitioners, relying on their own experience and knowledge of their patients, to make diagnoses, to determine dosages and the best treatment for each individual patient, and to take all appropriate safety precautions.

To the fullest extent of the law, neither the Publisher nor the authors, contributors, or editors, assume any liability for any injury and/or damage to persons or property as a matter of products liability, negligence or otherwise, or from any use or operation of any methods, products, instructions, or ideas contained in the material herein.

Library of Congress Cataloging-in-Publication Data
Names: Helbert, Matthew, author. | Nairn, Roderick. Immunology for medical students. Preceded by (work):
   Title: Immunology for medical students / Matthew Helbert.
Description: Third edition. | Philadelphia, PA : Elsevier, [2017] | Preceded by: Immunology for medical
   students / Roderick Nairn, Matthew Helbert. 2nd ed. c2007. | Includes index.
Identifiers: LCCN 2016008040 | ISBN 9780702068010 (pbk. : alk. paper)
Subjects: | MESH: Immune System Phenomena
Classification: LCC QR181 | NLM QW 504 | DDC 616.07/9—dc23 LC record available at http://lccn.loc.gov/
2016008040

Content Strategist: Lauren Willis
Senior Content Development Specialist: Joanie Milnes
Publishing Services Manager: Patricia Tannian
Senior Project Manager: Carrie Stetz
Design Direction: Ryan Cook

Printed in China

Last digit is the print number: 9 8 7 6 5 4 3 2 1

Working together
to grow libraries in
developing countries

www.elsevier.com • www.bookaid.org

■ PREFACE TO THE THIRD EDITION

This book continues to be focused on meeting the needs of medical students. I have concentrated on a simple, straightforward treatment of immunology, reflecting an acknowledgment of the time constraints in today's curricula.

Immunology is one of the most rapidly developing medical sciences and, to respond to this, considerable new material has been added to this book, including regulation of the immune system, T-cell subsets, and epigenetics. There is also new material on some of the recent technical developments, notably vaccines, biopharmaceuticals, and screening and diagnostic tests. These technologies are already widely adopted, and some familiarity will be important for all medical students. New clinical vignettes have been added that focus on everyday clinical material. Material that, over time, has lost some of its impact on clinical practice has been reduced in this edition (eg, allelic exclusion, gene rearrangement studies to diagnose lymphoma, tetramers).

Medical students face two specific problems with immunology. First, the immune system is complex because it has evolved to respond to a wide range of pathogens. Many students find themselves bogged down in the complexities of the molecules and cells of the immune system without having an understanding of how these components work together to fight infection. We begin our book with two overview chapters that explain what the immune system does and then how the components fit together. We recommend that students begin by reading these chapters. Further on in the text, there are more short, integrating overview chapters. These are not just for review, but to make sure that students understand how the material that they have read fits into the overall system. The second problem is that medical students do not always immediately see the relevance of immunology to day-to-day clinical practice. We have included clinical correlations throughout the text that explain how understanding the science of immunology can translate into understanding real clinical problems.

2016   M.H.

■ PREFACE TO THE SECOND EDITION

In preparing this edition, we have made improvements throughout to improve the clarity and accessibility of the material. We have updated all the sections, particularly the material dealing with Toll-like receptors, dendritic cells, regulatory T cells, and HIV. We have also introduced a final chapter on therapeutic immunomodulation, which is being increasingly utilized in clinical practice. This chapter also aims to review what readers will have learned about the immunopathogenesis of several diseases covered in earlier chapters. In response to user feedback, we have also enhanced the clinical vignettes, which form the final pages of most chapters. Although some of these vignettes describe rare diseases, we hope that this helps readers link their studies of immunology with real clinical experience.

2007   R.N. & M.H.

■ PREFACE TO THE FIRST EDITION

We have recognized the need for an immunology book that is primarily focused on the needs of medical students for as long as we have been teachers of immunology. This book has been written to fill this need. Immunology can fall into different medical school courses or modules. Often, immunology is taught in the Host Defense course, which integrates basic and clinical immunology (including allergy, immunopathology, etc). Some medical schools, however, teach basic immunology and clinical immunology in two separate courses. This book should be useful for either curriculum organization.

We have concentrated on a simple, straightforward treatment of the subject. The book is relatively short and contains the topics we considered important to understanding the human immune system and its role in protecting us from disease. This reflects our acknowledgment of the time constraints on today's medical student. With new topics and a growing amount of information considered to be essential, there are increasing demands on students. It is therefore important to have a concise, readable textbook, and that has been our primary aim. Most chapters contain the information needed for a typical 50-minute large class or small-group teaching/learning session. This, of course, means that details dear to the hearts of some immunologists are not covered!

We are aware of two specific problems that medical students have with immunology. First, the immune system is complex because it has evolved to respond to the wide range of pathogens. Many students find themselves bogged down in the complexities of the molecules and cells of the immune system without having an understanding of how these components work together to fight infection. We begin our book with two overview chapters that explain what the immune system does and then how the components fit together. We recommend that students begin by reading these chapters. Further on in the text, there are more short, integrating overview chapters. These are not just for revision, but are there to make sure that students understand how the material that they have read fits into the overall system. The second problem is that medical students do not always immediately see the relevance of immunology to day-to-day clinical practice. We have included clinical correlations throughout the text that explain how understanding the science of immunology can translate into understanding real clinical problems.

The book is a concise description of the science of immunology, a topic that defies a final complete description because there is much still to be learned. Hopefully, we will have succeeded in inducing an interest and appreciation of the relevance of immunology to medical students, to form the basis for a lifetime of learning about the immune system and its potential for use in improving the human condition. Most medical students today could still be practicing medicine in 40 to 50 years. Approximately 50 years ago, immunology was still in its infancy. For example, we did not know the chemical structure of antibody molecules in any detail, and treatments such as organ transplantation had not been carried out. The next 50 years will likely bring equally important advances in the field. History suggests that we would be foolish to try to predict what they will be. We hope that you enjoy participating in these advances in immunology and their application to human disease as much as we have in those that we have been privileged to observe in our careers.

2002   R.N. & M.H.

ACKNOWLEDGMENTS

I am grateful to the very helpful team at Elsevier. I thank Antonio Benitez for his kindness and support, without which writing this edition would have been impossible. My greatest debt is to the patients who have informed and inspired me over the last 30 years.

HOW TO USE THIS BOOK

Immunology for Medical Students is organized to be read comprehensively. The flow of the book is from genes and molecules to cells and organs, and finally to the immune system as an integrated system protecting the body from infection and helping to maintain the health of the body.

Section I introduces the basic concepts and is essential for an understanding of the language of immunology.

Section II continues with a discussion of the antigen recognition molecules, that is, antibodies, T-cell receptors, and the molecules encoded by the major histocompatibility complex.

Section III deals with immune physiology, the role of the cells and organs of the immune system in the response to a pathogen.

Section IV discusses the innate immune system and its connections to the adaptive immune system.

Section V considers hypersensitivity, allergy and asthma, autoimmunity, immunodeficiency, and transplantation and includes a new chapter on therapeutic immunomodulation.

Throughout the book, the core knowledge objectives are listed as Learning Points at the ends of chapters to aid in review. There are also several integrating overview chapters (eg, "Review of Antigen Recognition," "Brief Review of Immune Physiology") that focus the student on the major points of the pertinent topics. Each section is relatively freestanding. For example, Section V, "Immune System in Health and Disease," could be used in a clinical correlations course, independent of the remainder of the book. *Immunology for Medical Students* will be most useful in the comprehensive host defense–type courses that are growing in popularity in medical schools.

The icons used throughout are illustrated on the next page. You should become familiar with them to fully understand the illustrations. Several pathogens (listed on the next page) have been selected to use throughout the book as examples. Some basic aspects of the structure and mechanism of action of these organisms are described. You should reacquaint yourself with these organisms, which are commonly encountered in microbiology and infectious disease courses, and use the figure as a convenient reference as you encounter these pathogens in the examples used in this book.

In general, boxes have been clustered at the end of chapters to aid the flow of the text and understanding of the material.

Clinical Box

Clinical boxes throughout the text put immunology into a clinical context. The clinical material selected is current and relevant.

Technical Box

Technical boxes show how advances in the field have expanded our knowledge of how the immune system works and provided new means of preventing disease.

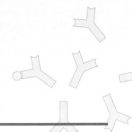

Icons in Immunology

Key molecules

DNA

Signaling molecule

Cytokine, chemokine, etc.

Receptor, surface molecule, ligand

MHC I

MHC II

Antigen

T-cell receptor (TCR)

Immunoglobulin (Ig)

Complement (C′)

Key cells

Professional antigen-presenting cell (APC)

Neutrophil, eosinophil, mast cell

Lymphocytes

Key colors

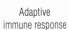

Adaptive immune response

Innate immune response

Antigen, microorganism, tumor, etc.

Key complexes

Bone marrow

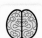
Thymus

Lymph node

Other (peripheral) tissue

In vitro

Medical intervention

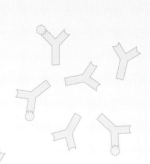

MICROORGANISMS MENTIONED IN THIS BOOK

This table shows some of the different types of microorganisms the immune system has to deal with. These microorganisms are used throughout the book to illustrate the diverse range of targets for the immune system. These select microorganisms cause about 10 million deaths per year around the world.

Microorganism		Type
HIV	RNA Virus	Small virus with a high mutation rate. Many different strains develop in one infected person, allowing the virus to escape the immune response.
Influenza virus	RNA virus	Spreads easily from person to person. Mutates gradually but also can exchange genes with other viruses.
Epstein-Barr virus (EBV)	DNA virus	Causes infectious mononucleosis. The EBV genome encodes proteins that help the virus escape the immune system.
Hepatitis B virus	DNA virus	Lives in hepatocytes. The immune response to the virus causes liver damage. Vaccination prevents infection.
Escherichia coli (E. coli)	Bacterium	One of many organisms normally living harmlessly in the gut. If it invades the body, it may trigger septic shock.
Mycobacterium tuberculosis	Bacterium	Transmitted by airborne droplets. Able to survive inside phagocytes. If not adequately controlled by the immune system, it causes tuberculosis.
Candida albicans	Fungus	Lives harmlessly on the skin but able to cause disease ("thrush") if not controlled by the immune system.
Plasmodium	Protozoan	Transmitted by insect bites and causes malaria. Has a complex life cycle that allows it to evade the immune system. Effective vaccines are now being developed.
Schistoma	Helminth	Invasive worm that attacks the liver and urinary tract.

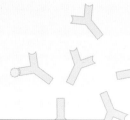

CONTENTS

CONTENTS

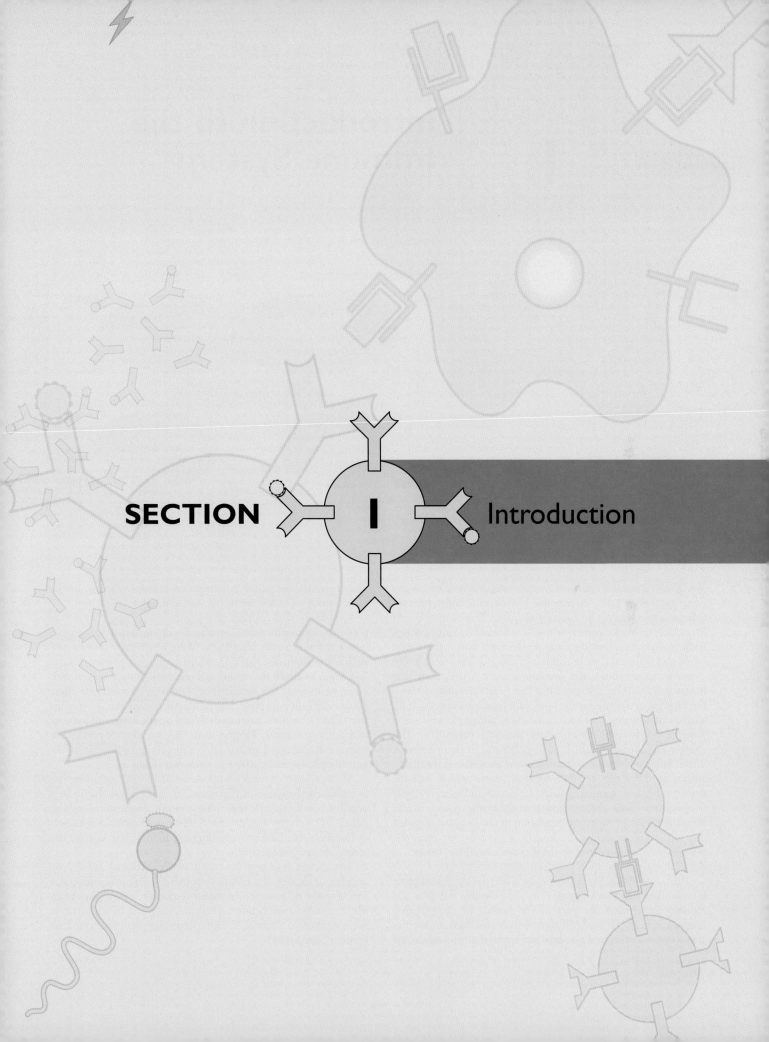

SECTION **I** Introduction

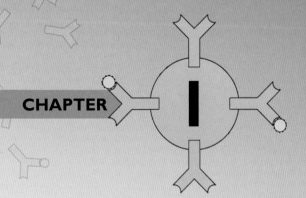

CHAPTER 1

Introduction to the Immune System

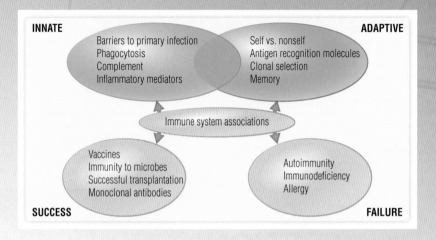

We inhabit a world dominated by microbes, many of which can cause harm (Box 1.1). The immune system is the body's primary defense system against invasion by microbes. This chapter briefly introduces the major components of the human immune system, what they do, and how they accomplish their host defense role.

As you will read later in this book, and as is illustrated in the overview figure above, the immune system is organized into innate and adaptive components. The *innate immune system* is the first line of defense for the body, and it uses nonspecific cells, such as phagocytes, and molecules, such as complement components, to attempt to eliminate invading organisms. This chapter first introduces the innate system and its characteristics. This is followed by an introduction to the antigen-specific mechanisms used by the *adaptive immune system*, which include, among others, antigen recognition molecules and specific sets of lymphocytes. This chapter also introduces the reader to the important ways in which manipulation of the immune response can aid us in ensuring the health of people—for example, through vaccination—and to the diseases caused by "failure" of the immune system, such as in autoimmunity.

The human body has evolved natural barriers to prevent entry by microbes (see also Chapter 20). For example, the skin and mucous membranes are part of the innate, or nonadaptive, immune system. However, if these barriers are broken, such as after a cut, microbes and potential pathogens (harmful microbes) can enter the body and can begin to multiply rapidly in the warm, nutrient-rich systems, tissues, and organs.

One of the first features of the immune defense system that a foreign organism encounters after being introduced through a cut in the skin is the phagocytic white blood cells (leukocytes, such as macrophages; Fig. 1.1), which congregate within minutes and begin to attack the invading foreign microbes (Chapter 21). Later, neutrophils are recruited into the area of infection. These phagocytic cells bear molecules called *pattern recognition receptors* that detect structures commonly found on the surface of bacteria and other pathogens. Phagocytosis, the ingestion of particulate matter into cells for degradation, is a fundamental defense mechanism against invading foreign microbes (Chapter 21).

Various other protein components of serum, including the complement components (Chapter 20), may bind to the invader organisms and facilitate their phagocytosis, thereby limiting the source of infection and disease. Other small molecules known as *interferons* mediate an early response to viral infection by the innate system (Chapter 20).

The innate immune system is often sufficient to destroy invading microbes. If it fails to clear infection rapidly, it activates the adaptive or acquired immune response, which takes over. Messenger molecules known as *cytokines* mediate the connection between the two systems. The interferons are part of the cytokine family (Chapter 24).

The effector cells of the adaptive immune defense system are also white blood cells, the T and B lymphocytes (Chapters 2, 12, 14, and 15). The B and T cells of the adaptive immune system are normally at rest, but they become activated (Chapters 2 and 11) on encountering an entity referred to as an *antigen*. Most antigens are derived from invading pathogens, but when things go wrong, an antigen can be a harmless foreign substance, as in hypersensitivity, or even a molecule derived from the self, as in autoimmunity. Adaptive immune responses are highly effective but can take 7 to 10 days to mobilize completely. A very important aspect of the adaptive immune response is the molecular mechanism used to generate specificity in the response. The immune system as a whole distinguishes self from nonself.

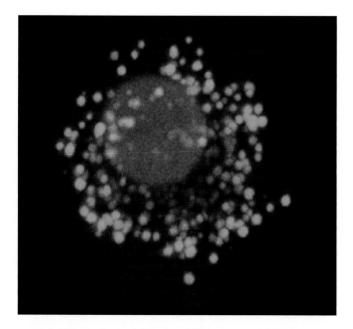

Fig 1.1 Confocal image of a human monocyte–derived macrophage harboring live M1T1 streptococci (green) as assessed by staining with a bacterial viability. (From Norrby-Teglund A, Johansson L. Beyond the traditional immune response: bacterial interaction with phagocytic cells. *Int J Antimicrob Agents.* 2013;42[suppl]:S13-S16.)

It is able to cope with the great diversity in nonself structures by anticipating these foreign antigens and creating a diverse repertoire of antigen receptors or antigen recognition molecules. These receptors bind to small areas of the molecular structures of the foreign antigens called *epitopes*. The genetic mechanisms used for generation of this diverse range of antigen recognition molecules are described in Chapters 6, 7, 8, 14, and 15. Several versions of these antigen receptors are used by the immune system; these are antibodies (B-cell antigen receptors), T-cell antigen receptors, and the protein products of a genetic region referred to as the *major histocompatibility complex* (MHC). All vertebrates appear to possess an MHC. The MHC genes of humans are referred to as *human leukocyte antigen* (HLA) genes, and their products are known as *HLA molecules* (Chapter 8).

In addition to being antigen receptors on B cells, antibodies are also found as soluble antigen-recognizing molecules in the blood (immunoglobulin or antibody). Both the B-cell and T-cell antigen receptors are clonally distributed (for B cells and antibodies; Fig. 1.2), which means that a unique antigen receptor is found on each lymphocyte. When a foreign antigen enters the body, it eventually encounters a lymphocyte with a matching receptor. This lymphocyte divides and, in the case of B cells, the daughter clones produce large amounts of soluble receptor. In the case of T cells, large numbers of specific effector cells bearing the appropriate receptor on their cell surface are generated. Different types of specialist T cells, such as T-helper (TH) cells, are produced for specific situations (Chapter 16). For example, TH1 T cells are usually produced in response to viral infections, TH2 T cells are produced in response to worms, and TH17 cells respond to fungi and extracellular bacteria.

B-cell and T-cell antigen receptors differ in one very important way: B-cell antigen receptors can interact directly with antigen, whereas T-cell antigen receptors recognize antigen only when it is presented to them on the surface of another cell by MHC molecules (Chapters 2, 7, and 8).

In addition to recognizing nonself antigens, the cells of the immune system also recognize alterations of self that result from certain disease processes—for example, modified self antigens found on tumor cells—and may eliminate the tumor cell once it has been recognized (Fig. 1.3; Chapter 35). The ability to recognize unaltered self antigen can, if unregulated, lead to

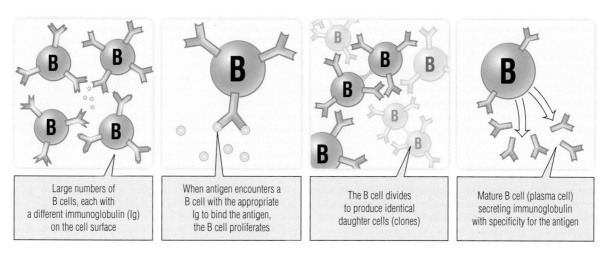

| Large numbers of B cells, each with a different immunoglobulin (Ig) on the cell surface | When antigen encounters a B cell with the appropriate Ig to bind the antigen, the B cell proliferates | The B cell divides to produce identical daughter cells (clones) | Mature B cell (plasma cell) secreting immunoglobulin with specificity for the antigen |

Fig 1.2 Clonal selection of B cells.

 MCH II   Cytokine, chemokine, etc.   Complement (C')   Signaling molecule

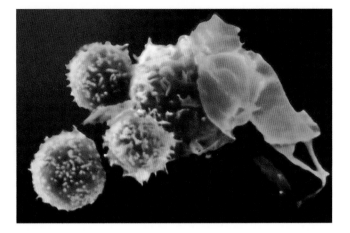

Fig 1.3 Scanning electron micrograph of T cells (*blue*) and a tumor cell (*red*). (From BSIP Lecaque and the Science Photo Library.)

TABLE 1.1 Comparison of Some Overall Features of the Innate and Adaptive Immune Systems

	Innate	Adaptive
Characteristics	Nonspecific response Fast response (minutes) No memory	Very specific Slow response (days) Memory
Components	Natural barriers, phagocytes, and secreted molecules Few pattern-recognition molecules	Lymphocytes and secreted molecules Many antigen recognition molecules

autoimmune disease, such as with some forms of diabetes mellitus (Chapter 28). Fortunately, the adaptive immune system contains a number of mechanisms to ensure that unaltered self antigens are tolerated, which prevents autoimmune disease in most people (Chapter 18).

A critically important feature of the adaptive immune response is that it displays memory of a previous encounter with a microbe (or antigen). This is the basis of protection from disease by vaccination with an attenuated form of the pathogen (Box 1.2; see also Box 2.1), but it is also the way in which the body is protected from reinfection. For example, we are regularly exposed to influenza viruses (Box 1.3). If we reencounter the same antigenic form of influenza virus, or even an antigenically similar (i.e., cross-reactive) form, the response is faster and greater in magnitude, and infection is limited or prevented. Unfortunately, because influenza virus is one of a class of organisms capable of radically changing its genetic structure (and antigenic makeup), new viruses are always around to cause new infections. Several overall characteristics of the innate and adaptive immune systems are summarized in Table 1.1.

The medical successes associated with advances in knowledge about the host defense system include improvements in public health that have arisen from vaccination against communicable diseases (see Box 1.2 and Chapter 25); success with organ transplantation, such as with kidneys and hearts (Box 1.4 and Chapters 8 and 34); treatments to alleviate hereditary defects in the immune system (Chapter 32); drugs to control the symptoms of allergy (Chapter 27) or hypersensitivity (Chapters 26 and 29 through 31); and a variety of technologic developments that, coupled with the ability to manufacture antibodies with precise specificities (monoclonal antibodies), have been adapted to be used for everything from pregnancy tests to treating cancer (Chapter 36).

Information obtained about the immune system has had an important role in our understanding and treatment of infection; therefore this subject is deserving of study in medical school. Moreover, the potential for studies of the immune system to result in therapies for common diseases such as cancer or diseases with an autoimmune component—including diabetes mellitus, rheumatoid arthritis, and multiple sclerosis—strongly requires the attention of future physicians.

BOX 1.1 World of Microbes

A newborn infant leaves the safe environment of the uterus and is exposed to a wide range of harmful bacteria, viruses, fungi, protozoa, and worms. The first year of life is the most dangerous, and most deaths are caused by infection. Over the next 5 years, this baby has a 1 in 8 chance of dying from infection. The largest threat is from water-borne **bacteria** causing severe diarrhea. Measles **virus** infects through the respiratory tract and kills up to 1 in 20 children in the developing world. **Fungi** are able to invade the child's mucosa. In addition, this child will encounter **protozoa** transmitted through insect bites and **worms** that can burrow through the skin.

What is the nature of the systems that protect children from such a wide range of infections? Figure 1.4 shows very different mortality rates (deaths in the first year of life), even for adjacent countries. Can our knowledge of immunology reduce infant mortality rates by simple public health measures such as vaccinations?

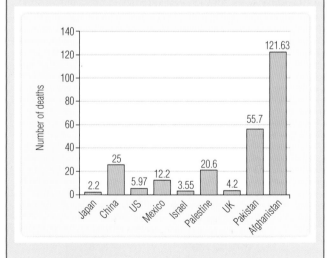

Fig 1.4 Mortality rates in the first year of life.

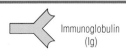 T-cell receptor (TCR)

Immunoglobulin (Ig)

 Antigen

 MCH I

BOX 1.2 Young Person With Jaundice

A medical student has been infected with hepatitis B virus (HBV) following a needle-stick injury from an infected patient. HBV is also spread sexually and from mother to child; in the developing world, it is a leading cause of death in adults. HBV multiplies in the liver. The immune response to HBV produces T cells, which, in most patients, can eliminate the virus. In some individuals, however, the virus persists, and the T cells cause damage to liver cells, which leads to inflammation (hepatitis), cirrhosis, and even cancer (hepatoma).

However, HBV infection is preventable. In recent years, hepatoma is no longer the problem it was in some parts of the world. This has been achieved through vaccines that prevent transmission of HBV. These vaccines work by stimulating B cells, which produce antibody against the virus. This book will help you to answer the question of how such a safe, simple intervention can have such a major impact on health.

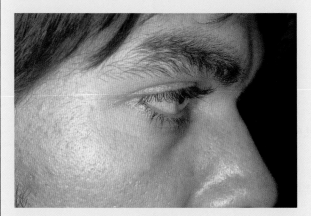

Fig 1.5 Jaundice. (From Savin JA, Hunter JA, Hepburn NC. *Diagnosis in Color: Skin Signs in Clinical Diagnosis.* Mosby-Wolfe; London; 1997.)

BOX 1.3 A Man Sneezing

Everyone knows what it is like to have influenza, and most people are infected every few years or so. In recent years, influenza has killed approximately 1 out of 200 people infected. In 1918, an influenza epidemic killed more than 40 million people around the world. When you have finished this book, you should be able to answer questions such as "Why do we fail to build up lifelong immunity to influenza?" "Why are some outbreaks of infectious agents such as influenza virus so lethal?" "What can be done to protect people against influenza?" Given concerns about a possible avian flu pandemic, it is important that you can answer questions such as "Why does the current flu vaccine not protect people from viruses such as avian flu?"

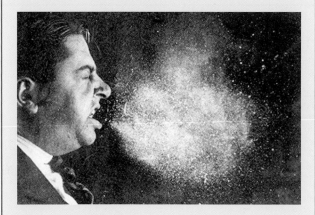

Fig 1.6 Sneezing spreads influenza virus. (Courtesy American Association for the Advancement of Science.)

BOX 1.4 Man With Kidney Failure

A man has irreversible kidney failure. Three times a week, he must undergo dialysis. As a consequence, he is unable to work, and his relationship has broken up as a result of his constant ill health. He recently became aware that his treatment costs more than $40,000 per year.

Every year several thousand people die in car accidents. Many of these people have perfectly healthy kidneys that could be transplanted into this patient. He wants to know why he is waiting so long for a transplant. He is also worried about the medication that he will need to take after the transplant because he has heard these drugs will suppress his immune system and predispose him to certain infections. Would you be able to answer his questions about his treatment? This book will help you respond to such questions from your patients.

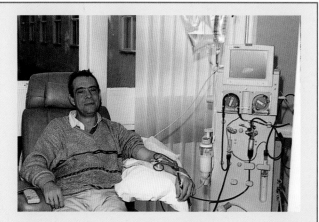

Fig 1.7 A patient receives dialysis for kidney failure. (Courtesy Dr. H.R. Dalton, Royal Cornwall Hospital, United Kingdom.)

 MCH II

 Cytokine, chemokine, etc.

 Complement (C′)

 Signaling molecule

LEARNING POINTS — Can You Now ...

1. List the main characteristics of the innate and adaptive immune systems?
2. List at least three examples of antigen recognition molecules?
3. Define clonal distribution with respect to antigen receptors on B and T cells?
4. Compare antigen recognition by T and B cells?
5. Compare the primary and the secondary immune response to an antigen?
6. List at least three reasons why the study of the immune system is important to you as a physician in training?

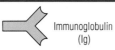 T-cell receptor (TCR)

 Immunoglobulin (Ig)

Antigen

 MCH I

Basic Concepts and Components of the Immune System

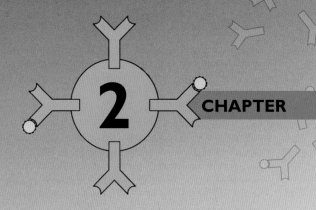

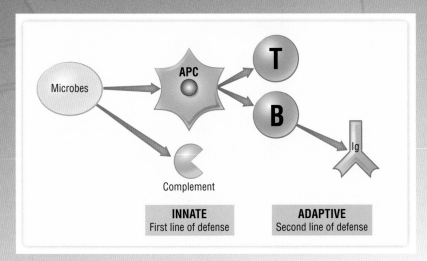

The essential features of the host defense system comprise an innate component that functions as a first line of defense and an adaptive component that takes longer to mobilize but confers specificity and exhibits memory. As shown in the overview figure above, the two components are not independent but are functionally interrelated in various critical ways, such as through the actions of soluble effector molecules called *cytokines*.

■ INNATE IMMUNITY

An innate immune system exists in some form in most organisms, and several important principles about the operation of the innate system apply. First, it is fast! Unlike the adaptive system, which may take days to mobilize, aspects of the innate system are extremely quickly mobilized. For example, phagocytic cells—in particular, macrophages resident in tissues—will recognize infection via pattern recognition molecules that detect structural motifs on invading microbes. Toll-like receptors (TLRs) are one type of pattern recognition molecule used by innate immune system cells. TLRs recognize a variety of substances found on a range of microbes but not on host cells. Another example of a pattern recognition molecule is the *mannan-binding lectin* (MBL) of the complement system, which recognizes sugar molecules containing mannose on the surface of bacteria, fungi, and viruses and helps activate the complement

cascade (Chapter 20). MBL is present in solution in the plasma. This use of non–pathogen-specific recognition molecules is a key feature of the innate system.

The innate system uses phagocytic cells, chiefly neutrophils and macrophages, in addition to molecules such as the serum proteins of the complement system, which can interact directly with certain microbes to protect the host. Other cells important in the innate response are the natural killer (NK) cells (Chapter 22), which can detect and kill certain virally infected cells by inducing programmed cell death (apoptosis). Another group of important soluble molecules that is part of the innate defense system is the interferons (Chapter 20). Viral infection triggers interferon production by the infected cell. Interferon inhibits the replication of many viruses and is not pathogen specific.

Many innate system components—for example, complement, interferon, and cytokines or cells such as macrophages—can affect cells of the specific adaptive system. This is another important observation. The innate and adaptive systems are interconnected and overlapping. The adaptive system is usually triggered by the innate system, and it only comes into play if the innate system fails to overwhelm the invading microbes or if the invading microbe has found a way to avoid interaction with the innate system. The innate and adaptive systems are compared throughout this book, and the mechanisms that pathogens use to avoid detection by the immune system are the subject of a later discussion.

■ ADAPTIVE IMMUNITY

An adaptive immune system is first observed in the evolutionary tree at the level of vertebrates. The adaptive immune system is capable of specifically distinguishing self from nonself. This is accomplished by creating an anticipatory defense system of recognition molecules that interact with foreign, nonself antigen. Vertebrate genomes contain several genes that encode many millions of antigen recognition molecules. These gene families include antigen receptors capable of recognizing any given antigen (Fig. 2.1).

Immature adaptive immune system cells "cut and paste" (recombine) segments of the receptor genes to produce this huge diversity of receptors (Chapter 6). In addition, a molecular mechanism enables some of the receptors (antibodies) to be modified at the somatic level during the immune response to create receptors with a better fit; that is, the binding is more specific.

The ability of vertebrates to generate anticipatory defense systems against nonself entities was enhanced by duplication of those genes in the germline that encoded proteins that had binding sites and could function as receptors (Fig. 2.2).

The products of these gene duplications are the gene families that encode the antigen recognition molecules: antibodies, T-cell receptors (TCRs), and major histocompatibility complex (MHC) proteins. A major step forward in understanding how this system works came with the idea that each lymphocyte expresses a unique antigen receptor. Once an antigen encounters a lymphocyte bearing the receptor that best fits the antigen, this preexisting cell divides and gives rise to many daughter cells (clones). Thus the lymphocyte is clonally expanded, making available more of the receptor specific for the antigen encountered. In other words, as the repertoire of receptors is expressed clonally on lymphocytes and on binding antigen, a preexisting clone is triggered selectively to generate more of the precise receptor required to interact with the antigen encountered (see Fig. 2.1).

One complication of an anticipatory system with preexisting receptors is that antiself receptors can be generated (Fig. 2.3),

and the cells that carry these potentially damaging receptors must be deleted or inactivated. When mistakes occur and potentially antiself cells are allowed to remain active, autoimmune (antiself) disease can occur (Chapter 28).

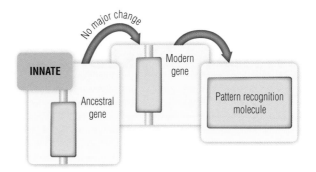

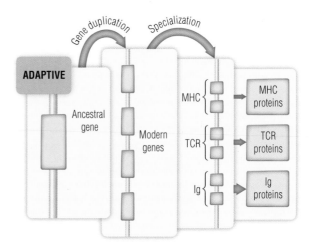

Fig 2.2 Evolution of antigen recognition molecules and pattern recognition molecules. *Ig,* immunoglobulin; *MHC,* major histocompatibility complex; *TCR,* T-cell receptor.

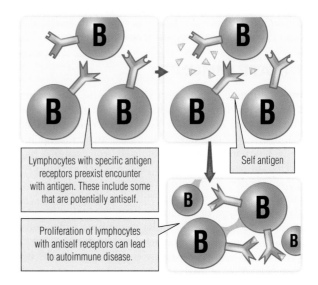

Fig 2.1 Lymphocytes with specific antigen receptors exist before an encounter with antigen.

Fig 2.3 Proliferation of antiself response.

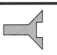 T-cell receptor (TCR)   Immunoglobulin (Ig)   Antigen   MCH I

This model for understanding the development of the capacity to recognize and respond specifically to nonself molecules is known as the *clonal selection theory* (see Fig. 1.3). Aspects of this theory are developed further in Chapters 6, 7, 14, and 15.

■ COMPONENTS OF THE IMMUNE SYSTEM

The major features of an adaptive immune response are specificity, diversity, and memory. The response is *specific* in that it discriminates among various molecular entities; it is *diverse* in that it has the capacity to respond to almost any antigen that may be encountered; and it has *memory* in that it can recall previous contact with antigen and show a stronger response the second time. The last feature is the basis of vaccination, illustrated in Box 2.1.

The immune system uses cells (Fig. 2.4) and soluble molecules as effectors to protect the host. It consists of a number of different cell types, all leukocytes, specialized to perform different functions. For example, phagocytic cells such as neutrophils and macrophages are used nonspecifically to destroy invading microbes.

Mature cells can occur in blood or in tissues, such as lymphocytes in blood and dendritic cells in tissue. Lymphocytes (B and T cells) provide specific immunity. The products of B cells—antibodies—are soluble molecules sometimes referred to as the *humoral immune system.* Extracellular pathogens are eliminated chiefly by antibodies, whereas intracellular pathogens require T cells and macrophages for elimination. In contrast to humoral or antibody-mediated immunity, the function of T cells is sometimes referred to as *cell-mediated immunity.* Antigen-presenting cells (APCs), such as dendritic cells and macrophages (Fig. 2.5), are critical in initiating the activation of B and T cells.

Antigen processing and presentation is presented in Chapter 10. Briefly, APCs such as macrophages take up antigens and subject them to proteolytic degradation in various compartments of the cell. These events are called *antigen processing,* and they are required because although B-cell antigen receptors bind directly to antigen, T-cell receptors for antigen recognize only processed antigen displayed on APCs. The peptide antigens are displayed in the peptide-binding groove of MHC molecules (Chapter 8).

Some organisms try to evade the immune system, but the immune system has developed methods of fighting back (Box 2.2).

■ ACTIVE AND PASSIVE IMMUNITY

Two further divisions of immunity exist. *Active immunity* occurs when the individual plays a direct role in responding to the antigen—for example, after an encounter with a virus (see Box 4.1). This is in contrast to *passive immunity,* wherein immunity is transferred from one individual to another by transferring immune cells or serum from an immunized individual to an unimmunized individual (e.g., when antirabies antibody is provided after a dog bite; see Box 4.2). The antibodies to rabies virus are developed in other individuals and are administered to confer protection more rapidly than can be achieved by the injured individuals making the necessary antibodies themselves.

■ PHASES OF AN IMMUNE RESPONSE

An active immune response consists of several steps or phases (Fig. 2.6). First is the *cognitive phase,* when antigen is recognized. Antigen encounters a cell bearing a receptor that fits the antigen. This cell is activated and proliferates (Chapter 11). Next, more and more of the same clone of cells is produced; this is the *activation phase.* The cells undergo various changes, known as *differentiation,* to enable a response. For example, various developmental steps occur in a B cell (Chapter 14); this leads to a whole new cell, called a *plasma cell,* that synthesizes and secretes large amounts of antibody molecules. At this point, the antibodies help eliminate the antigen. This is the third phase, referred to as the *effector phase.* Various steps take place to downregulate the response once the antigen is eliminated. These steps are designed to regulate the response and prevent it from continuing after the antigen or microbe is neutralized or eliminated.

■ TYPES OF IMMUNE RESPONSE

Invading pathogens can be categorized zoologically into viruses, bacteria, fungi, protozoa, or worms or by their habitat. For example, the luminal surface of the gut or respiratory system can be invaded by worms, and the surface of the skin can be attacked by arthropods. The extracellular spaces between cells can be invaded by bacteria or fungi. On the other hand, viruses, some bacteria, and parasites live inside cells. Broadly speaking, the components of the immune system make three different types of immune response, depending on the habitat of the invading pathogen. Table 2.1 summarizes these three types of response. Importantly, these three types of immune response can each cause very common diseases. You will read a lot more about the three types of response as you progress.

 MCH II   Cytokine, chemokine, etc.   Complement (C′)   Signaling molecule

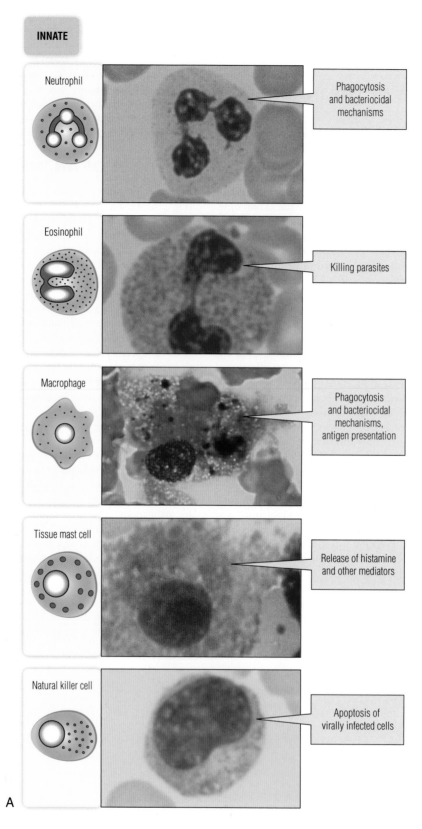

INNATE

Neutrophil — Phagocytosis and bacteriocidal mechanisms

Eosinophil — Killing parasites

Macrophage — Phagocytosis and bacteriocidal mechanisms, antigen presentation

Tissue mast cell — Release of histamine and other mediators

Natural killer cell — Apoptosis of virally infected cells

A

Fig 2.4 Major cells of the immune system. **A,** Innate.

 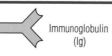 T-cell receptor (TCR)   Immunoglobulin (Ig) Antigen   MCH I

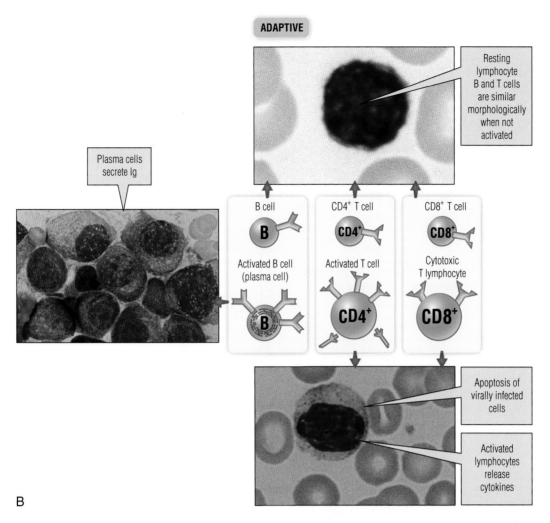

ADAPTIVE

Resting lymphocyte B and T cells are similar morphologically when not activated

Plasma cells secrete Ig

B cell

Activated B cell (plasma cell)

CD4⁺ T cell

Activated T cell

CD8⁺ T cell

Cytotoxic T lymphocyte

Apoptosis of virally infected cells

Activated lymphocytes release cytokines

B

Fig 2.4, cont'd B, Adaptive. *Ig,* immunoglobulin.

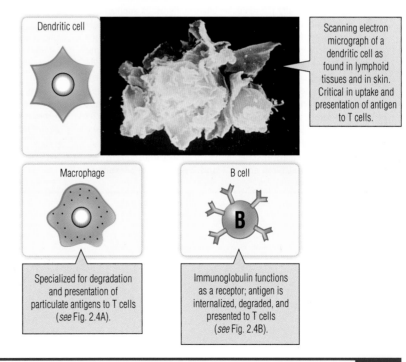

Dendritic cell

Scanning electron micrograph of a dendritic cell as found in lymphoid tissues and in skin. Critical in uptake and presentation of antigen to T cells.

Macrophage

Specialized for degradation and presentation of particulate antigens to T cells (*see* Fig. 2.4A).

B cell

Immunoglobulin functions as a receptor; antigen is internalized, degraded, and presented to T cells (*see* Fig. 2.4B).

Fig 2.5 Antigen-presenting cells. (Scanning electron micrograph of dendritic cell courtesy Dr. Stella Knight, London, United Kingdom.)

 MCH II

 Cytokine, chemokine, etc.

Complement (C′)

 Signaling molecule

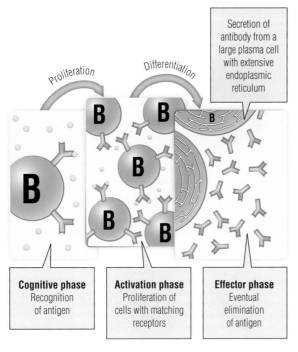

Fig 2.6 Phases of an immune response illustrated for B cells and leading to antibody production.

TABLE 2-1 Types of Immune Response

	Type 1: Intracellular Pathogens	Type 2: Surface Pathogens	Type 3: Extracellular Pathogens
Examples of pathogens	Mycobacteria (eg, tuberculosis), viruses, protozoa	Helminths, arthropods	Bacteria (eg, *Staphylococcus*), fungi (eg, *Candida*)
Innate immune system components	Interferon, macrophages, natural killer cells	Mast cells, eosinophils	Neutrophils
Adaptive immune system components	TH1 T cells Cytotoxic T lymphocytes IgM, IgG, IgA	TH2 T cells IgE	TH17 T cells
Immunopathology	Autoimmune disease	Allergy	Autoimmune disease

Ig, *immunoglobulin;* TH, *T helper.*

BOX 2.1 Vaccination With Hepatitis B

Hepatitis B virus (HBV) infection can cause short-term illness, typically jaundice, or chronic illnesses such as cirrhosis, liver cancer, or death. In the United States, approximately 1.25 million people are afflicted with chronic hepatitis B every year, and approximately 5000 people die from it. Also in the United States, HBV is spread through contact with the bodily fluids of an infected person. A vaccine is available that is a recombinant protein (hepatitis B surface antigen [HBsAg]) expressed from a plasmid in yeast cells. In the vaccine, the recombinant HBsAg protein assembles itself into viruslike particles (VLPs). To the host immune system, VLPs resemble HBV, but of course, they do not contain viral genes and are unable to reproduce.

The typical vaccination schedule is three intramuscular injections, usually given at birth and at 1 and 2 months. In persons at high risk of exposure, such as medical students, blood samples are taken after vaccination to ensure that sufficient antibody to HBsAg is present in the vaccine recipient's blood. A level of 10 mIU/mL of antibody to HBsAg is necessary for protection. Figure 2.7 shows a graph of conversion to protected status after the three-dose schedule. If an individual does not have 10 mIU/mL or more of antibody to HBsAg, the vaccine schedule is repeated.

Figure 2.7 also illustrates the difference in antibody response between a primary and a secondary, or subsequent, exposure to antigen. The initial, primary response is relatively slow and low level. On subsequent immunization, the response is faster and of greater magnitude.

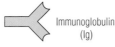 T-cell receptor (TCR)

 Immunoglobulin (Ig)

Antigen

 MCH I

BOX 2.1 Vaccination With Hepatitis B—cont'd

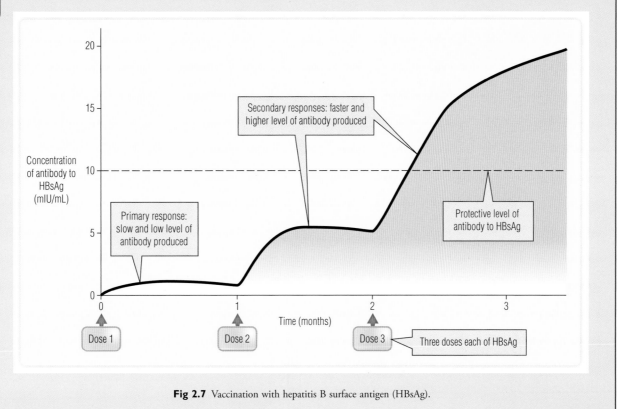

Fig 2.7 Vaccination with hepatitis B surface antigen (HBsAg).

BOX 2.2 Dealing With Sneaky Pathogens

Microbes evolve in numerous ways to evade the immune system, and the immune system has developed equally numerous ways to fight back. The innate immune system includes two populations of cells that combat special types of evasion mechanisms.

Parasitic worms have adapted to live inside the host at mucosal surfaces, notably the gut. These surfaces are out of reach of many immune system mechanisms, and the large, multicellular worms are difficult to attack. Mast cells and eosinophils are innate immune system cells that reside or are recruited to mucosal surfaces and can recognize worms. In doing so, they stimulate secretion of mucus and smooth muscle contraction in the affected organ, whereupon the worm loses its grip and is expelled from the host.

At the other extreme, some viruses have evolved mechanisms for evading recognition by T cells of the adaptive immune system. For example, herpesviruses can switch off expression of major histocompatibility complex (MHC) molecules in infected cells. Because T cells use MHC molecules to detect antigen, herpesvirus infection can go unrecognized. Natural killer (NK) cells have evolved to gauge the level of MHC expression on cells. If MHC expression on a cell is reduced, the NK cells are able to kill the cell. NK cells thus help overcome the evasion mechanism used by herpesviruses.

Mast cells, eosinophils, and NK cells are all described in detail in Chapter 22.

LEARNING POINTS Can You Now...

1. Describe at least three characteristics of the innate and adaptive immune response systems?

2. Describe at least three ways in which the innate and adaptive systems are interrelated?

3. Explain the concept of an anticipatory immune defense system?

4. Describe the phases of an immune response and the critical role of clonal selection in achieving a specific response?

5. Describe the fundamental properties of an adaptive immune response system?

6. List the major cells involved in the innate and adaptive immune response?

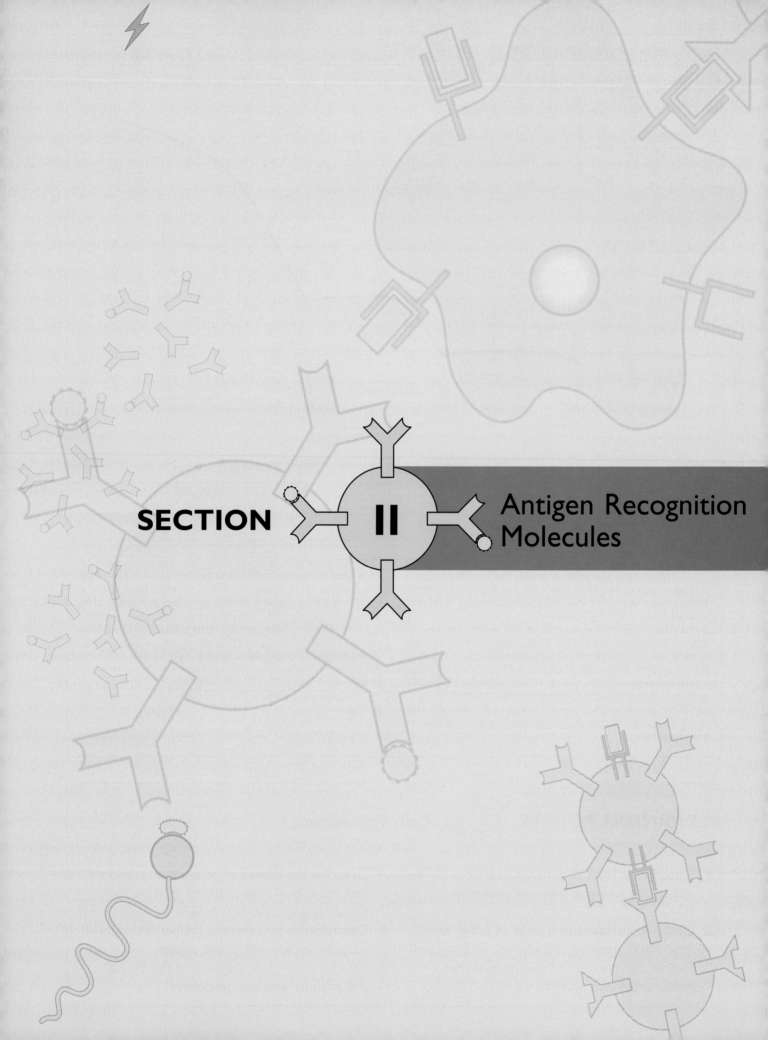

SECTION II Antigen Recognition Molecules

Introduction to Antigen Recognition

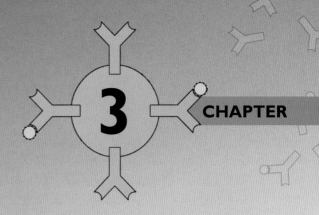

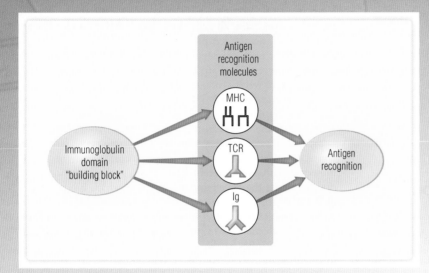

As described in Chapters 1 and 2, two main systems allow humans to identify foreign (nonself) materials: the *innate immune system* and the *adaptive immune system*.

The innate immune system is characterized by the presence of phagocytic cells and blood proteins, which recognize invading microbes using pattern recognition molecules. Mannan-binding lectin (MBL) and Toll-like receptors (TLRs) are examples of pattern recognition molecules. These recognize and bind types of molecules present in microbes but not host cells. MBL, for example, binds mannan on the surface of bacteria, viruses, and fungi. Mannan is not present on the surface of healthy host cells but is present on the surface of damaged cells. Thus MBL recognizes and binds both microbes and damaged host cells but not normal cells. Although MBL is able to distinguish between health and disease, it is described as being "nonspecific" because it cannot distinguish bacteria from viruses, nor can it distinguish different types of bacteria. This lack of specificity is the key feature of the pattern recognition molecules of the innate immune system.

The innate immune system relies on preexisting molecules and cells that nonspecifically attack invaders; this system protects us well against a wide range of infections. In general, the innate system protects against infection by removing the infectious agent. However, it is unable to respond *specifically* to

microbes or other foreign material (antigen). Microbes evolve much more rapidly than vertebrates, thus enabling them to evade nonadaptive defense systems by changing their structure. This is one reason vertebrates developed an adaptive immune system, which depends on gene rearrangement to generate a large number of preexisting receptors (repertoire), expressed on lymphocytes, that can identify essentially any antigen.

ANTIGEN RECOGNITION MOLECULES

Three groups of molecules specifically recognize foreign antigen for the adaptive immune system. The first two are the cell surface–located receptors found on B and T cells. The B-cell receptor (BCR) is also secreted from differentiated B cells (plasma cells) to create a soluble antigen receptor, known as *antibody*. The third group of antigen receptors is encoded in the major histocompatibility complex (MHC). This cluster of genes is known as *human leukocyte antigen* (HLA) in humans. The MHC molecules function to present antigenic peptides to T cells. T-cell receptor (TCR), BCR, and MHC molecules have similar structures and are part of the family of protein molecules that uses the immunoglobulin fold; this family is known as the *immunoglobulin superfamily* (Chapter 9). Figure 3.1 summarizes how the three types of antigen receptor differ.

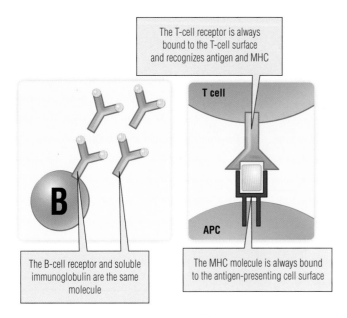

The T-cell receptor is always bound to the T-cell surface and recognizes antigen and MHC

T cell

APC

The B-cell receptor and soluble immunoglobulin are the same molecule

The MHC molecule is always bound to the antigen-presenting cell surface

Fig 3.1 The B-cell receptor, T-cell receptor, and major histocompatibility complex (MHC) molecule are all members of the immunoglobulin superfamily and have similar structures. Note how their functions differ. *APC,* antigen-presenting cell.

■ B-CELL AND T-CELL RECEPTORS

As described in Chapter 2, adaptive immunity depends on clonal selection for its efficient operation. Each B cell or T cell expresses a unique antigen receptor on its cell surface. On encountering foreign antigen, the cell that expresses a receptor that best fits the antigen divides and produces daughter cells (clones) that have the same receptor. Diversity of receptors is generated by gene rearrangement (Chapters 6 and 7). This allows a vast repertoire of receptors to be made from a limited number of genes that rearrange and combine to give the diversity needed. Thus the B-cell and T-cell antigen receptors are inherited as gene fragments. The gene fragments are joined together to form a complete antigen receptor gene only in individual lymphocytes as they develop. The process of rearranging and joining fragments of antigen receptor genes creates a diverse array of receptors. Theoretically, the number of different antibody molecules that could be made by the B lymphocytes in an individual could be as high as 10^{11}. This is why it is thought that there are sufficient B-cell and T-cell antigen receptors to identify all the antigens—such as microbes—in our environment. Keep in mind that receptors for every antigen in a microbe need not exist as long as one or a few exist. The immune system needs to identify only one of the many potential antigens in a microbe to protect the host by interfering with the ability of the microbe to grow and divide.

The genes that encode B-cell antigen receptors also undergo a process during the immune response called *hypermutation* to create receptors that are an even better fit for the foreign antigen. This process of rapid mutation of sequences that encode the binding site for antigen creates many more unique receptors and an even more specific and diverse repertoire.

In addition to being generated via similar genetic mechanisms, the antigen receptors of B cells and T cells are also similar with respect to their protein structures. They have a protein structure feature known as the *immunoglobulin fold,* which is common to several receptor families, where parallel strands of amino acids fold into a compact globular domain, including the antigen receptors found on immune cells.

■ MAJOR HISTOCOMPATIBILITY COMPLEX MOLECULES

Proteins encoded by the MHC genes represent the third group of antigen receptor molecules. There are two main classes of molecules, initially named because of their role in tissue (histo-) graft rejection (compatibility). Class I MHC molecules are found on essentially all cells, and class II MHC molecules are found chiefly on antigen-presenting cells (B cells, macrophages, and dendritic cells). The main function of both class I and class II MHC molecules is to present antigen peptides to T cells. A second role of MHC is to regulate natural killer (NK) cells.

The *structure* of the MHC molecules is described in greater detail in Chapter 8, and their *function* is described in Chapter 10. In brief, the TCR can recognize a foreign antigen only if it is presented as a complex with an MHC molecule. The TCR contacts residues on both the foreign peptide and the MHC molecule. This is a different kind of antigen recognition from that involving the B-cell antigen receptor, which binds directly to the antigen. The dual-recognition requirement distinguishes TCR molecules from BCR molecules. The physiologic function of MHC molecules is to capture and display antigens from cell-associated microbes, such as viral proteins made in the host cell, for identification as foreign by T cells.

The genes that encode MHC molecules are the most variable genes we know of in the human genome. They are said to be extensively polymorphic, which denotes existence of multiple alleles or forms of the same gene. Their diversity, however, exists in the population as a whole, not in the individual. Figure 3.2 compares MHC diversity with immunoglobulin and TCR diversity. Every person has approximately six different class I and II MHC gene products. Given that their parents likely have completely different HLA genes, most people have 12 different class I and II MHC molecules on the surfaces of their cells. Unlike B-cell or T-cell receptors, which differ in every lymphocyte in an individual, all of the MHC alleles are the same in an individual, but they are different among individuals. Thus in the population as a whole, some MHC molecules can bind antigenic peptides from a given microbe; however, potentially, any given individual may not bind a peptide from that microbe. This means that some individuals in the population may be more susceptible to a given microbe-induced disease than others. For example, if the structure of your MHC molecules makes it impossible for you to recognize and bind any peptide antigen from a given virus, you will not be able to activate a T-cell response to cells infected with that virus. Consequently, you would be susceptible to that virus-induced disease. However, the broad specificity of the peptide-binding groove in MHC molecules (described in Chapters 8 and 10) makes it unlikely that *no* peptides from any given microbe would fit the peptide-binding groove of an individual's MHC molecules.

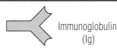 T-cell receptor (TCR)

 Immunoglobulin (Ig)

 Antigen

 MCH I

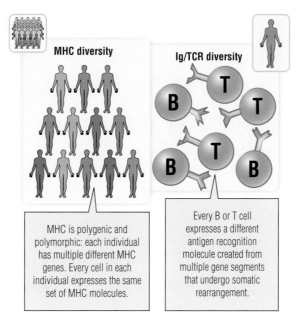

Fig 3.2 Diversity mechanisms of major histocompatibility complexes (MHCs) compared with immunoglobulin (Ig) and T-cell receptors (TCRs).

Labels within figure:

MHC diversity

Ig/TCR diversity

MHC is polygenic and polymorphic: each individual has multiple different MHC genes. Every cell in each individual expresses the same set of MHC molecules.

Every B or T cell expresses a different antigen recognition molecule created from multiple gene segments that undergo somatic rearrangement.

BOX 3.1 Advantages of Human Leukocyte Antigen Diversity: Human Leukocyte Antigen and HIV-1

Some genetic polymorphisms confer an advantage over infections. The most well-known example is sickle cell trait and protection against malaria. People with sickle cell trait are heterozygous for an abnormal hemoglobin β-chain. Homozygotes for this abnormal gene have severe sickle cell disease and have severe hematologic problems. On the other hand, heterozygotes with sickle cell trait only have mild hematologic problems. In addition, heterozygosity for the abnormal gene makes red cells resistant to parasitization with malaria; thus sickle cell trait reduces the risk of severe malaria by 90%. Malaria remains an important infection is some parts of the world, such as in sub-Saharan Africa. Many people of African heritage continue to carry the abnormal hemoglobin gene, whereas this has become very rare in other ethnic groups. The relationship between malaria and sickle cell trait has shaped human evolution and is an example of pathogen-mediated selection.

Major histocompatibility complex (MHC) genes behave differently, but their huge diversity is also driven by pathogens. Individual MHC alleles vary in their ability to present antigens from particular infections; therefore a specific MHC allele might predispose an infected individual to a more or less favorable disease outcome. This has been shown for HIV and hepatitis B virus

(HBV) infections. Different mechanisms contribute to pathogen-mediated selection of MHC as follows:

- *Heterozygote advantage.* If individuals in a population tend to be heterozygous for MHC alleles, they are more likely to have protective alleles.
- *Rare allele advantage.* A new infection may evolve and succeed because it evades the prevalent MHC alleles in a population. In this situation, individuals with rare MHC alleles are more likely to survive.

Both these models favor genetic diversity for MHC alleles. In other words, the more different MHC alleles available in a population, the more likely the population is to survive a new infection.

Although MHC diversity reduces the risk of human populations being wiped out by emerging infections, it causes significant problems in transplantation. As you will see in Chapter 34, successful transplantation requires the donor and recipient to have MHC alleles that are as similar as possible. As a result of MHC diversity, any given patient only has a 1 in 100,000 chance of being identical at all MHC alleles for any random kidney that becomes available.

LEARNING POINTS Can You Now ...

1. List the main categories of antigen recognition molecules?
2. Explain how T-cell and B-cell receptor diversity is achieved?
3. Explain MHC polymorphism and why it is advantageous?

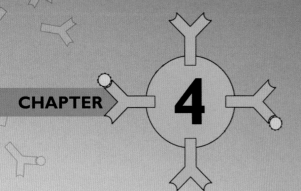

CHAPTER 4

Antigens and Antibody Structure

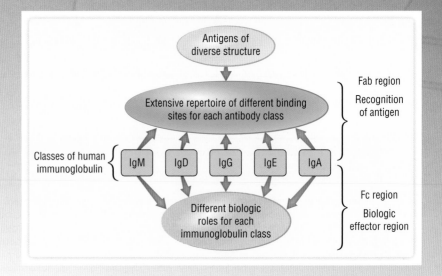

The first part of this chapter describes the various types of antigen and which antigens elicit the best immune responses. The second part describes the general structure of the various classes of human antibodies (immunoglobulins) and selected molecular and biologic properties of antibodies. Chapter 5 explores in more depth the nature of antibody-antigen interaction, and Chapter 6 explains how antibody diversity is generated.

Antigens that cause a strong immune response can have an extensive variety of chemical structures. Antibodies are the antigen-specific proteins produced by B cells in response to contact with antigen. Antibodies circulate in the blood and lymph as plasma components. Each individual has the capacity to synthesize a vast number of different antibody molecules, each capable of specifically interacting with an antigen.

■ ANTIGENS

Types of Antigens

In Chapter 1, antigens were introduced as substances recognized by the receptors of the adaptive immune system. Antigens can be classified as to how well they induce an immune response and also by their origins.

An *immunogen* is a substance that by itself causes an immune response, such as production of an antibody. Effective immunogens are fairly large, generally with a molecular weight greater than ≈6000, and they are chemically complex; for example, proteins made up of 20 different amino acid residues are better immunogens than nucleic acids made up of four different nucleotide bases. An example of an immunogen is the surface antigen of the hepatitis B virus (Box 4.1).

Haptens, by comparison, are compounds capable of being bound by immunologic receptors, but they do not necessarily elicit an immune response by themselves. For example, a relatively simple chemical compound such as penicillin cannot by itself induce an antibody response. If the hapten is coupled to a macromolecule, such as a protein, antibodies can be generated that bind very specifically to the hapten (Fig. 4.1).

A third type of antigen is a *tolerogen.* These molecules are recognized by the adaptive immune system, but the adaptive immune system has been programmed not to respond.

Antigens have different origins. Those derived from pathogens usually act as immunogens or haptens and elicit a strong immune response. Proteins derived from other people—such as a different major histocompatibility complex (MHC) allele present on a kidney transplant—can act as an *alloantigen* against triggering a strong immune response. In most people antigens

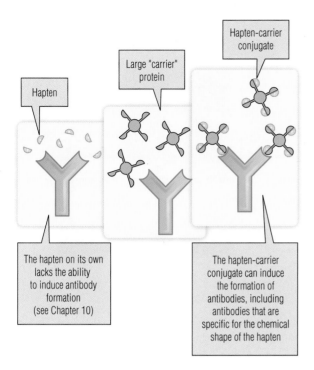

Fig 4.1 Hapten-carrier conjugate.

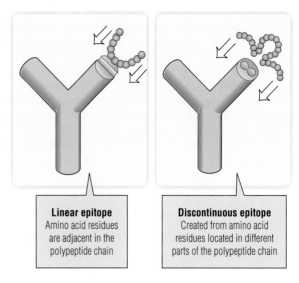

Linear epitope
Amino acid residues are adjacent in the polypeptide chain

Discontinuous epitope
Created from amino acid residues located in different parts of the polypeptide chain

Fig 4.2 Linear and discontinuous epitopes.

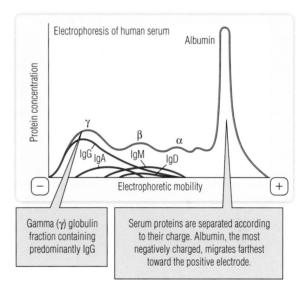

Fig 4.3 Electrophoresis of total human serum. *Ig,* immunoglobulin.

derived from foods such as peanuts act as tolerogens. When tolerizing programming goes wrong, these antigens may act as *allergens,* triggering a harmful immune response. Failures in tolerization can also lead to normal host molecules becoming *autoantigens.*

Epitopes

An epitope is part of a much larger antigen, such as a viral protein, with which an antibody can react. A viral protein may contain a large number of epitopes capable of interacting with many different specific antibodies or T-cell receptors. The two types of epitope, shown in Figure 4.2, are *discontinuous* or *conformational epitopes,* which result from bringing together amino acid residues from noncontiguous areas of the polypeptide chain into a three-dimensional (3-D) shape, and *continuous* or *linear epitopes,* which are contiguous areas of sequence such as amino acids 12 through 22 in a polypeptide chain.

Immunologic receptors on T cells recognize linear epitopes because of the way in which processed antigen is presented to them (associated with MHC molecules; see Chapter 10). As indicated in Figure 4.2, antibodies can recognize both types of epitope.

■ ANTIBODIES

Antibody Isolation and Characterization

Antibodies are proteins that react specifically with the antigen that stimulated their production. Two key characteristics of antibodies are that they are usually very specific, binding only on a particular antigen, and that they have a high affinity, meaning they bind antigen very strongly.

Antibodies make up approximately 20% of the plasma proteins. They were initially detected by analytic techniques such as electrophoresis, which is used to separate individual blood proteins based on their electric charge and molecular weight. During electrophoresis, antibodies are separated into the γ-zone and are sometimes referred to as the *gamma globulin* fraction of serum (Fig. 4.3).

More often, the antibody-bearing fraction of serum is referred to as *immunoglobulin.* Because normal serum immunoglobulins are the heterogeneous products of many clones of B cells (polyclonal immunoglobulin [Ig]), the immunoglobulins in serum constitute a highly heterogeneous spectrum of proteins rather than a single molecular species (see Fig. 4.3). Antibodies that arise in response to a single complex antigen, such as a bacterial protein with multiple epitopes, are heterogeneous in chemical structure and specificity because they are formed by several

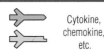 MCH II   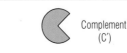 Cytokine, chemokine, etc.   Complement (C′)   Signaling molecule

different clones of B cells, each expressing an immunoglobulin capable of binding to a different epitope on the antigen (Chapters 6 and 14). This initially made biochemical studies of immunoglobulins very difficult because pure molecules of one specificity could not easily be isolated. One finding that helped in this regard was the observation that after electrophoresis of serum, the immunoglobulin region in patients with a B-cell malignancy called *myeloma* (Chapter 35) was often a band covering a very narrow range of electrophoretic mobility (Fig. 4.4).

In this disease, a single clone of B cells may proliferate, and these multiple cells secrete a homogeneous immunoglobulin that accumulates in the serum at relatively high concentration. These immunoglobulins became a source of relatively pure protein for biochemical studies early in the investigation of their structure.

Antibody Structure

All antibodies have the same basic molecular structure (Fig. 4.5). They are made up of light (L) and heavy (H) chains, terms that refer to their relative molecular weights. The *light chains* have a molecular weight of approximately 25,000, and the *heavy chains* have a molecular weight of approximately 50,000 to 70,000. In the basic immunoglobulin molecule, two heavy and two light chains are linked together by intermolecular disulfide bonds as shown in Figure 4.5. The five different classes of human heavy chains have slightly different structures, designated by lowercase Greek letters: μ (mu) for IgM, δ (delta) for IgD, γ (gamma) for IgG, ε (epsilon) for IgE, and α (alpha) for IgA (Table 4-1). Light chains are divided into two types, κ (kappa) or λ (lambda). Both types of light chain are found in all five classes of immunoglobulin, but any one antibody contains only one type of light chain. Any one IgG molecule consists of identical H chains and identical L chains organized into the Y-shaped structure shown in Figure 4.5.

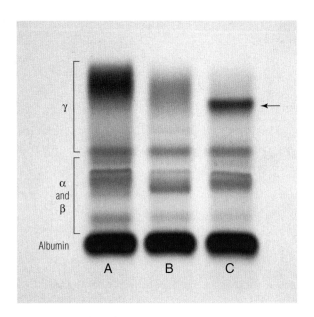

Fig 4.4 Gel electrophoresis of serum from different patients. The center sample (B) is from a healthy control. The serum sample from each patient is placed on a gel. An electric charge is applied across the gel for several hours, after which the different proteins are stained blue. The darkest zone corresponds to albumin, which is the most plentiful protein in the serum. The albumin zone is the same for all three samples. The α and β zones contain clotting proteins, some immunoglobulins, and some proteins produced in response to infection (see Box 20.1). The γ region is almost pure immunoglobulin. Sample A is from a patient with an infection and has increased levels of protein in zones α, β, and γ. The increased amount of immunoglobulin in the γ zone stains as a diffuse smear because the patient is producing many different immunoglobulins of different molecular weight and electric charge. Sample C shows a monoclonal expansion of B cells with an immunoglobulin spike *(arrow)* from a patient with a B-cell malignancy. The monoclonal B cells all produce exactly the same immunoglobulin molecule, reflected by a well-defined spike or band on electrophoresis.

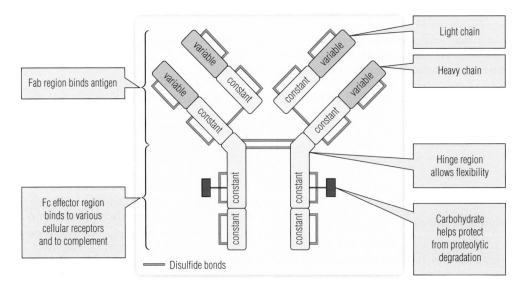

Fig 4.5 Basic antibody structure.

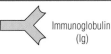 T-cell receptor (TCR)   Immunoglobulin (Ig)   Antigen   MCH I

TABLE 4-1   Selected Properties of Human Immunoglobulins

	IgM	IgD	IgG	IgE	IgA
Heavy chain symbol	μ	δ	γ	ε	α
Mean serum concentration (mg/mL)	0.4-2.5	<0.03	7-18	<0.0005	0.8-4
Serum half-life (days)	7	2	21	2	7
Activates complement	++	−	+	−	−
Placement transfer	−	−	+	−	−
Cell binding via Fc receptors	−	−	Mononuclear cells and neutrophils	Mast cells and basophils	Mononuclear cells and neutrophils

The basic immunoglobulin contains molecular parts with distinctive functions. This has been shown by a number of biochemical studies. If the basic immunoglobulin molecule (IgG) is subjected to proteolytic cleavage, several fragments are produced (Fig. 4.6). For example, if the enzyme papain is used to cleave IgG, two major types of fragment are obtained. One fragment binds antigen and is referred to as *fragment antigen binding* (Fab). The other fragment is *fraction crystallizable* (Fc); it does not bind antigen, but rather activates a molecular pathway known as *complement* (Chapter 20). Fc has various biologic effector functions, such as the ability to bind to Fc receptors found on macrophages and various other cells. If the proteolytic enzyme pepsin is used, the two Fab fragments remain linked (F[ab′]$_2$), but the Fc fragment is digested to small fragments and the effector functions are lost. These findings suggested that the different molecular parts of the Ig molecule have different functions; one is responsible for binding antigen and one performs other biologic effector functions.

Further biochemical studies, initially involving amino acid sequencing of the L and H chains of a number of different antibody molecules, demonstrated that the L and H chains can be differentiated into regions that are highly variable in sequence (V$_L$ and V$_H$) and regions that are essentially constant (C$_L$ and C$_H$). If, for example, several different λ-chains from different immunoglobulins are subjected to amino acid sequencing, there will be a region of considerable similarity in sequence but also a region of approximately 110 amino acid residues at the N-terminus of the L chain where substantial sequence differences are observed between different λ-chains (Fig. 4.7).

The same is true for H chains. The C regions carry out the biologic effector functions, such as the ability to bind complement proteins, and the V regions bind antigen. The variable regions are critical for the ability to respond to a vast number of different antigen structures.

Additional 3-D structure determination has revealed that the immunoglobulins are composed of folded, repeating segments called *domains*. An L chain consists of one variable domain and one constant domain, and an H chain consists of one variable and three or more constant domains. Each domain is approximately 110 amino acid residues long and is connected to other

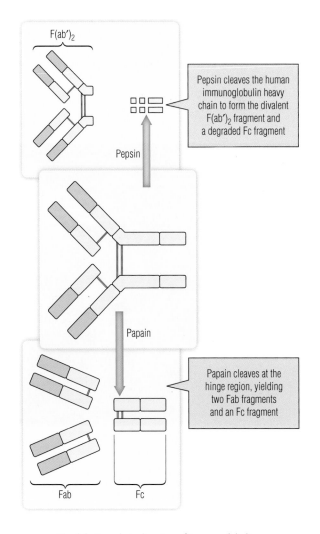

Pepsin cleaves the human immunoglobulin heavy chain to form the divalent F(ab′)$_2$ fragment and a degraded Fc fragment

Papain cleaves at the hinge region, yielding two Fab fragments and an Fc fragment

Fig 4.6 Proteolytic digestion of immunoglobulin.

 MCH II

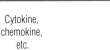 Cytokine, chemokine, etc.

 Complement (C′)

 Signaling molecule

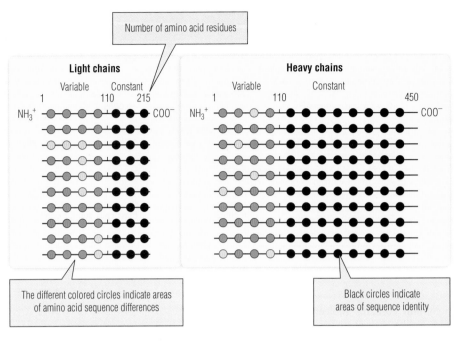

Fig 4.7 Immunoglobulin amino acid sequences: variable and constant regions.

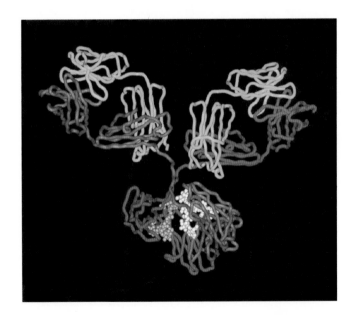

Fig 4.8 Three-dimensional domain structure of an immunoglobulin molecule. (From Kumar et al: *Robbins and Cotran Pathologic Basis of Disease,* 7th ed. Philadelphia: Elsevier; 2005.)

domains by short segments of more extended polypeptide chain, as shown in Figure 4.8.

Other molecules of the immune system have similar folded polypeptide domains, giving rise to the term *immunoglobulin superfamily* to describe this group of related proteins.

Selected Features and Biologic Properties of the Immunoglobulin Classes

Antibodies can occur as soluble proteins in the circulation, or they can be displayed on the surface of B cells. The primary function of all antibodies is to bind antigen, which can result in the inactivation of a pathogen—for example, by *agglutinating* bacteria, clumping them together and thus preventing their entry into host cells. If bacteria are coated with antibody, the likelihood that they will be engulfed by phagocytic cells (*opsonized*) is enhanced. Antibodies can also activate complement (Chapter 20) and can initiate a lytic reaction that destroys the cell to which the antibody is bound. The five classes of antibody have different functions that are a consequence of differences in structure (Fig. 4.9).

- **IgM** is the predominant antibody early in an immune response. It has a pentameric structure composed of five H_2L_2 units, each similar to an IgG, held together by a joining (J) chain. It has 10 potential antigen-binding sites; because of this, it is the most efficient antibody at agglutinating bacteria and activating complement.
- **IgD** is chiefly found on the surface of B cells as a receptor molecule and is involved in B-cell activation.
- **IgG** is the most prevalent antibody molecule in serum (see Table 4-1). It also survives intact in serum for the longest time (i.e., it has the longest half-life) and is able to cross the placenta to allow maternal protection of the newborn.
- **IgE** originally evolved to protect against parasitic infections. Binding of antigen to IgE coupled to an Fc receptor on mast cells and basophils triggers an allergic reaction (Chapter 27) by the activation of the mast cell and release of mediators such as histamine.

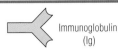 T-cell receptor (TCR)    Immunoglobulin (Ig)   Antigen   MCH I

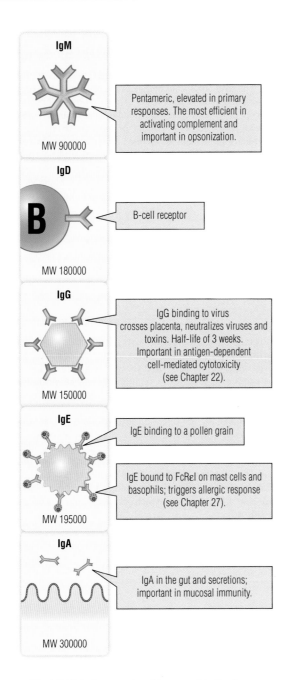

Fig 4.9 Biologic properties of immunoglobulin classes.

• **IgA** is the main immunoglobulin in secretions such as saliva, breast milk, and tears. It is also heavily represented in the mucosal epithelia of the respiratory, genital, and intestinal tracts. The IgA found in secretions (sIgA) consists of two molecules of IgA, a J chain, and one molecule of secretory component. The secretory component appears to protect the molecule from proteolytic attack and facilitates its transfer across epithelial cells into secretions.

As shown in Table 4-1, immunoglobulins interact with a variety of cell types via the presence of Fc receptors of various kinds on the cell. This interaction recruits the cells (e.g., inflammatory macrophages), which then secrete cytokines to become a part of the protective host response to foreign antigens.

BOX 4.1 Active Immunity

Vaccination, or active immunization, has greatly reduced the incidence of a number of infectious diseases, including smallpox and polio. The key principle (Chapter 2) is that previous exposure to a pathogen induces a protective response if the pathogen is ever encountered again. Active immunization may involve the use of antigens prepared by recombinant DNA techniques; for example, hepatitis B surface antigen (HBsAg) very successfully protects individuals from this infection. Hepatitis B virus (HBV) is a major cause of hepatitis, which is associated with considerable morbidity and mortality. This eliciting of antibodies by immunization with a vaccine of this type confers resistance to infection in over 90% of people who receive the vaccine. In many countries, hepatitis B vaccine is now given in infancy. In other countries, it is given only to specific groups, such as health care workers (see also Boxes 2.1 and 25.3). HBV uses HBsAg to bind to a receptor on hepatocytes. Once the virus is bound to the cell, it can gain entry. The vaccine induces the production of antibodies against HBsAg, and these antibodies prevent the interaction between HBsAg and its receptor (Fig. 4-10).

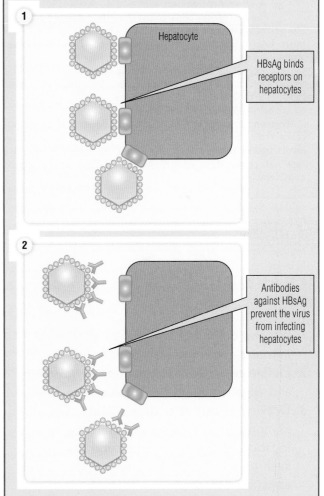

Fig 4.10 Antibodies against hepatitis B surface antigen (HBsAg) prevent the hepatitis B virus from infecting hepatocytes. Antibodies produced as a result of vaccination (active immunity) or given as passive immunity work the same way.

 MCH II

 Cytokine, chemokine, etc.

 Complement (C′)

 Signaling molecule

BOX 4.2 Passive Immunity

During routine blood tests, a pregnant woman is found to be infected with hepatitis B virus. The blood tests indicate she has a high level of virus present in her blood and that the baby is at high risk of infection. In many countries, this type of vertical transmission is the most frequent way in which babies become infected with this virus, which then establishes lifelong infection. In the case of our patient, the baby is given hepatitis B immune globulin (HBIG) 6 hours after birth. Subsequently, she also received hepatitis B vaccine. Testing at 1 year of age confirmed she had no evidence of infection.

HBIG is manufactured from plasma from donors who have been vaccinated with hepatitis B vaccine and have produced large quantities of antibodies against hepatitis B surface antigen (HBsAg). It is over 70% effective in preventing vertical transmission of hepatitis B. It is also used as postexposure prophylaxis, such as in people who have had needle-stick injuries. This antibody preparation confers instant protection from the virus without requiring the body to develop a response (passive immunity). The protection lasts only as long as the antibody persists; the serum half-life is 21 days. Passive immunity is also used to prevent other infections and has been tried with Ebola virus.

BOX 4.3 Therapeutic Antibodies

A 78-year-old woman with mild dementia is brought to the emergency department after she collapsed at home. She normally takes digoxin and a diuretic for atrial fibrillation and heart failure. She has sinus bradycardia of 47 beats/min; her attending physician wonders whether this may be the result of the patient taking too many of her digoxin tablets. Her blood digoxin level is 7.2 nmol/L, which is well above the therapeutic range (1.2 to 2 nmol/L). The diagnosis is sinus bradycardia due to accidental digoxin overdose.

Digoxin has a long half-life of 36 hours. Because of the serious bradycardia, the patient's physician decides to give her Fab fragments against digoxin. Four hours after this is given, the pulse rate has returned to normal, and the patient has improved considerably.

Antidigoxin Fab fragments are produced by vaccinating sheep with digoxin combined with a carrier protein. The carrier protein is required because digoxin acts as a hapten. Once the sheep is producing good levels of antibody, a large blood sample is taken. The immunoglobulins are separated out of the sheep serum and are treated with papain to produce Fab fragments, which are then ready for injection into patients. The antidigoxin Fab fragments are successful because they have two characteristics of antibodies. Fab fragments have a higher *affinity* for digoxin than digoxin has for its pump receptor, allowing the Fab fragments to displace digoxin, thus reducing its cardiotoxic effect. Fab fragments are also very *specific* and do not bind onto anything else in the body, which reduces the risk of them causing side effects.

LEARNING POINTS Can You Now...

1. List the origins of antigens to which the immune system may respond?
2. Define *antigen, immunogen, hapten, tolerogen,* and *epitope* and give examples of each?
3. Draw the basic structure of the immunoglobulin molecule, indicating the location of the major structural features, such as variable regions, hinge regions, and constant domains?
4. Recall what useful fragments of immunoglobulin may be produced by proteolytic digestion?
5. Recall the structural features and biologic properties of the different immunoglobulin classes?
6. Define *monoclonality* and *polyclonality* with respect to antibodies?
7. Understand the difference between passive and active immunity, using examples?

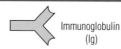 T-cell receptor (TCR)    Immunoglobulin (Ig)   Antigen   MCH I

Antibody-Antigen Interaction

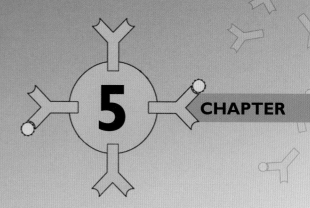

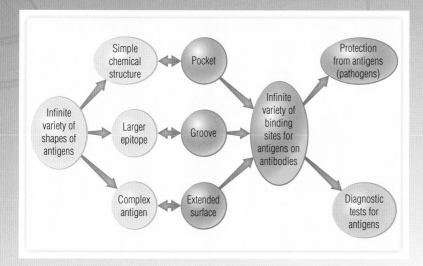

The above figure illustrates the topics for this chapter, which describes how antibodies interact with an almost infinite variety of shapes of antigens and how this interaction protects us from pathogens. This chapter also reviews the development of very specific diagnostic tests for the presence of antigens or antibodies. The most striking features of antibody-antigen interactions are their specificity and affinity. Otherwise, antibody-antigen interactions are much like other receptor-ligand interactions. Physicochemical forces are involved in the interaction between an antibody and an antigen that are similar to those between an enzyme and its substrate (or competitive inhibitor) or between a receptor, such as an insulin receptor, and a ligand, such as insulin. These forces derive from four sources: (1) electrostatic interactions between charged side-chains, (2) hydrogen bonds, (3) van der Waals forces, and (4) hydrophobic interactions.

When a good fit is present between antigen and antibody, the sum of these typically weak, noncovalent interactions can be a relatively strong interaction, and the antibody is described as having a high affinity.

The extraordinary specificity and affinity of antibodies has led to their widespread use in diagnostic testing. The latter part of this chapter describes several of the most important applications of antibody-antigen interaction in diagnosing disease.

ANTIGEN-BINDING SITES OF ANTIBODIES

Many experimental approaches have been used to define the structure of the antibody-binding site for antigen. By far the most detailed and valuable information has come from x-ray crystallographic studies of antigen-antibody complexes. One conclusion from analyses of the three-dimensional (3-D) structure of several antigen-antibody complexes is that the size and shape of the antigen-binding site can vary greatly. For example, the combining site can be a long, shallow crevice or a wider, more open cleft-type structure (Fig. 5.1). For small chemical compounds, the site on the antibody for binding antigen is analogous to an enzyme active site. For antibodies prepared against intact larger protein molecules, where the antibody will be specific for an epitope, a part of the protein antigen—namely, the combining site on the antibody—may be an extended surface rather than a cleft or crevice (see Fig. 5.1). In all cases, chemical complementarity exists between the residues of the antigen and the residues of the combining site of the antibody. The walls of the combining site are formed from the amino acid residues of regions of the variable segments of the heavy and light chains (VH and VL), known as the *hypervariable regions*

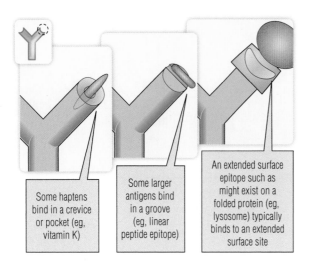

Fig 5.1 Antigen-binding sites vary in size and shape according to the type of molecule or epitope they bind.

Some haptens bind in a crevice or pocket (eg, vitamin K)

Some larger antigens bind in a groove (eg, linear peptide epitope)

An extended surface epitope such as might exist on a folded protein (eg, lysosome) typically binds to an extended surface site

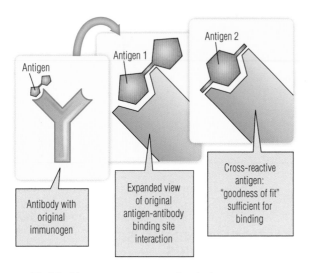

Fig 5.2 Schematic representation of antibody cross-reactivity.

Antigen

Antigen 1

Antigen 2

Antibody with original immunogen

Expanded view of original antigen-antibody binding site interaction

Cross-reactive antigen: "goodness of fit" sufficient for binding

(*hV regions;* see Chapter 6). Antibody specificity results from the precise molecular complementarity between chemical groups in the antigen and chemical groups in the antigen-binding site of the antibody molecule.

Cross-Reactivity

An antibody occasionally binds to more than one antigen, which is referred to as *cross-reactivity* or *multispecificity*. The antibody is specific for antigen 1, but a different molecule, antigen 2, fits well enough to create a stable binding interaction (Fig. 5.2). Cross-reactivity happens because a sufficient number of chemical interactions exists between the antigen and the antibody to create a stable structure regardless of the total "goodness of fit." It is important to note that cross-reactivity can have clinical consequences (Box 5.1).

■ DIAGNOSTIC TESTS FOR ANTIBODY OR ANTIGEN

Several routinely used diagnostic tests are based on the specificity and high affinity of antibodies. The remainder of this chapter provides examples of how different tests are used and describes the general principle of each test. In general, these tests are used both qualitatively and quantitatively and can be helpful to determine the presence of either antigen or antibody.

Enzyme-Linked Immunosorbent Assay

The enzyme-linked immunosorbent assay (ELISA) is a very sensitive and simple test that uses a covalent complex of an enzyme linked to an antibody either to detect antigen directly or to bind to an antibody-antigen complex (Fig. 5.3). The test uses plastic plates that have the relevant antigen bound onto the insides of "wells." Patient serum is incubated in these wells, and any of the relevant antibody will subsequently bind to antigen. The plate is washed to dispose of serum that contains irrelevant antibodies; but because of its high affinity, antibody bound to antigen will not be disturbed. Finally, a second antibody derived from an animal and conjugated to an enzyme is added and will bind to patient antibody. This anti–human immunoglobulin will bind to antibody still present in the well. The enzyme chosen is one capable of catalyzing a reaction to generate a colored product from a colorless substrate (eg, alkaline phosphatase or horseradish peroxidase [HRP]; see Fig. 5.3). The amount of antibody bound to antigen is then proportional to the amount of colored end product that can be visualized. Box 5.2 shows how ELISA can be used to screen for infectious disease.

Lateral Flow Test

A lateral flow test is a simple test to determine whether a protein, antigen, or antibody is present in a body fluid. It has some similarities to the ELISA test but has been engineered to be very simple to use, not require any special equipment, and be relatively cheap. The most widely used type of lateral flow test is a pregnancy test, which confirms the presence or absence of human chorionic gonadotropin (hCG) in the urine of a pregnant woman.

The pregnancy test stick is made of an absorbent paperlike material. A urine sample placed at one end of the stick will be drawn along by capillary action and encounter different reagents during its course along the strip (Fig. 5.4). The first reagent is a mouse antibody conjugated to a colored microbead against an epitope of hCG., The urine mixes with this when it is first placed on the stick, and if there is any hCG present the urine becomes part of an hCG-antibody-bead complex. Although these are dispersed, these complexes remain invisible and continue their flow along the stick.

The urine-antibody mixture next reaches an area where a second antibody against a different epitope of hCG has been immobilized onto the paper. This antibody will bind and capture any hCG-antibody-bead complexes. If sufficient hCG is present, a colored line will form where the bead particles aggregate.

The pregnancy test needs to include a control to indicate that the test is performing satisfactorily. For example, urine flow along the stick must be ensured, as well as the presence of the

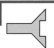 T-cell receptor (TCR)

 Immunoglobulin (Ig)

 Antigen

 MCH I

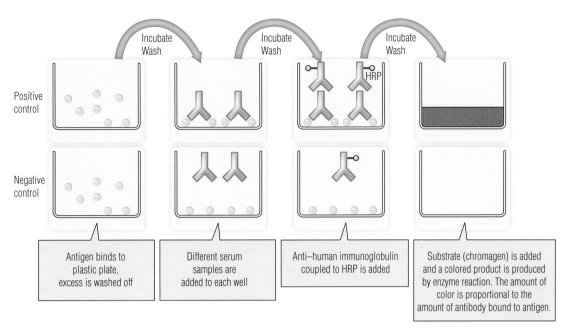

Fig 5.3 Enzyme-linked immunosorbent assay (ELISA). The illustration shows what is taking place in the positive and negative control wells, which are used to confirm the test is working. In this example, the ELISA is being used to detect antibody against syphilis. In the first step, cardiolipin (see Box 5.2) is bound to the bottom of each well. In the next step, serum is added. The top row shows serum from a donor who has syphilis antibody as a result of infection and is the positive control. The bottom row shows serum from a patient who has not been vaccinated and does not have the antibody. *HRP,* horseradish peroxidase.

antibody-bead complex. In this example the urine next encounters an area with a third antibody produced in sheep and specific for mouse immunoglobulin. This will capture the last few beads and will produce a control line indicating the test has worked.

Figure 5.5 shows pregnancy tests with positive and negative results as well as a failed test (eg, when insufficient urine has been used).

Immunofluorescence

Immunofluorescence uses antibodies to which fluorescent compounds (fluorochromes) have been covalently attached. One fluorescent compound widely used by immunologists is fluorescein isothiocyanate (FITC), which couples to free amino groups on proteins. FITC emits a greenish light when exposed to ultraviolet (UV) light. Fluorescence microscopes equipped with UV sources are used to examine specimens that have been exposed to fluorescent antibodies. This test is used extensively to detect antigens in cells or tissue sections. It is also used to screen for

autoantibodies to cell or tissue antigens (Chapter 28). Either the test antibodies are directly linked to the fluorescent compound (direct test) or a ligand that can identify the antibody is linked to the fluorescent compound (indirect test; Fig. 5.6). Often the fluorescent ligand is a second antibody that is specific for the test antibody (eg, goat anti–human immunoglobulin). Box 5.2 provides an example of a clinical use of the indirect immunofluorescence assay.

Flow Cytometry

Flow cytometry is a technique used to enumerate cells that express an antigen. The cells are stained with antibody specific for the cell-surface antigen. The antibody is coupled to specific fluorescent reagents, such as FITC (several other different colored fluors are available), and is then passed through the flow cytometer. The number of stained cells can be counted, such as the number of CD4+ T cells (Fig. 5.7; see Chapter 35 for another example).

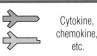 MCH II

 Cytokine, chemokine, etc.

Complement (C')

 Signaling molecule

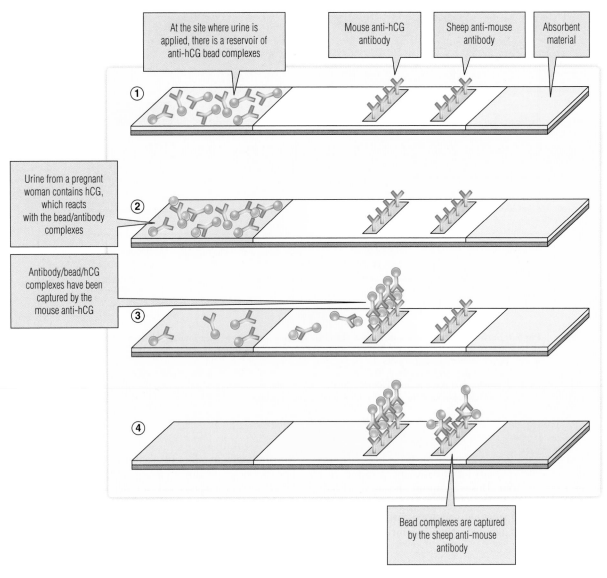

At the site where urine is applied, there is a reservoir of anti-hCG bead complexes

Mouse anti-hCG antibody

Sheep anti-mouse antibody

Absorbent material

Urine from a pregnant woman contains hCG, which reacts with the bead/antibody complexes

Antibody/bead/hCG complexes have been captured by the mouse anti-hCG

Bead complexes are captured by the sheep anti-mouse antibody

Fig 5.4 Sequence of events in a positive pregnancy stick test. *hCG*, human chorionic gonadotropin.

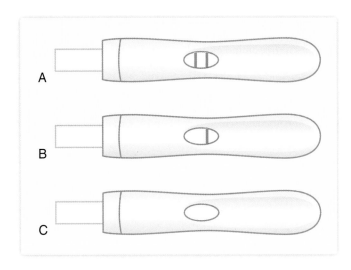

A

B

C

Fig 5.5 A, Positive pregnancy test with two lines. **B,** Negative test with a single line. **C,** Failed test with no lines.

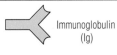 T-cell receptor (TCR)

Immunoglobulin (Ig)

 Antigen

 MCH I

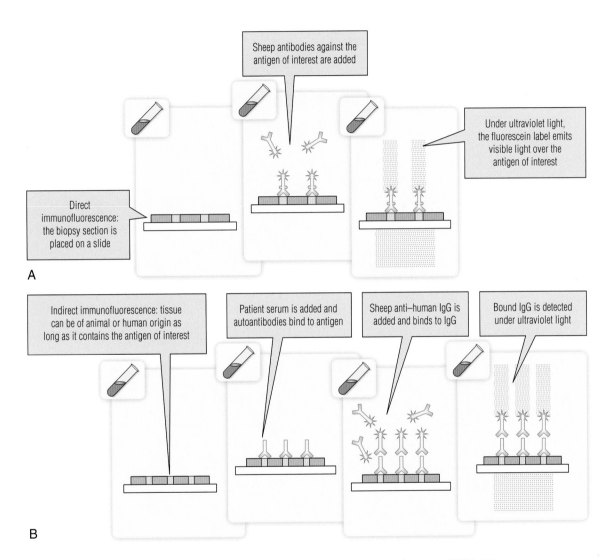

Fig 5.6 Direct (**A**) and indirect (**B**) immunofluorescence using fluorescein isothiocyanate (FITC). Other fluorochromes can be used with different colors. *IgG,* immunoglobulin G.

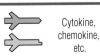 MCH II

 Cytokine, chemokine, etc.

Complement (C′)

 Signaling molecule

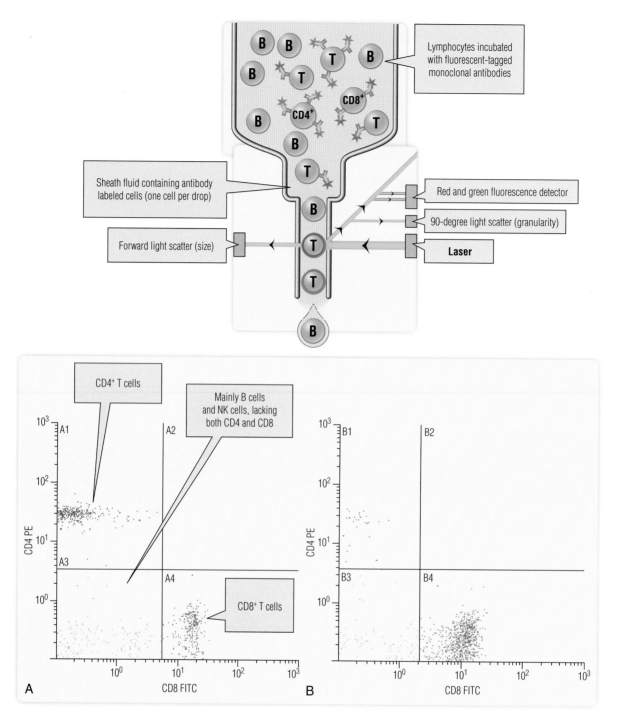

Fig 5.7 Flow cytometry "dot plots." **A,** Cells stained with the red CD4 antibody account for 59% of all lymphocytes; this is a normal sample. **B,** In this sample from a patient with HIV infection, a reduction is seen in the number of red-staining CD4⁺ T cells. *CD,* cluster of differentiation; *PE,* phycoerythrin (emits red light); *FITC,* fluorescent isothiocyanate (emits green light); *NK,* natural killer. (**A** and **B,** Courtesy John Hewitt, Manchester Royal Infirmary.)

T-cell receptor (TCR)   Immunoglobulin (Ig)   Antigen   MCH I

BOX 5.1 Drug Allergy–Immunoglobulin E Cross-Reactivity

A 58-year-old woman has been diagnosed with pneumonia and needs antibiotics urgently. However, about 20 years ago, she was prescribed penicillin for a sore throat, and within 30 minutes of taking the first capsule, she developed a widespread rash, had difficulty breathing, and went into shock. Her attending physician decides that this was probably an episode of penicillin allergy. The physician knows that people with penicillin allergy should not receive penicillin again and have about a 5% to 10% risk to reacting to other antibiotics of the β-lactam group, such as some cephalosporins and carbapenems. He decides to treat the patient with erythromycin, which has a very different molecular structure. The patient responds well and has no side effects with this antibiotic.

Adverse immunologic reactions to drugs, particularly antibiotics, can be a significant medical problem. For example, people die from anaphylactic reactions to penicillin (see also Chapter 27). Penicillin can form a hapten-carrier conjugate with a self protein that can then act as an immunogen that generates an immunoglobulin E (IgE) antibody (see Fig. 4.1). Unfortunately, the antipenicillin IgE antibodies also cross-react with a number of other antibiotics. This can complicate the treatment of bacterial infections in these patients because they are unable to take the antibiotics necessary to combat the infection.

Penicillin is a β-lactam antibiotic, so called because it contains the four-membered β-lactam ring structure, as shown in Figure 5.3. Some antipenicillin IgE antibodies can react with other antibiotics with similar structures. The precise specificity may vary, but there is enough "goodness of fit" (cross-reactivity) to allow significant binding to these other antibiotics and to create treatment problems (Fig. 5-8).

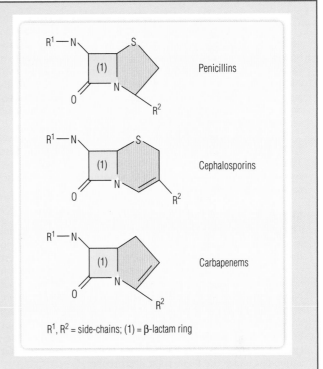

R^1, R^2 = side-chains; (1) = β-lactam ring

Fig 5.8 Structures of penicillin and related antibiotics. The β-lactam ring is yellow.

BOX 5.2 Screening for Infectious Disease

Blood donors are screened for infections that can be passed via blood components, and part of the screening is to ask donors to exclude themselves if they are at risk of these infections. One example is men who have sex with men, who may be excluded in some countries because of the risk of HIV, syphilis, or viral hepatitis in this group. Blood tests are also done to rule out infection. These tests look for antibodies against pathogens that are produced after infection or after vaccination, as in the case of hepatitis B virus.

Figure 5.9 shows an enzyme-linked immunosorbent assay (ELISA) screening test for syphilis. The ELISA plate contains two control wells and samples from 94 potential blood donors. The first well is a positive control using serum from a patient who has had syphilis. The second well contains serum from someone who has never had syphilis, which is used a negative control. The two controls are incorporated to make sure the test has worked normally. One additional well is colored yellow, which indicates a positive result.

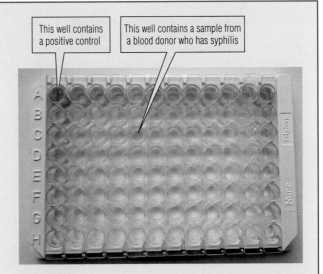

This well contains a positive control

This well contains a sample from a blood donor who has syphilis

Fig 5.9 A plate used to run 94 blood samples in an enzyme-linked immunosorbent assay (ELISA) test screening for syphilis. The first two wells are positive and negative controls.

Continued

 MCH II

  Cytokine, chemokine, etc.

Complement (C′)

 Signaling molecule

BOX 5.2 Screening for Infectious Disease—cont'd

Syphilis is an infectious disease caused by a bacterium called *Treponema pallidum*. It is transmitted sexually, in utero, and by blood transfusion. The screening test detects antibodies against a phospholipid antigen called *cardiolipin* and is called the Venereal Disease Research Laboratory (VDRL) test. Although nearly all patients with syphilis produce these antibodies, they are also produced by people with other types of infections or with autoimmunity. Thus the VDRL test for syphilis is sensitive but not very specific.

To confirm whether a potential blood donor actually has syphilis, the serum is used in a specific immunofluorescent test. This is also positive, confirming this donor does actually have syphilis. Her blood cannot be used for transfusion, and she is also referred for treatment of her syphilis.

SPECIFIC SEROLOGIC TESTS FOR SYPHILIS

The spirochete *Treponema pallidum* causes syphilis. This bacterium is a flexible, spiral rod (Fig. 5.10). To obtain the picture shown in this figure, a fluorescent treponemal antibody absorbed test (FTA-ABS) was carried out. A test serum was first absorbed with nonpathogenic treponemes to remove cross-reacting antibodies. Next, the absorbed test serum was reacted with *T. pallidum* organisms on a microscope slide. Then, as per the indirect immunofluorescence assay described in Figure 5.6, any antibodies bound to the *T. pallidum* were detected with fluorescein isothiocyanate (FITC)–conjugated anti–human immunoglobulin G (IgG) antibodies under the fluorescent microscope.

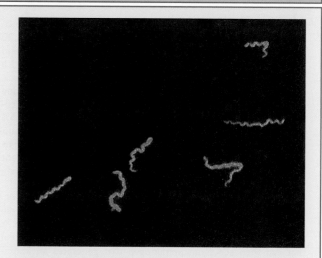

Fig 5.10 *Treponema pallidum* visualized by a fluorescent treponemal antibody absorbed test. (Courtesy Dr. S.A. Cavalieri, Department of Pathology, and Dr. R.A. Bessen, Department of Medical Microbiology and Immunology, Creighton University School of Medicine, Omaha, NE.)

BOX 5.3 New Technology for the Clinical Diagnostic Laboratory: Fluorescent Microsphere-Based Immunoassay

A new approach to diagnostic testing that appears to be very valuable, especially when multiple tests must be done on a small sample volume, is known as *Luminex xMAP* technology. This technology utilizes aspects of both enzyme-linked immunosorbent assay (ELISA) and flow cytometry. In essence, polystyrene microspheres are internally color coded with two fluorescent dyes that can be detected after laser illumination. By mixing different dyes, each bead in a set of up to 100 can be given a unique identity ("spectral signal") that can be detected in a flow cytometer (see Fig. 5.7). Each bead can also be coated with different compounds—such as antibodies, oligonucleotides, and enzymes—that can collect molecules from a test sample. By using a sandwich assay with a different-colored fluorescent reporter tag, as illustrated in Figure 5.11, the amount of a compound (eg, antibodies to hepatitis virus) can be measured with a second laser. The microspheres are in solution in a microtiter well or test tube, and multiple beads can be present in a single container. Each bead can be derivatized with a different reactant, and up to 100 different compounds can be assayed for with a set of 100 beads. The beads are transported in fluid into the analyzer and are subjected to laser illumination, much like individual cells in a flow cytometer (see Fig. 5.7). This technology can be used to carry out multiple tests, called *multiplex testing*, from a small volume of sample in a very short amount of time. The assay method has been shown to be sensitive and specific and to have some advantages over other assay formats, such as ELISA.

An example of a situation where the test could be used is as follows. Your patient has developed jaundice shortly after a trip overseas. The patient claims no history of high-risk behavior during travel, and you request testing for antibodies to hepatitis virus. A blood sample is collected, and the serum is used to assay for the presence of antibodies to hepatitis viruses A, B, and C. As shown, the patient's serum contains antibodies that bind to the Luminex beads that express hepatitis A antigen and not to the beads that express hepatitis B or C antigens. The patient receives treatment for hepatitis A, and the jaundice resolves.

One advantage of the microsphere bead assay is being able to test simultaneously for multiple reactants, such as a panel of viral antigens or a panel of cytokines.

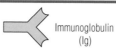 T-cell receptor (TCR)   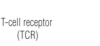 Immunoglobulin (Ig)   Antigen   MCH I

BOX 5.3 New Technology for the Clinical Diagnostic Laboratory: Fluorescent Microsphere-Based Immunoassay—cont'd

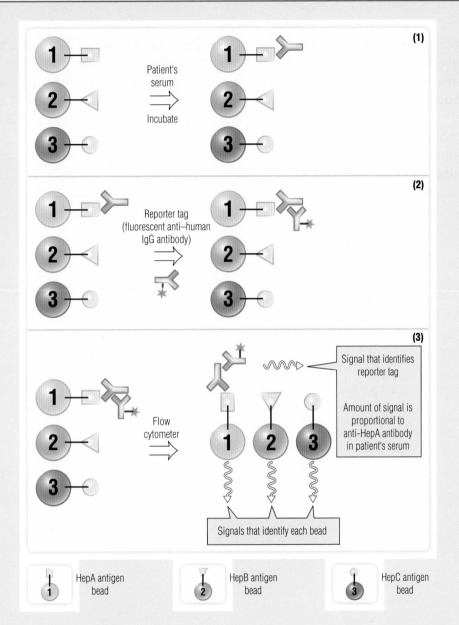

Fig 5.11 Fluorescent microsphere–based immunoassay for antibodies to hepatitis (Hep) virus (Luminex xMAP technology). *IgG,* immunoglobulin G.

 MCH II   Cytokine, chemokine, etc.   Complement (C′)   Signaling molecule

LEARNING POINTS — Can You Now....

1. Describe antigen-antibody interaction as a subset of receptor-ligand interactions?
2. Draw the structure of the antigen-binding site of antibodies for various types of antigen?
3. Explain antibody cross-reactivity in terms of "goodness of fit" of the antigen in the combining site?
4. Describe a range of diagnostic tests based on antigen-antibody interaction, indicating the general principle of each test?
5. List at least three examples of diseases for which immunologic tests are useful in diagnosis?

 T-cell receptor (TCR)

 Immunoglobulin (Ig)

Antigen

 MCH I

Antibody Diversity

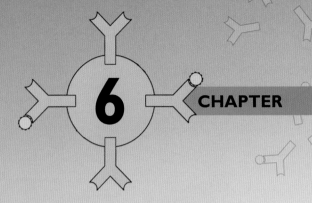

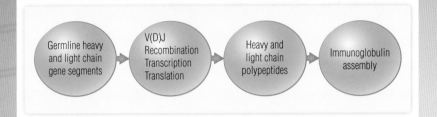

Germline heavy and light chain gene segments → V(D)J Recombination Transcription Translation → Heavy and light chain polypeptides → Immunoglobulin assembly

The human body appears to be capable of generating an almost infinite number of antibody (immunoglobulin [Ig]) molecules—perhaps at least one for every antigen in the universe! Some calculations suggest that there could be as many as 10^{11} different antibody molecules available in the human antibody repertoire, the collection of antibodies of different specificity. This chapter describes the various mechanisms used in B cells to achieve this diversity. Similar mechanisms are used in T cells to generate T-cell receptor (TCR) diversity, but so far they have not been detected in other genes. These various mechanisms are collectively referred to as the *generation of diversity*. The overview figure above illustrates the various steps on the pathway to assembling a complete Ig molecule, and this chapter provides a description of the pathway of Ig assembly in B cells.

■ IMMUNOGLOBULIN GENES

As described in Chapter 4, immunoglobulins have two kinds of polypeptide chains, heavy and light. Each chain has a variable (V) and a constant (C) region. Ig polypeptide chains are encoded by gene segments (Fig. 6.1) that are rearranged during B-cell development (Fig. 6.2) to assemble a functional gene that encodes either a light or a heavy chain (Fig. 6.3). These gene segments include leader (L), joining (J), and diversity (D) gene segments in addition to the V and C gene segments. Gene segments exist in sets, or groups, that are arrays of different versions of that gene segment. For example, five different J_k gene segments constitute the J_k set. Figure 6.1 illustrates the organization of the human light and heavy chain gene segments and enumerates the different gene segments for Igs.

During the development of B cells (Chapter 14), the Ig gene segments are rearranged and brought next to each other to form a contiguous functional gene (see Fig. 6.3). The process of rearrangement is known as *somatic recombination,* and it occurs even in the absence of antigen to create a repertoire of potential antibody (antigen receptor) molecules. Once complete light and heavy chain genes have been assembled, the Ig light and heavy chains can be synthesized, and the polypeptide chains are assembled as an Ig molecule. This molecule is either expressed at the surface of the B cell or is secreted from a differentiated B cell known as a *plasma cell* (see Fig. 6.6 and Chapter 14).

The V regions of the chains constitute the antigen-binding site, and the C regions contribute specialized effector functions, such as binding to cellular receptors or complement proteins. Antibody diversity is created by recombining different gene segments to create different V regions. This considerably reduces the number of genes that would otherwise be needed to encode the very large number of different antibody molecules, and it reduces the amount of the genome that would otherwise be given over to genes for antibody molecules.

Assembly of Variable Regions by Somatic Recombination

After the initial gene rearrangements have occurred (see Fig. 6.2), the entire gene is transcribed, including the *exons* (coding sequences) and the *introns* (noncoding sequences), into a primary RNA transcript (see Fig. 6.3). RNA splicing then takes place, whereby RNA processing enzymes remove the intron sequences to produce a messenger RNA (mRNA) that can be translated into protein. The leader (L) peptide sequence is then removed by proteolytic enzymes (see Fig. 6.3).

The V region of light chain genes is composed of V and J segments, and that of heavy chains is assembled from three

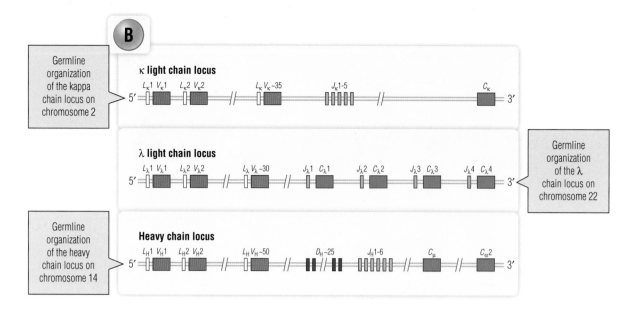

Fig 6.1 Genomic organization of the immunoglobulin loci.

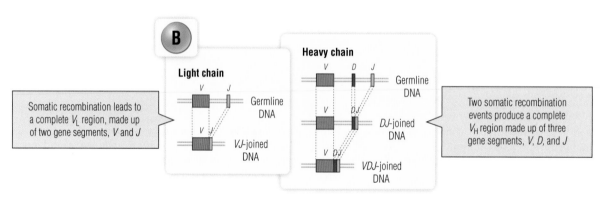

Fig 6.2 Immunoglobulin variable regions are constructed from gene segments by recombination.

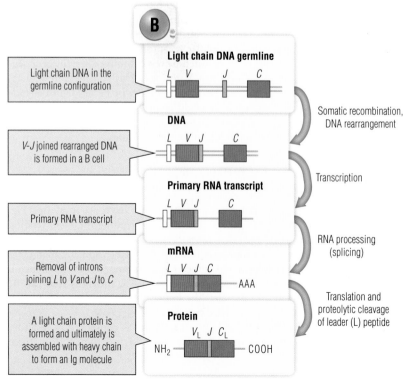

A

Fig 6.3 Major steps in the synthesis of light (**A**) and heavy (**B**) immunoglobulin (Ig) chains.

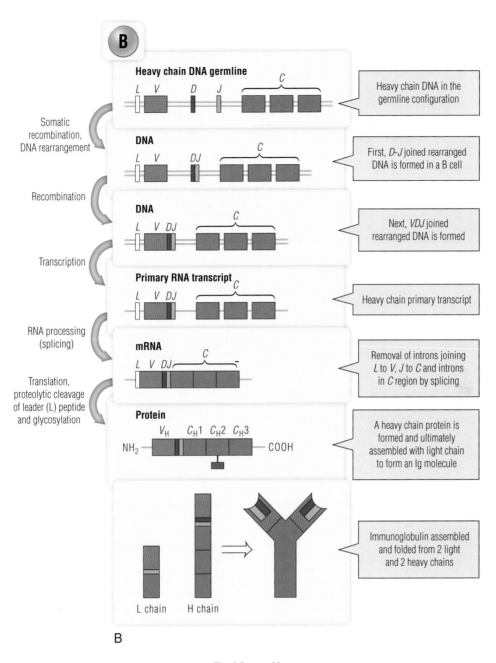

Heavy chain DNA germline

Heavy chain DNA in the germline configuration

Somatic recombination, DNA rearrangement

DNA

First, *D-J* joined rearranged DNA is formed in a B cell

Recombination

DNA

Next, *VDJ* joined rearranged DNA is formed

Transcription

Primary RNA transcript

Heavy chain primary transcript

RNA processing (splicing)

mRNA

Removal of introns joining *L* to *V*, *J* to *C* and introns in *C* region by splicing

Translation, proteolytic cleavage of leader (L) peptide and glycosylation

Protein

A heavy chain protein is formed and ultimately assembled with light chain to form an Ig molecule

Immunoglobulin assembled and folded from 2 light and 2 heavy chains

L chain   H chain

B

Fig 6.3, cont'd

segments: *V*, *D*, and *J* (see Fig. 6.2). For a complete *V* region to be transcribed, the *V* region gene segments (*V* and *J* or *V*, *D*, and *J*) have to be "cut out" and then joined together by enzymes responsible for DNA recombination. For example, one *J* segment from the array of *J* segments is combined with one *V* segment from the array of *V* segments to form a V_L region. Similarly, one *V*, one *D*, and one *J* segment are rearranged to make a V_H region. First the *D* and *J* segments are joined, then a *V* gene segment is joined to the *DJ* segment to create a complete V_H exon (see Fig. 6.2). Because there are multiple *V*, *D*, and *J* gene segments (see Fig. 6.1), many different complete variable regions can be created. For example, *V1* combined with *J2* forms a different V_L region with a different specificity for antigen than that formed when *V6* combines with *J2*.

The complex of enzymes involved in somatic recombination in lymphocytes is known as the *V(D)J recombinase*. These enzymes are responsible for the cleavage and rejoining of the DNA involved in rearrangement. Two of these enzymes, products of the recombination activating genes *RAG1* and *RAG2*, are responsible for the first cleavage step involved in somatic recombination of Ig genes. The RAG-1 and RAG-2 enzymes are only found in lymphocytes, and defects in these enzymes lead to blockage of lymphocyte development (see Box 7.1).

Thus B cells recombine genes from either chromosome 2 (κ light chain) or chromosome 22 (λ light chain) plus chromosome 14 (heavy chain) to produce immunoglobulin. Each cell has two of each of these genes, one inherited from each parent. One copy of each gene needs to be silenced: for example, if the variable

 MCH II

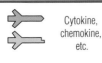 Cytokine, chemokine, etc.

 Complement (C′)

Signaling molecule

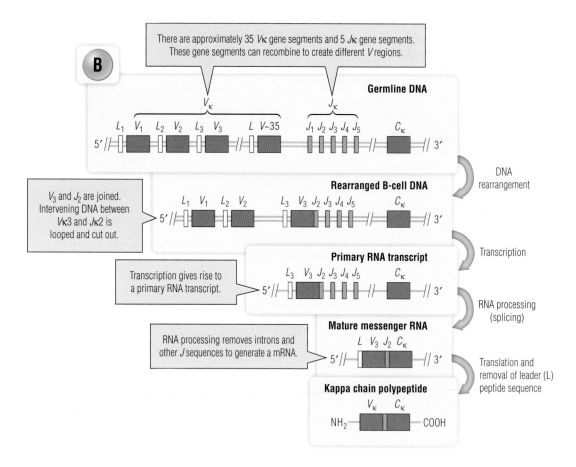

Fig 6.4 Details of κ light chain synthesis.

segments from both maternal and paternal genes were processed at the same time, a B cell could produce two different antibody specificities. The process of silencing either a parental or maternal gene is known as *allelic exclusion*.

Gene Organization and Synthesis

Human Light Chain

As described in Chapter 4, the two types of light chain are kappa (κ) and lambda (λ). The events leading to synthesis of a κ light chain are shown in Figure 6.4 and are described below. The process is essentially the same for λ light chain synthesis.

In the germline of humans, approximately 35 different V_k genes are found in the κ locus on chromosome 2. Each V_k gene encodes the N-terminal (95 amino acid residues of a κ variable region). Downstream of the V_k region (ie, 3′) are five J_k exons. Each J_k segment encodes amino acids 96 through 108 of the κ variable region. After a long intron, the κ locus ends in the one C_k exon that encodes the constant region of the κ light chain.

To synthesize a κ light chain, a cell early in the B-lymphocyte lineage (Chapter 14) selects a V_k exon (eg, V_k3), and after a process of DNA rearrangement involving the V(D)J recombinase, it joins it to a *J* segment (eg, J_k2). The intervening DNA, in this example from approximately the 3′ end of V3 to the 5′ end of J2, is deleted by looping it and cleaving it out for ultimate degradation. From this rearranged DNA, a primary RNA transcript is made (see Fig. 6.4). This primary RNA transcript

undergoes RNA splicing reactions to bring, for example, the V_k3, J_k2, and C_k exons together as a mature mRNA. Splicing removes all the intervening sequences (eg, J3, J4, and J5), thereby allowing the RNA to be translated into a κ polypeptide chain in the endoplasmic reticulum of the cell. The process is similar for λ chain genes, except that λ is found on chromosome 22 in humans, and about 30 V_λ and four J_λ genes exist. Each of the J_λ genes is associated with a different C_λ gene (see Fig. 6.1). Consequently, four different subtypes of λ light chain are possible in humans.

Human Heavy Chain

Approximately 50 V_H, 25 D_H, and 6 J_H gene segments are present in the heavy chain locus on chromosome 14 in the human genome (see Fig. 6.1). The diversity (D) segment, like the J segment, encodes amino acids in the third hypervariable (hv3) region of the heavy chain. The term *hypervariable region* is used in discussions of both Ig and TCR diversity (Chapter 7).

The mechanism of heavy chain synthesis (Fig. 6.5) is very similar to those described for κ light chains except that three segments, rather than two, are required for assembly of the V_H exon and that multiple C_H exons are present in the heavy chain locus.

First, the D and J segments are joined, then the V segment joins to the combined DJ segments to form the complete V_H exon. C region exons are spliced to the V_H exon during processing of the heavy chain RNA transcript.

T-cell receptor (TCR)

Immunoglobulin (Ig)

Antigen

MCH I

introduce point mutations at a very high rate into the *V* regions of heavy and light chains. Some of the mutations produce antibody molecules that are a better fit for antigen than the "original" antibody. These new antibodies tend to bind antigen with a higher affinity, and B cells that express them are preferentially selected for maturation into plasma cells (Chapter 14). This phenomenon is sometimes referred to as *affinity maturation* of the population of antibody molecules in an individual.

When B cells respond to a persistent infection, the amount of antibody measured by an enzyme-linked immunosorbent assay (ELISA) gradually increases. This is in part because as the months pass, more B cells are being produced, which results in higher quantities of antibody being secreted. But in addition, somatic hypermutation is taking place, so the quality of the antibody being produced is improved, with higher affinity. Once the infection is cleared, some B cells survive as memory B cells. These are derived from the B cells that secreted the best immunoglobulin as a result of affinity maturation.

■ IMMUNOGLOBULIN CLASSES

Class Switching

As described in Chapter 4, the five classes of human immunoglobulin are IgM, IgD, IgG, IgE, and IgA. There are C_H genes for each of these Igs (see Fig. 6.5), and the same V_H exon can be rearranged to associate with a different C_H exon at different times in the course of an immune response. For example, early in the immune response to an antigen, a B cell will always express IgM. Later, in response to the same antigen, the assembled *V* region may be expressed in an IgG antibody. This change involves DNA recombination between specific regions, called *switch regions*. Using a different constant region creates additional diversity, because different effector functions are associated with different *C* regions.

Class switching enables B cells to tailor an antibody to specific circumstances. For example, IgM is a particularly useful antibody for dealing with infections in the blood, but its high molecular weight prevents it from diffusing into tissues. For this reason, the B cells will undergo class switching to produce predominantly IgG when responding to tissue infection, such as an abscess. On the other hand, the immune system has evolved IgA to respond to infections at mucosal surfaces, such as in the gut. B cells will class switch from IgM to IgA in response to gut infection. The clinical box in this chapter describes how this knowledge can also help diagnose infections.

Membrane-Bound and Secreted Immunoglobulin

B cells can produce immunoglobulins in membrane-bound or secreted forms. The membrane-bound form of Ig has approximately 30 additional amino acid residues at the C-terminus of the heavy chain. These residues include a stretch of approximately 25 hydrophobic amino acids that anchor the Ig in the cell membrane, where it can act as a receptor (see Chapter 11). The two different forms are encoded in different C_H exons, and alternative RNA processing (see Fig. 6.6) is used to generate either the secreted or the membrane-bound form. Again, the mechanism of regulation of this alternative RNA processing or choice of polyadenylation site is not fully understood. Presumably, signals generated by antigen binding and/or interaction with T cells are involved (see Chapter 16).

BOX 6.1 Using Antibodies to Diagnose Acute Hepatitis B Infection

A 29-year-old woman presents with a 4-week history of mild fever, weight loss, and jaundice. She has a history of unprotected sex with multiple partners and also has a number of homemade tattoos. In addition to markedly abnormal liver function tests, her virology results are used to make the diagnosis of acute hepatitis B virus infection as the cause of her jaundice.

Her blood work is negative for antibodies against hepatitis A and hepatitis C virus, making these infections highly unlikely as the cause of her jaundice. She is positive for antibodies against hepatitis B surface antigen (HBsAg). This could be consistent with vaccination, but she is not sure if she has been vaccinated. In this case, two other scenarios could rule this out:

1. She is positive for HBsAg. The *antigen*, rather than the *antibody*, is only detectable after hepatitis B infection not after vaccination. She is also positive for viral DNA, which can only be present after infection.
2. She has antibodies against hepatitis B core antigen (anti-HBc). Hepatitis B core antigen (Fig. 6.7A) is not present in

the vaccine, so antibodies against it are not produced in response to vaccination. Because HBc is present in hepatitis viruses, antibodies against it are produced after infection.

The likely diagnosis is that the cause of jaundice in our patient is hepatitis B infection. However, people with chronic hepatitis B infection often have normal liver function. These individuals test positive for immunoglobulin G (IgG) anti-HBc. However, this patient has IgM anti-HBc, indicating the infection took place in the past few weeks (Fig. 6.7B, C, and Table 6.2). This makes the diagnosis of acute hepatitis B infection quite likely.

The patient gradually felt better without any specific treatment. Her HBsAg and viral DNA tests became negative, indicating her body was bringing the infection under control. Her anti-HBc class switched from IgM to IgG. However, only time will tell if she becomes a chronic carrier and whether she will develop more problems related to hepatitis B infection in the future (see Chapter 23).

Continued

 MCH II

 Cytokine, chemokine, etc.

 Complement (C')

 Signaling molecule

BOX 6.1 Using Antibodies to Diagnose Acute Hepatitis B Infection—cont'd

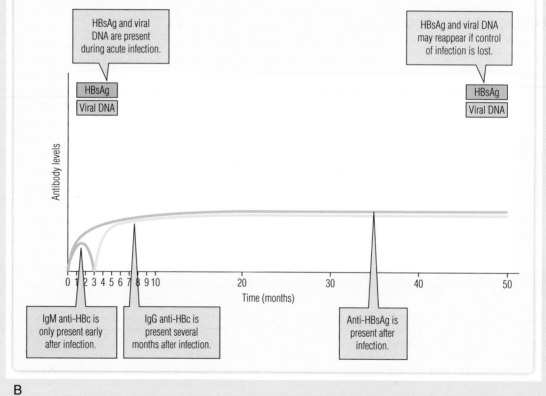

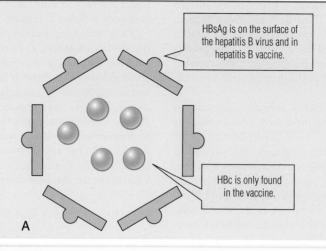

A

B

Fig 6.7 A, Structure of the hepatitis B virus. **B,** Tests that can be used at the different stages of the hepatitis B virus infection. *HBC,* hepatitis B core (antigen); *HBsAg,* hepatitis B virus surface antigen.

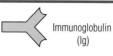 T-cell receptor (TCR)　　 Immunoglobulin (Ig)　　 Antigen　　MCH I

BOX 6.1 Using Antibodies to Diagnose Acute Hepatitis B Infection—cont'd

TABLE 6.2   Profile of Test Results Helps Diagnose Different States of Immunity to Hepatitis B Virus

	Anti-HBsAg	HBsAg	Hepatitis B DNA	Anti-HBc
Nonvaccinated healthy individual	−	−	−	−
After hepatitis B vaccination	+	−	−	−
Acute hepatitis B infection	+	+	+	IgM+
Chronic hepatitis B infection, well controlled	+	−	−	IgG+
Chronic hepatitis B infection, poorly controlled	+	+	+	IgG+

HBc, *hepatitis B core;* HBsAg, *hepatitis B surface antigen;* Ig, *immunoglobulin.*

LEARNING POINTS   Can You Now...

1. Explain how rearrangement of gene segments generates an antibody repertoire?
2. Draw a diagram of Ig light chain gene organization and synthesis?
3. Draw a diagram of Ig heavy chain gene organization and synthesis?
4. Describe the various mechanisms that contribute to the generation of antibody diversity, for example, rearranging multiple gene segments?
5. Draw a diagram of the process of class switching?
6. Draw a diagram of the process used to generate membrane-bound and secreted forms of Ig?

 MCH II   Cytokine, chemokine, etc.   Complement (C')    Signaling molecule

7

The T-Cell Receptor

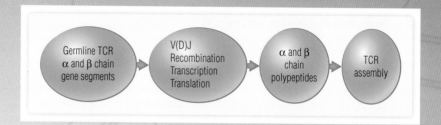

This chapter describes the antigen recognition molecule of T cells, the T-cell receptor (TCR). The figure above indicates the main steps on the pathway to TCR assembly that are outlined here. As described in Chapter 2, TCRs recognize peptide antigens only when they are displayed by self major histocompatibility complex (MHC) molecules—that is, they have a dual specificity. This is quite unlike the B-cell antigen recognition molecule (antibody), which binds various kinds of peptide and nonpeptide antigen directly. The end of this chapter discusses how the interaction between the TCR and antigen MHC forms part of the immunologic synapse. Despite the different mechanism of antigen recognition used, the TCR is structurally similar to immunoglobulin (Fig. 7.1). The TCR, like the B-cell antigen receptor, is clonally distributed. Every clone of T cells expresses a different antigen receptor molecule.

■ STRUCTURE OF THE T-CELL RECEPTOR

The TCR is a heterodimeric membrane protein. The two types of receptor are those with αβ chains, present on approximately 95% of human T lymphocytes, and those with γδ chains, found on approximately 5% of human T lymphocytes. Each of these chains has a molecular weight in the range of 40,000 to 60,000. The extracellular portion of each chain is composed of two domains (see Fig. 7.1). The overall structure is similar to that of a membrane-bound antigen-binding fragment (Fab) of immunoglobulin (Ig). The TCR domains farthest away from the membrane are similar to Ig variable (V) region domains, and the domains closest to the membrane are similar to Ig constant (C) region domains. Antigen binds to a site created by the V domains of the αβ or γδ chains. The three-dimensional (3-D) structure

of the extracellular portion of the TCR has been determined (Fig. 7.2) and has a great deal of similarity with that of Ig.

Protein and nucleic acid sequence data have been obtained for many TCRs with different specificities. Analyses of these sequences suggest the existence of three hypervariable (hv) regions in the variable region. Determination of 3-D structure shows that these hypervariable regions are arranged as a relatively flat surface (see Fig. 7.2) that contacts amino acid residues of both the MHC molecule and the peptide antigen.

The αβ T-Cell Receptor

The αβ TCR is the predominant (95%) human TCR found on MHC-restricted T cells. In general, when we refer to the TCR, we are referring to an αβ TCR. The different types of helper T cells are αβ T cells, as are most of the cytotoxic T lymphocytes that kill virally infected cells. The αβ TCR recognizes peptide antigens presented by MHC molecules (Chapters 2, 3, 9, and 10).

The γδ T-Cell Receptor

The γδ TCR is found on a few (5%) human T cells. These cells are derived in the thymus as a separate cell lineage from those cells that express αβ TCR molecules (Chapter 15). In some epithelial tissues, γδ T cells have been found to be more numerous, which has led to the hypothesis that they are a first line of defense and may initiate responses to those microbes frequently encountered at epithelial boundaries, such as the skin. Also, γδ T cells differ from αβ T cells in two important ways. First, they can recognize lipid molecules as well as peptides; second, they do not always recognize MHC and are not MHC restricted.

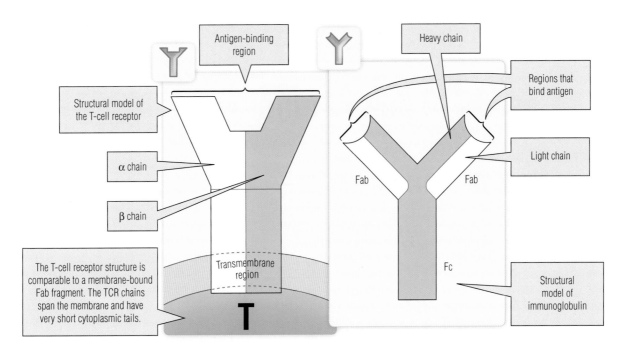

Fig 7.1 Structure of the T-cell receptor (TCR) compared with immunoglobulin. *Fab*, antigen-binding fragment; *Fc*, crystallizable fraction.

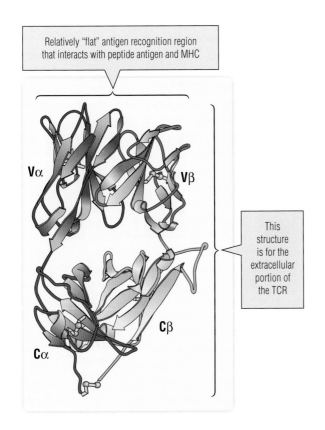

Fig 7.2 The three-dimensional structure of the T-cell receptor (TCR). *MHC*, major histocompatibility complex; *V*, Ig variable. (Modified from Garcia KC, Degano M, Stanfield RL, et al. An αβ T cell receptor structure at 2.5 A and its orientation in the TCR-MHC complex. *Science.* 1996;274:209.)

GENERATION OF DIVERSITY OF THE T-CELL RECEPTOR GENES

The organization of the gene segments that encode the TCR chains is very like that for Ig heavy and light chain gene segments. As shown in Figure 7.3, genes for the α and γ chains are like the genes for Ig κ and λ light chains in that they use only *V* and *J* segments. The genes for the β and δ chains are like Ig heavy chain genes in that they use *V, D,* and *J* gene segments. A difference from the Ig genes is that there are fewer TCR C-region genes. For example, there is only one *Cα* gene, and although there are two *Cβ* genes, they appear to be functionally identical. This is in contrast to Igs in which the C regions include the μ, δ, γ, ε, and α classes and the λ-subtypes (λ1 through λ4), among others.

The mechanisms that generate diversity before antigenic stimulation of T cells are, in essence, the same as those already described for generation of diversity in B cells (Chapter 6). After stimulation by antigen, however, the pathway in T cells is quite different from that in B cells. Whereas Ig genes continue to diversify after antigenic stimulation—such as by somatic hypermutation and by class switching, attaching a V region to a different C region—the genes for the TCRs remain unchanged.

TCR genes rearrange in the thymus (Chapter 15). The basic molecular steps in synthesis of the TCR chains are very similar to those described for Ig light and heavy chains (Fig. 7.4). As for Ig genes in B lymphocytes, the V(D)J recombinase, including the RAG-1 and RAG-2 enzymes, is involved in TCR gene rearrangements; therefore defects in these functions will affect B and T cells (Box 7.1). For the α chain, a *V* gene segment (eg, $V_α 2$) and a *J* gene segment (eg, $J_α 5$) are recombined to form a V-region exon (eg, $V_α 2\ J_α 5$). Transcription of the *V* region,

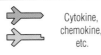 MCH II

Cytokine, chemokine, etc.

 Complement (C′)

 Signaling molecule

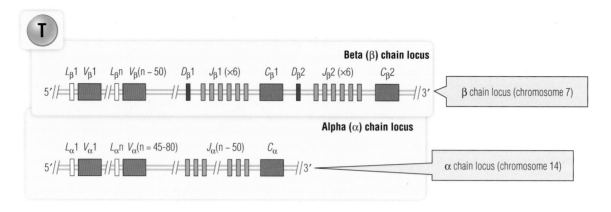

Fig 7.3 Organization of human genes for T-cell receptors.

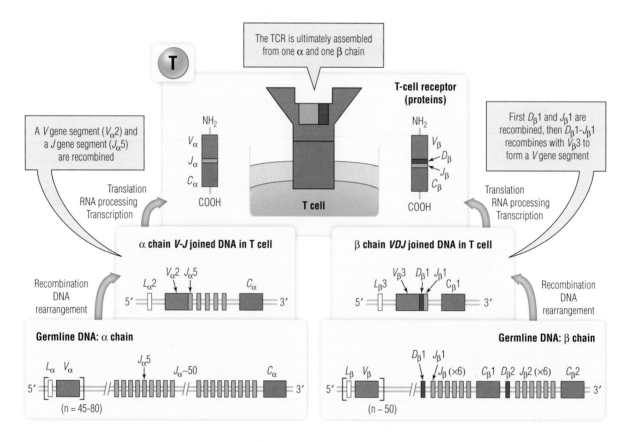

Fig 7.4 Synthesis and expression of a human αβ T-cell receptor (TCR).

along with the Cα exon, yields a primary RNA transcript. Splicing of this RNA yields a messenger RNA (mRNA) that on translation produces a TCR α chain protein (see Fig. 7.4) in a manner similar to that described for Ig light chains in Figure 6.3A and in Figure 6.4.

Assembly of the β chain is similar to assembly of the Ig heavy chain in that first a D and a J gene segment are combined, followed by combination of this DJ unit to a V gene segment, such as $D_\beta 1$, $J_\beta 1$, and $V_\beta 3$ as shown in Figure 7.4. The complete V region exon is then transcribed along with $C_\beta 1$ to form a primary RNA transcript. RNA splicing yields an mRNA, which on

translation yields the β chain of the TCR (see Fig. 7.4) in a manner similar to that described for Ig heavy chains in Figures 6.3B and 6.5. The α and β chains are translated in the rough endoplasmic reticulum, and like other membrane-bound glycoproteins, they are processed through the endoplasmic reticulum and Golgi compartments before expression at the cell-surface membrane.

As with the immunoglobulins, TCR diversity is generated by (1) the existence of multiple V-region genes, (2) junctional diversity created by imprecise joining and addition of nucleotides by the terminal deoxynucleotidyl transferase (TdT)

 T-cell receptor (TCR)

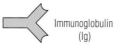 Immunoglobulin (Ig)

 Antigen

 MCH I

enzyme, and (3) random combination of chains. Unlike Ig, there is no somatic hypermutation in TCR genes. However, the total potential B- and T-cell antigen receptor repertoires are similar in size because the lack of somatic hypermutation is offset by a greater potential for junctional diversity in TCR genes (Chapter 9 provides a summary). Theoretically, the TCR repertoire may be as high as 10^{16} to 10^{18}, with much of the repertoire contributed by junctional diversity. One illustration of the importance of junctional diversity to TCR diversity is that there are more than 10 times as many *J* segments available for TCR α chains as for the Ig κ and λ light chains.

RECOGNITION OF ANTIGEN

The TCRs occur only on the cell surface; T cells do not have the potential to express an alternative secreted form like the B-cell antigen receptor. Figure 7.5 shows how the TCR interacts with peptide antigen presented by self MHC molecules. Most peptide antigens after processing (Chapter 10) are displayed in the MHC groove (Chapters 2, 3, and 8) for binding to the TCR. A few, known as *superantigens,* can activate T cells independent of antigen processing and presentation. These superantigens bind simultaneously to MHC class II molecules and to certain TCRs with particular β chains. In doing so, they activate all T cells bearing this Vβ region and give rise to a massive immune response (Box 7.2).

A 3-D structural analysis has been carried out on the trimolecular TCR-peptide-MHC complex; one example of this for MHC class I (HLA-A2), a viral peptide and a specific TCR, is shown in Figure 7.6. This figure shows that the hypervariable sequences of this TCR V region create a "flat" surface that interacts with residues of the peptide antigen and with some of the polymorphic amino acid residues located in the α1 and α2 domains of the MHC molecule.

OTHER ACCESSORY MOLECULES INVOLVED IN T-CELL FUNCTION

As shown in Figure 7.7, several molecules contribute to T-cell function. These molecules form one side of the *immunologic synapse,* which T cells use to communicate with other cells. This chapter has primarily focused on the TCR $\alpha\beta$ and $\gamma\delta$ chains, which bind antigen. The TCR cannot function as a receptor without the CD3 complex, which consists of four different transmembrane protein chains: γ, δ, ϵ, and ζ (zeta). CD3 molecules are necessary for a signal to be transduced to the cytoplasm after the TCR binds antigen (Chapter 11), thus allowing T-cell activation. Several additional molecules—such as integrins like CD11a, also known as *leukocyte function–associated antigen 1* (LFA-1)—function in adhesion of the T cell to its target cell (see Fig. 7.7), and yet others function both in adhesion and in signal transduction. The most important of the latter are CD4 and CD8, which enhance the response of specific T cells, both by stabilizing the TCR-peptide-MHC complex through binding to the class II or class I MHC molecules, respectively, and

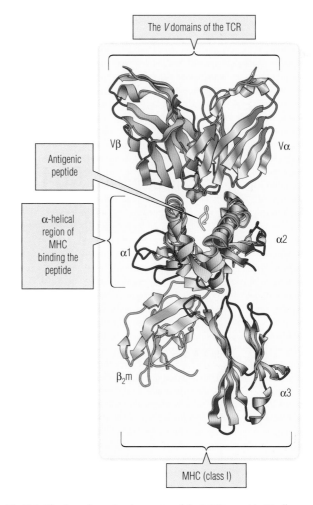

Fig 7.6 The three-dimensional structure of the MHC–peptide–T-cell receptor (TCR) complex. *MHC,* major histocompatibility complex. (Modified from Bjorkman PJ. MHC restriction in three dimensions: a view of T cell receptor/ligand interactions. *Cell.* 1997;89:167.)

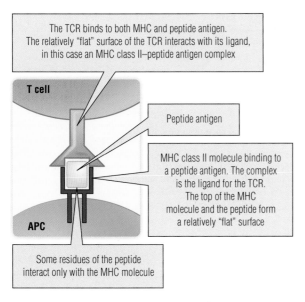

Fig 7.5 Interaction of the T-cell receptor (TCR) with the peptide and major histocompatibility complex (MHC). *APC,* antigen-presenting cell.

 MCH II

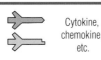 Cytokine, chemokine, etc.

 Complement (C′)

 Signaling molecule

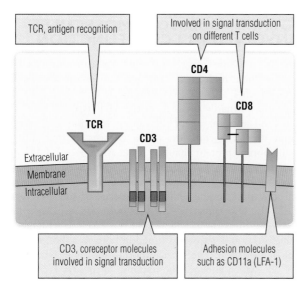

TCR, antigen recognition

Involved in signal transduction on different T cells

CD4

CD8

TCR

CD3

Extracellular
Membrane
Intracellular

CD3, coreceptor molecules involved in signal transduction

Adhesion molecules such as CD11a (LFA-1)

Fig 7.7 Accessory molecules involved in T-cell function. *LFA-1,* leukocyte function–associated antigen 1; *TCR,* T-cell receptor.

by bringing a tyrosine kinase—Lck, a member of the Src family—into the proximity of the cytoplasmic tails of the CD3 and ζ proteins, thereby facilitating signal transduction and cell activation. T cells that carry CD4 are known as *T-helper cells,* in that they usually promote the responsiveness of other cells. However, one subset of T-helper cells, called *regulatory T cells* (Tregs), inhibits other T cells. T cells that carry CD8 have killing functions, such as inducing apoptosis of virally infected cells, and are also known as *cytotoxic T lymphocytes* (CTLs).

The *immunologic synapse* differs from a *neurologic synapse* in that it is a very temporary structure. For example, when a T cell recognizes a peptide antigen on an antigen-presenting cell (APC), a synapse forms for several hours. During this time, two-way communication exists between the two cells. Once the T cell is responding to the antigen, the synapse breaks down and releases the T cell to interact with other cells, with which the response to the antigen will take place (Fig. 7.8). These processes are described further in Chapter 16.

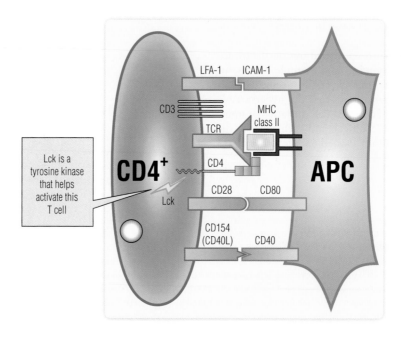

LFA-1   ICAM-1

CD3

MHC class II

TCR

CD4

CD4⁺

APC

Lck is a tyrosine kinase that helps activate this T cell

Lck

CD28   CD80

CD154 (CD40L)   CD40

Fig 7.8 This figure shows an immunologic synapse between a CD4⁺ T cell and an antigen-presenting cell. The interaction between the T-cell receptor (TCR) and the antigen provide the specificity for the synapse. CD4 and CD3 are linked to Lck, which triggers signaling in the T cell. The other pairs of molecules, leukocyte function–associated antigen 1 (LFA-1)–intracellular adhesion molecule 1 (ICAM-1; CD28/CD80) and CD154 (CD40L-CD40), stabilize the synapse and will also trigger signals in the participating cells. *APC,* antigen-presenting cell; *MHC,* major histocompatibility complex.

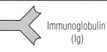 T-cell receptor (TCR)

 Immunoglobulin (Ig)

Antigen

 MCH I

BOX 7.1 Autosomal-Recessive Severe Combined Immunodeficiency Due to Defects in the Recombination Activating Gene (RAG-1, RAG-2) Products

A 3-week-old girl is brought to the hospital by her parents. The infant has lost 10% of her body weight since delivery and is struggling with breathing. The parents are noted to be first cousins, but there is nothing else of note in the history. On examination, the baby has extensive *Candida* infection of the skin and is also found to be in respiratory failure; a chest radiograph shows features of *Pneumocystis jiroveci* pneumonia, and the lymphocyte count is very low. When flow cytometry (Chapter 5) is carried out to count the various types of lymphocytes, T cells and B cells are found to be completely absent. There are a few natural killer (NK) cells. Genetic tests are used to confirm autosomal-recessive severe combined immunodeficiency (AR-SCID) caused by mutations in the *RAG1* and *RAG2* genes. The baby is referred for stem cell transplantation.

The recombination activating gene (RAG) enzymes initiate immunoglobulin gene rearrangements in B cells (Chapters 6 and 14). As stated earlier in this chapter, they are also essential in T cells for T-cell receptor gene rearrangements (Chapter 15). Further evidence of their importance comes from the fact that deficiencies in RAG-1 or RAG-2 lead to AR-SCID. The form of

AR-SCID that results from *RAG1* and *RAG2* mutations is different from other forms of the disease in that there is a complete absence of both T and B cells. However, NK cells are found in the circulation. Hence this form of the disease is known as *TB-SCID*.

TB-SCID is a rare syndrome that is invariably fatal by 2 years of age without bone marrow transplantation (BMT) from a human leukocyte antigen (HLA)-compatible donor. The disease presents in infants during the first few weeks of life as lymphopenia with recurrent infections. Only a very small thymus can be detected. These babies have recurrent episodes of pneumonia, otitis, and skin infections along with persistent infections with opportunistic organisms such as *Candida albicans* and *P. jiroveci*. For the parents and the pediatrician, this is a dire emergency situation because such children are at great risk. However, if BMT is performed early enough, more than 80% of children survive. SCID as a syndrome is rare, and TB-SCID is even more rare. However, several hundred individuals are alive today after BMT to correct various forms of SCID. BMT is further discussed in Chapter 34.

BOX 7.2 Superantigens and Toxic Shock Syndrome

A 23-year-old woman is brought to the emergency department after collapsing at work. She is found to have a widespread red rash, a high temperature (38.9°C), and low blood pressure (systolic pressure of 86 mm Hg). She is noted to be menstruating with a tampon in situ. Emergency blood tests show evidence of acute renal failure and liver inflammation. A preliminary diagnosis of toxic shock syndrome is made. The tampon is removed, and the patient is resuscitated with fluids and makes a good recovery. Over the next few days, blood cultures are shown to be negative, and 2 weeks later she experiences desquamation of the skin on her palms. These features enable the retrospective diagnosis of toxic shock syndrome to be confirmed.

Certain proteins produced by some bacteria and viruses are recognized by αβ T-cell receptors (TCRs) that express T cells without processing. They have been shown to bind directly (but outside the antigen recognition site) to numerous TCR Vβ sequences and to directly activate T cells. They also bind to the outside surface of major histocompatibility complex (MHC) class II molecules (Fig. 7.9). By virtue of their binding to Vβ regions of TCRs found on many T cells, the superantigens are capable of activating 1% to 20% of T cells and can cause the presence of high levels of cytokines in the blood. The very high levels of cytokines are sometimes called a *cytokine storm* and will contribute to the low blood pressure and multiorgan failure that

characterize toxic shock syndrome. Note how a local infection, in this case an infected tampon, can cause widespread, life-threatening symptoms. Septic shock is another cause of cytokine storm and low blood pressure (Chapter 21). In the case of septic shock, the infection is usually widespread, and blood cultures are typically positive.

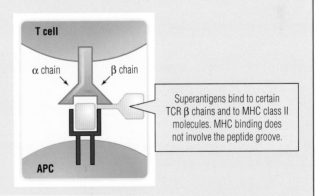

Superantigens bind to certain TCR β chains and to MHC class II molecules. MHC binding does not involve the peptide groove.

Fig 7.9 Superantigen binding to major histocompatibility complex (MHC) class II and the T-cell receptor (TCR). *APC,* antigen-presenting cell.

 MCH II   Cytokine, chemokine, etc.   Complement (C′)   Signaling molecule

BOX 7.3 Cluster of Differentiation Molecules

In immunology, cell surface molecules are designated *CD*, such as CD3. This abbreviation stands for cluster of differentiation, a term first used when these molecules were being discovered. Several hundred CD molecules have been described so far. Probably the most well known is CD4, which is the cellular receptor for HIV attachment to T cells. The numbers of CD4$^+$ T cells are measured to assess disease progression in HIV-mediated immunodeficiency disease (Chapter 33).

LEARNING POINTS Can You Now...

1. Draw the biochemical structure of the antigen recognition proteins of the TCR?
2. Explain the roles of the various proteins in the TCR complex and list the major accessory molecules involved in T-cell recognition?
3. Recall the structural relationship between Ig and the TCR?
4. Differentiate between the αβ and γδ TCRs and recall their different functional roles?
5. Draw the TCR gene organization (αβ and γδ)?
6. Describe the genetic mechanisms involved in the generation of TCR diversity, such as junctional diversity?
7. Compare the generation of diversity for Ig and the TCR?
8. Compare the recognition of antigen and superantigen by the TCR?
9. Describe the processes involved in toxic shock syndrome?

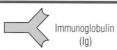
T-cell receptor (TCR)

Immunoglobulin (Ig)

Antigen

MCH I

Major Histocompatibility Complex

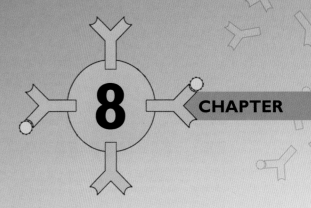

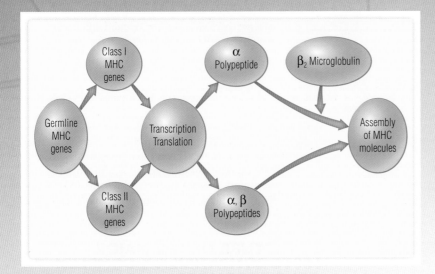

The major histocompatibility complex (MHC) is a region of DNA that encodes a group of molecules that recognize antigen. The MHCs of different organisms have specific names. The human MHC, found on human chromosome 6, is known as *human leukocyte antigen* (HLA). When referring specifically to HLA, we use the terms *HLA genes* or *HLA molecules* (eg, *HLA-A* genes encode HLA-A molecules). As described in Chapter 3, HLA molecules are antigen recognition molecules, just as antibodies and T-cell receptors (TCRs) are antigen recognition molecules. However, it was not until the three-dimensional (3-D) structure of an HLA molecule was obtained that the role of HLA molecules as antigen recognition molecules became clear. As shown in the above figure, the main topics for this chapter are the genetic organization of the MHC and the structure and assembly of the MHC gene products. The role of MHC molecules in antigenic peptide display relative to T cells is also described in more detail.

GENETIC ORGANIZATION

Figure 8.1 shows the organization of the genes encoded in the human MHC. Only the major loci are shown. It should be noted that some 224 loci have been identified in the HLA region. Also, note the breakdown of loci into three major classes:

class I, class II, and class III. As shown in Figure 8.2, extensive polymorphism (existence of a large number of alleles in a healthy population) is apparent in the MHC. Indeed, this is the most polymorphic locus known. The alleles are also unusual in that they differ in approximately 10 to 20 amino acid residues rather than just one or a few residues. Figure 8.3 shows another unusual feature of this genetic region: blocks of alleles (haplotypes) are inherited together, and they are identical in families. This is largely because of a lack of genetic recombination in the MHC. Genetic recombination involves crossover, and relatively few crossover events take place that involve the chromosomal segment that includes the MHC.

REGULATION OF GENE EXPRESSION

An important difference between the HLA class I (A, B, and C) and class II (DP, DQ, DR) gene products (see Fig. 8.1) and the immunoglobulin and TCR gene products is that the MHC molecules are codominantly expressed. This means that both the maternally and the paternally derived allelic forms are expressed as cell-surface proteins. By contrast, immunoglobulin and TCR gene products exhibit allelic exclusion; that is, only one form is expressed on each cell (Chapter 6). This is illustrated in Figure 8.3 for a human family. Therefore, except for the rare

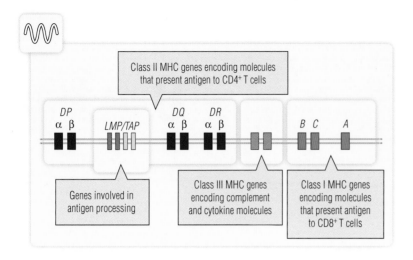

Fig 8.1 Genetic organization of major histocompatibility complex (MHC). You will read about large multifunctional protease (LMP) and transporter associated with antigen presentation (TAP) in Chapter 10.

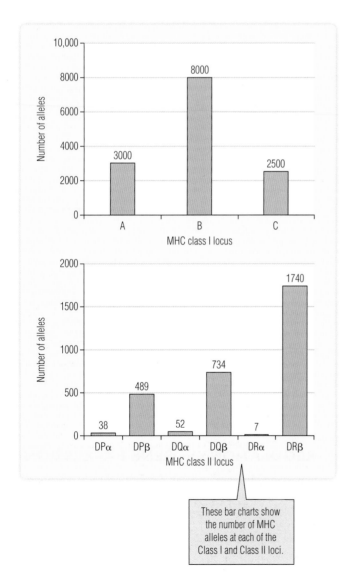

Fig 8.2 Polymorphism in the major histocompatibility complex (MHC) (data from Immuno Polymorphism Database).

recombinant, children express the haplotypes they inherited from their parents.

Class I molecules are found on all nucleated cells. As described later, this means all nucleated cells can display antigens derived from intracellular pathogens. This is in contrast to class II molecules, which are examples of differentiation antigens. The class I molecules are found on antigen-presenting cells (APCs) and include B cells, macrophages, and dendritic cells. They can be induced on human T cells.

STRUCTURE OF THE MAJOR HISTOCOMPATIBILITY COMPLEX GENE PRODUCTS

Class I

Figure 8.4 shows the structure of the protein products of the class I genes. The class I molecules are noncovalently associated heterodimers of an approximately 45,000–molecular weight transmembrane glycoprotein (the β chain, encoded in the MHC) with an approximately 12,000–molecular weight chain (β₂ microglobulin) encoded on a completely different chromosome (chromosome 15 in humans). The β_2 microglobulin is a soluble protein that complexes with the α chain during synthesis and assembly in the endoplasmic reticulum. It is essential for the peptide-binding function of the MHC-encoded "heavy chain." Unlike the α chain, β_2 microglobulin is not polymorphic: exactly the same β_2 microglobulin molecule is used in each MHC class I molecule.

DNA and protein sequences obtained for a number of HLA molecules show that they are structurally homologous to one another—that is, they have very similar sequences. HLA-A molecules have sequences very similar to HLA-B or HLA-C molecules. Alleles (alternative forms) of HLA-A, HLA-B, or HLA-C are even more similar to one another. Thus two different *HLA-A* alleles might have an approximately 90% sequence identity with each other.

The HLA class I genes have an exon-intron structure that is typical of genes that encode eukaryotic membrane proteins. HLA class I genes do not undergo gene rearrangements, such as

 T-cell receptor (TCR)   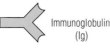 Immunoglobulin (Ig)   Antigen   MCH I

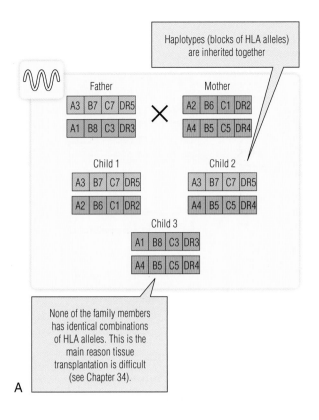

Haplotypes (blocks of HLA alleles) are inherited together

None of the family members has identical combinations of HLA alleles. This is the main reason tissue transplantation is difficult (see Chapter 34).

A

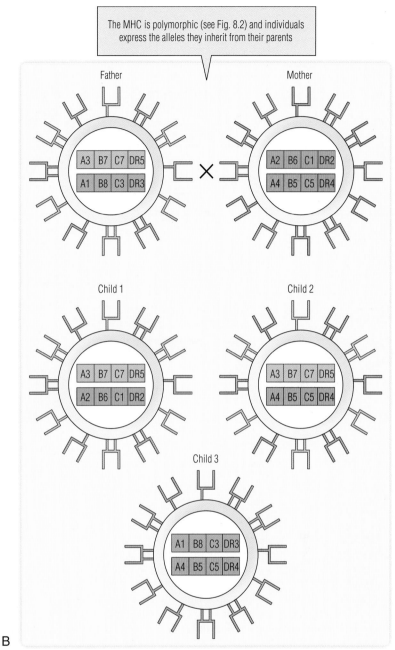

The MHC is polymorphic (see Fig. 8.2) and individuals express the alleles they inherit from their parents

B

Fig 8.3 A, Haplotype inheritance, a simplified example with only one class II locus. **B,** Codominant expression of major histocompatibility complex (MHC) molecules, illustrated for the family combination. The MHC class I and II molecules are codominantly expressed; that is, no allelic exclusion is present, and all inherited alleles are found in all expressing cells. *HLA,* human leukocyte antigen.

occurs in immunoglobulin (Ig) or TCR genes. Individuals inherit a set of HLA class I genes from their parents, and they can express a maximum of six different class I HLA-A, -B, or -C molecules. However, the population as a whole is extensively polymorphic, and large numbers of alleles, approximately 700 at *HLA-B,* for example, exist in the human population.

Figure 8.4 also shows a ribbon-structure representation of the 3-D structure of an HLA class I molecule. Once the structure was determined, it was clear that a binding groove was present in the molecule for peptide (antigen). This binding groove is formed entirely by the α chain in class I molecules. The amino

acid residues that make up the groove are the chief sites of polymorphism. That is, different *HLA-A* alleles produce different amino acids in the antigen-binding groove; therefore they can bind a different range of peptide antigens. The 3-D structure also shows a β-pleated sheet platform structure (with homology to Ig) that supports the α helical binding site. The peptide antigen has been said to fit into the groove like a "hot dog in a bun." Peptides of about 8 to 11 amino acid residues fit into the class I binding site. The precise sequence of the peptide is less important than the presence of certain amino acids, referred to as *anchor residues,* at particular positions.

 MCH II

 Cytokine, chemokine, etc.

 Complement (C′)

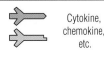 Signaling molecule

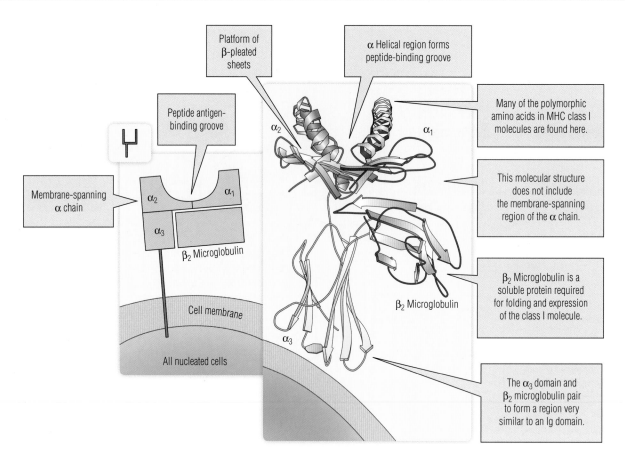

Fig 8.4 Structure of major histocompatibility complex (MHC) class I molecules. *Ig*, immunoglobulin. (Modified from Roitt I, Brostoff J, Male D. *Immunology*, ed 6. London: Mosby; 2001.)

Class II

The class II MHC molecules are noncovalently associated transmembrane heterodimers, where both chains are encoded in the MHC. The molecular weight of the α chain is approximately 33,000, and that of the β-chain is approximately 29,000 (Fig. 8.5). Both are polymorphic transmembrane glycoproteins.

As for the class I genes, there is no evidence that gene recombination is used to generate diversity (polymorphism), and the class II genes have the typical exon-intron structure of membrane proteins. No variable and constant region gene clusters are present, as there are for Ig and TCR. When collections of gene and protein sequences for the many alleles at a class II locus are compared, however, there is evidence for regions of greater and lesser diversity. These regions of diversity are called *polymorphic regions,* and they come together in the folded molecule to form the antigen-binding groove. As shown in Figure 8.5, the 3-D structure of a class II molecule has a β-pleated sheet platform structure on top of which is a β helical binding site for peptides. The binding groove in class II molecules is created by both the α and β chains.

The overall 3-D structures of the class I and II molecules differ, although similarities are also apparent. The class II binding site for peptides is more "open" than the class I site, and longer peptides (30 amino acid residues or longer) can fit into the site and overlap at either end. Again, as is true for MHC class I

molecules, the precise sequence of the peptide antigen is less important than the fact that it contains particular residues at certain positions. Therefore any given MHC molecule can accommodate a wide range of peptides, one at a time. Hence, the likelihood is very low that any given complex antigen, such as a virus, would *not* contain a peptide antigen that could be efficiently recognized by, and bind to, at least one MHC molecule in an individual. However, that is possible; such an individual is said to be a nonresponder or low responder to that antigen. Control of immune responsiveness is therefore also one of the genetic traits associated with the MHC because of the role that MHC molecules have of binding antigens and presenting them to TCRs prior to initiation of an immune response.

■ RESTRICTION OF ANTIGEN RECOGNITION

The discovery of an antigen-binding groove in MHC molecules helped to explain the concept of MHC restriction, which had been discovered earlier. It had been observed that T cells are specific for both MHC and antigen and that the MHC molecule must be self MHC. Whereas the B-cell receptor can recognize antigen directly, the TCR recognizes only nonself antigen in association with self MHC; that is, there is a dual recognition process. Figure 8.6 illustrates the observations that were made.

 T-cell receptor (TCR)   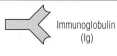 Immunoglobulin (Ig)   Antigen   MCH I

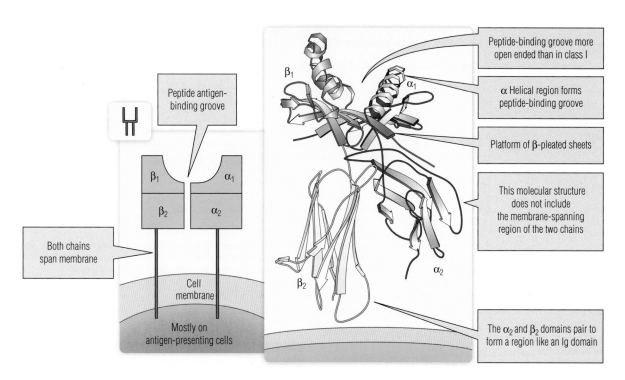

Fig 8.5 Structure of major histocompatibility complex (MHC) class II molecules. *Ig*, immunoglobulin. (Modified from Roitt I, Brostoff J, Male D. *Immunology*, ed 6. London: Mosby; 2001.)

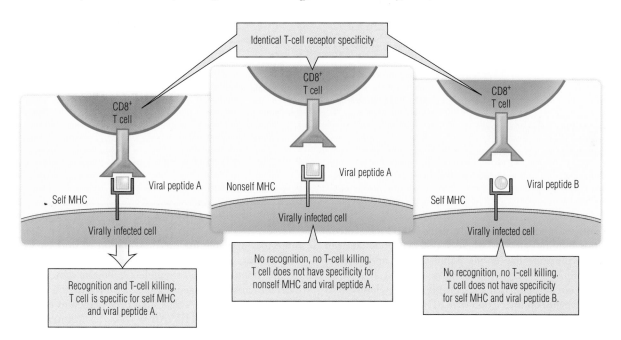

Fig 8.6 T-cell recognition of antigen is major histocompatibility complex (MHC) restricted.

T cells must recognize foreign antigen and self MHC. The function of MHC is to be both a binding site for nonself peptides and a ligand for the TCR. How the peptide antigens recognized by TCRs are derived from complex nonself antigens, such as viruses, and how they become associated with MHC molecules is the subject of Chapter 10. Table 8.1 contrasts the two types of MHC receptor with the T-cell and B-cell receptors.

Models of the Major Histocompatibility Complex–Antigen–T-Cell Receptor Complex

Figure 8.7 shows a schematic model of the recognition complex involving an MHC class I molecule, a nonself peptide antigen, and a TCR. The TCR contacts both amino acids from the MHC class I molecule and amino acids from the peptide antigen. Figure 8.7 also helps to illustrate how certain amino acids in the

 MCH II

 Cytokine, chemokine, etc.

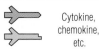 Complement (C′)

 Signaling molecule

TABLE 8.1   Organization of Antigen Recognition Molecule Genes

	B-Cell Receptor	T-Cell Receptor	MHC Class I	MHC Class II
Structure	Light and heavy chains	α and β TCR chains	α MHC chain and β₂ microglobulin	α and β MHC chains
Genetic recombination involved?	Yes	Yes	No	No
Multiple loci?	No	No	Yes; HLA-A, -B, and -C	Yes; DQ, DP, and DR
Multiple alleles?	No	No	Yes	Yes
Present on	B cells	T cells	All nucleated cells	APCs: macrophages, dendritic cells, and B cells
Function	Activates B cells after recognizing antigen	Activates T cells after recognizing antigen presented in MHC	Displays antigenic peptide from intracellular pathogens	Displays antigenic peptide from extracellular pathogens

APC, *antigen-presenting cells*; HLA, *human leukocyte antigen*; MHC, *major histocompatibility complex*; TCR, *T-cell receptor.*

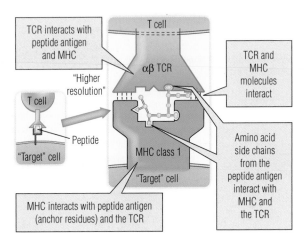

Fig 8.7 Structure of major histocompatibility complex (MHC)–antigen–T-cell receptor (TCR) complex.

TABLE 8.2   Correlations Between Various Diseases and HLA Alleles

Disease	HLA Type
Ankylosing spondylitis	B27
Goodpasture syndrome	DR2
Insulin-dependent diabetes mellitus	DQ2
Multiple sclerosis	DR2
Pemphigus vulgaris	DR4
Rheumatoid arthritis	DR4
Systemic lupus erythematosus	DR3

HLA, *human leukocyte antigen.*

peptide antigen bind to amino acids of the MHC molecule in the peptide-binding groove, whereas other peptide antigen amino acids protrude out of the MHC groove and interact with the TCR.

The repertoire of TCRs that is selected during development in the thymus depends on interaction with MHC molecules; that is, T cells "learn" self MHC in the thymus during development, and those that cannot bind appropriately to self MHC molecules are eliminated or made anergic (ie, nonresponsive; see Chapter 15). This also helps to explain the phenomenon of MHC restriction; that is, that the T-cell receptors are specific for self MHC.

■ POPULATION ADVANTAGES OF POLYMORPHISM IN THE MAJOR HISTOCOMPATIBILITY COMPLEX

The existence of multiple different HLA class I and II genes means that there are numerous different peptide antigen-binding molecules available for the presentation of antigen to T cells. This appears to be a selective advantage to the individual and to the population as a whole. A heterozygote can present more different pathogen-derived peptides than a homozygote. Homozygosity at HLA class I has been shown to be a disadvantage with respect to HIV/AIDS (Box 3.1). Similarly, evidence suggests that homozygosity at HLA class II increases the risk of hepatitis B virus infection persisting. Having a very rare HLA allele may also be advantageous when an epidemic sweeps through a population. Therefore evidence is accumulating that polymorphism in the MHC may indeed confer some advantage in responding to infections by pathogens.

■ DISEASE CORRELATIONS

Many human diseases appear to be linked to possession of certain *HLA* alleles. These diseases are often inflammatory or

 T-cell receptor (TCR)   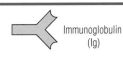 Immunoglobulin (Ig)   Antigen   MCH I autoimmune in nature. Extensive HLA typing of families has revealed correlations of varying extents with possession of certain *HLA* alleles. For example, a form of joint disease called *ankylosing spondylitis* is highly associated with the *HLA-B27* allele (Box 8.3). Another disease strongly correlated with HLA is insulin-dependent diabetes mellitus (IDDM), which is associated with (linked to) *HLA-DQ2*. Up to 75% of people with IDDM have

DQ2, depending on the ethnic group being studied. Some other high correlations are listed in Table 8.2. These observations remain to be fully explained. They could be related to the role of MHC molecules in binding peptides to present to T cells, or they could be the result of another gene linked to HLA. In the example of systemic lupus erythematosus, there is a linkage with complement genes (class III MHC; see also Chapters 28 and 30).

BOX 8.1 Transplantation Antigens and Graft Rejection

The products of major histocompatibility complex (MHC)-encoded genes were initially detected as transplantation antigens; that is, antigens recognized as nonself when tissue was exchanged between individuals as a graft (eg, kidney transplants). Transplantation antigens are the principal cause of graft rejection between nonidentical individuals (Chapter 34). As shown in Figure 8.8, grafts between genetically identical (syngeneic) individuals succeed. All others eventually fail in the absence of other interventions, such as immunosuppressive drugs (eg, cyclosporine). This is the fundamental law of transplantation. Transplantation antigens, chiefly molecules encoded in the MHC, do not exist merely to frustrate the efforts of transplant surgeons. They are important antigen recognition molecules that "display" antigen for "review" by T cells.

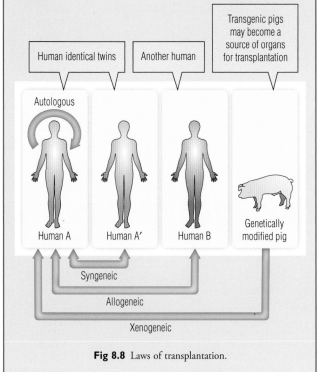

Fig 8.8 Laws of transplantation.

BOX 8.2 Who's the Murderer?

A 28-year-old woman has been found murdered at her home. The forensic science team finds evidence that she has been strangled, and her boyfriend is the prime suspect. However, the scientists find some skin under her fingernails and six hairs trapped in her hands. There is just enough tissue to extract DNA that can be used to check the human leukocyte antigen (HLA) type of the cells in the skin and hair. These show the following HLA type: A3 A1, B7 B8, C7 C3, DR5, DR3. Her boyfriend's HLA type is A3 A8, B7 B27, C7 C4, DR7, DR7. This indicates that the tissues found at necropsy could not have come from the victim's boyfriend, and someone else must have been involved.

In this case, HLA typing has been used to rule out a suspect. Even if the HLA type found in the tissues and the boyfriend happened to be the same, this could not be used as evidence to conclude that he was there at the time of murder. There is always a very small chance that the murderer and the boyfriend shared the same HLA type.

HLA typing can also be used for paternity testing to see who fathered a particular child. In this case, the lab will need to HLA type the mother and baby first. One haplotype is inherited from the mother, and the other haplotype is inherited from the father. The same logic applies in this scenario as in the one of the murderer above: if the baby's paternal haplotype is different from either haplotype possessed by the "suspect" father, he cannot be the "perpetrator."

BOX 8.3 Association Between HLA-B27 and Ankylosing Spondylitis

Both genetic and environmental factors contribute to autoimmune disease. Among the genes associated with autoimmune disease, the strongest associations are with major histocompatibility complex (*MHC*) genes (see Table 8.2). One of the strongest such associations is between *HLA-B27* and the presumed autoimmune disease ankylosing spondylitis. Patients with this disease develop inflammation of the vertebral joints. For example, a patient with ankylosing spondylitis may initially present with lower back pain and stiffness that leads to difficulty in walking. Eventually the spine may become bowed. Antiinflammatory drugs often alleviate the symptoms of the disease.

Individuals who possess *HLA-B27* are approximately 90 times more likely to develop ankylosing spondylitis than other individuals in the population. Neither the mechanism of the disease nor the basis for its association with *HLA-B27* is known. However, environmental factors, perhaps infection, contribute at least as much to the likelihood of contracting the disease as does HLA type. For example, only a small proportion of the people who express *HLA-B27* ever develop ankylosing spondylitis.

 MCH II   Cytokine, chemokine, etc.   Complement (C′)   Signaling molecule

LEARNING POINTS   Can You Now ...

1. Draw a diagram of the genetic organization of the human MHC, HLA?
2. Describe the main structural features of the class I and class II MHC gene products?
3. Explain the genetic basis of MHC polymorphism and its significance for the functioning of the immune system?
4. Describe the concept of MHC restriction and draw a model of MHC-peptide-TCR interaction?
5. Compare peptide antigen binding to class I and class II molecules?
6. List some diseases associated with *HLA* alleles?

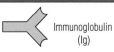 T-cell receptor (TCR)

 Immunoglobulin (Ig)

Antigen

 MCH I

Review of Antigen Recognition

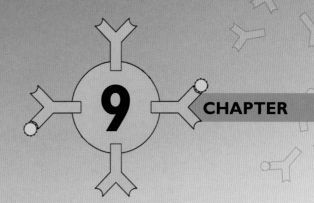

9 CHAPTER

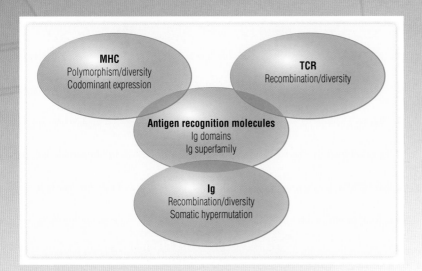

This section of the book has focused predominantly on the process of antigen recognition and the molecules involved in this process, which are key to understanding the immune system. The genes that encode the antigen recognition molecules influence the function of the entire adaptive immune system. The preceding chapters have described the structure of various antigen recognition molecules: B-cell receptors and antibodies (immunoglobulins), T-cell antigen receptors (TCRs), and major histocompatibility complex (MHC) molecules. The genetic mechanisms involved in generating diversity in antibodies and TCRs were also described. The generation of diversity in the genes for immunoglobulins (Igs) and TCRs involves similar mechanisms, chiefly somatic recombination of gene segments in each individual before exposure to antigen. MHC class I and II molecules are, by contrast, diverse through polymorphism. Many alternatives (alleles) exist in the human population as a whole, but the individual bears a restricted number. For example, there are six different MHC class I alleles—two each of human leukocyte antigens (HLAs) A, B, and C. Chapters 3 through 8 discussed the various three-dimensional shapes of the antigen recognition molecules and how they interact with antigen.

▌ IMPORTANT STRUCTURAL FEATURES

Immunoglobulin Domain Fold

As discussed in Chapter 4, the basic building block of the antibody molecule is a polypeptide chain of approximately 110 amino acid residues, folded to create an antiparallel β-pleated sheet structure and held in shape by intrachain disulfide bonds. This domain structure is shared by several other molecules, collectively referred to as the *immunoglobulin superfamily*. Most of the molecules in the superfamily are involved in recognition processes in the immune system, such as Ig, TCR, MHC class I and II molecules, killer cell immunoglobulin-like receptor (KIR), CD4, and CD8. Notice also how the members of the immunoglobulin superfamily, illustrated in Figure 9.1, have an extended structure; this allows these molecules to form ligand pairs to bridge the immunologic synapse (see Fig. 7.8).

Antigen Recognition Sites

As previously discussed in Chapters 5 through 8, x-ray crystallographic analyses of several types of antigen recognition

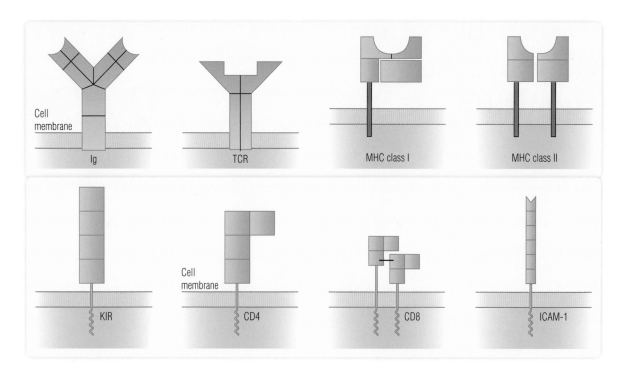

Fig 9.1 Representative members of the immunoglobulin (Ig) superfamily. *ICAM-1,* intercellular adhesion molecule 1; *KIR,* killer cell immunoglobulin-like receptor; *MHC,* major histocompatibility complex; *TCR,* T-cell receptor.

molecules show that the antigen-binding site in antibodies can vary considerably in shape, whereas the TCR site for interaction with peptides presented by MHC molecules tends to be a flat surface area (see Fig. 7.2), at least in the TCR variable regions that have been analyzed so far. The peptide-binding grooves of MHC class I and II molecules are similar in being formed from the α helical regions of the polymorphic domains of the MHC molecules. The groove in class II molecules is open ended, which allows longer peptides (approximately 9 to 30 amino acid residues) to "hang over" the groove, whereas the class I peptide groove is closed and only allows binding of peptides of a fixed size (approximately 8 to 11 residues).

Molecular analyses of the antigen recognition molecules highlight the fundamental difference between recognition by B- or T-cell receptors: Ig binds antigen directly, whereas the T-cell receptor interacts with peptide antigens presented by MHC molecules. The ligand for the B-cell receptor is antigen alone, but the ligand for the T-cell receptor is a peptide antigen–MHC molecule complex (see Fig. 7.5).

■ GENERATION OF DIVERSITY

An enormous number of organisms have evolved to live on Earth, and all of them need to be recognized by the adaptive immune system. For example, 1000 different species of microorganisms live in the gut, and another 200 species live on the skin. Even the simplest of these organisms produces several different antigens, each of which may contain many different potential epitopes (recognition sites).

Several mechanisms have evolved to generate a wide range of antigen recognition molecules—a full repertoire capable of

TABLE 9.1 Mechanisms Used to Generate Diversity in Immunoglobulin and T-Cell Receptors

	Immunoglobulin	T-Cell Receptor
BEFORE EXPOSURE TO ANTIGEN		
Multiple V region gene segments	+	+
Somatic recombination of gene segments	+	+
Junctional variability	+	+
Multiple combinations of chains (light/heavy, α/β)	+	+
AFTER EXPOSURE TO ANTIGEN		
Somatic hypermutation	+	−
Class switching	+	−

interacting with antigen. With respect to MHC, the MHC molecules are polygenic and polymorphic; that is, multiple copies of similar genes are present. For example, the MHC class I locus is represented by the *HLA-A, HLA-B,* and *HLA-C* loci in the human. Also present in the human population are a large number of alleles at these loci. This is *polymorphism,* the existence of multiple alleles at a locus in the population. This

T-cell receptor (TCR)

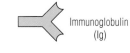
Immunoglobulin (Ig)

Antigen

MCH I

TABLE 9.2   Generation of Diversity: Contribution of Various Mechanisms

Mechanisms	Immunoglobulin	T-CELL RECEPTOR	
		$\alpha\beta$	$\gamma\delta$
V segment recombination (V, D, J)	$\sim2.5 \times 10^5$	$\sim2 \times 10^3$	$\sim10^2$
Estimated total repertoire	$\sim10^{11}$	$\sim10^{16}$	$\sim10^{18}$

polymorphic diversity in MHC was created by gene conversion mechanisms, not by the somatic recombination mechanisms used by immunoglobulin and TCR genes. Gene conversion does not occur widely in the immune system; therefore it will not be explained further here.

The Ig and TCR genes are extremely diverse. Again, like MHC alleles—which exist before exposure to antigen—the repertoire of Ig and TCR genes largely precedes contact with antigen. The same enzymes are involved in gene segment recombination in B and T cells; namely, the V(D)J recombinase that includes RAG-1 and RAG-2. These enzymes do not appear to function in other cells. Most Ig and TCR diversity is a result of junctional diversity created during the recombination of V region gene segments (eg, D to J, V to DJ, V to J). The various genetic mechanisms that contribute to diversity in Ig and TCR genes are listed in Table 9.1. Junctional diversity is created by imprecise joining and by insertion and addition of nucleotides by the enzyme terminal deoxynucleotidyl transferase (TdT) as gene segments are recombined; this is clearly a major contributor to this diversity (Table 9.2). Another point that should be highlighted is that although "improvement" of the immunoglobulin binding site for antigen is extensive after exposure to antigen, the TCR repertoire does not continue to change after antigenic exposure (see Table 9.1).

 MCH II

 Cytokine, chemokine, etc.

Complement (C')

 Signaling molecule

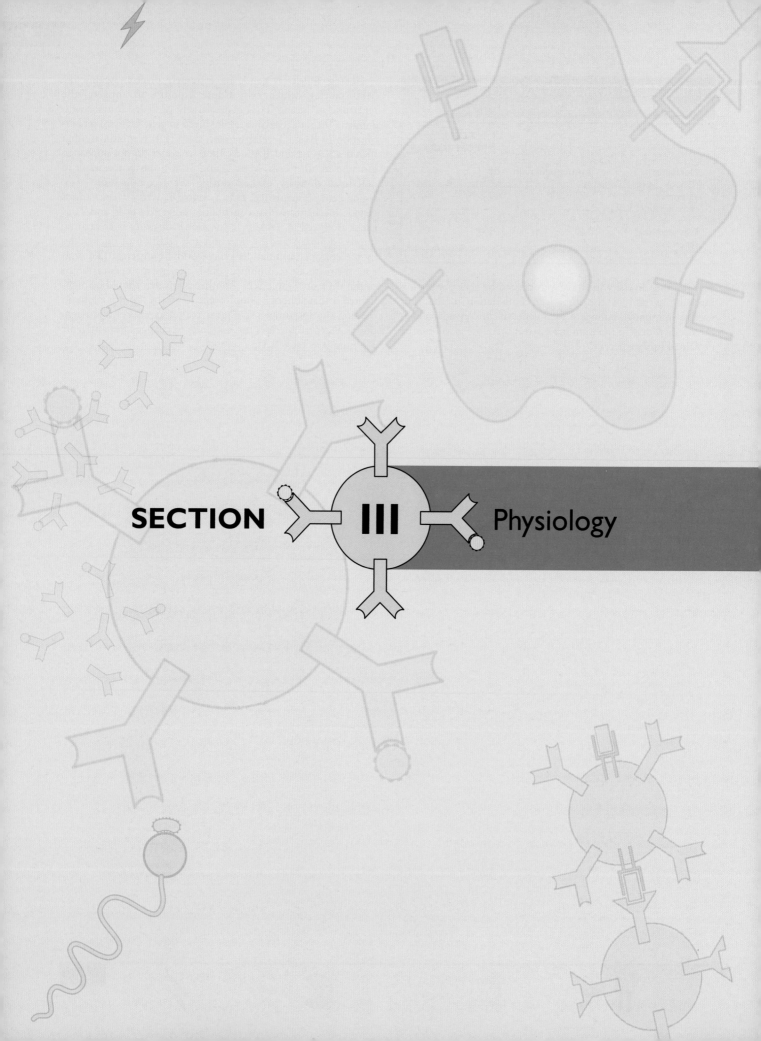

SECTION III Physiology

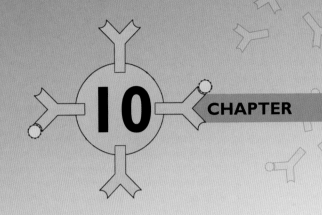

Antigen Processing and Presentation

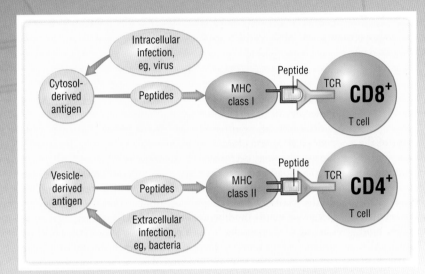

This chapter discusses *antigen processing,* which leads to the formation of the major histocompatibility complex (MHC)–foreign antigen complexes, and *antigen presentation* to the αβ T-cell receptor (TCR). As depicted in the above figure, extracellular antigens travel in cells via a different pathway than intracellular-derived antigens. The nature of these pathways and the processes by which antigens complex with either MHC class I or class II molecules are described.

As discussed earlier, the body has developed very effective barriers to prevent foreign antigens, such as bacteria or viruses, from gaining entry and inducing disease. If a foreign organism or antigen, such as a toxin, gains entry, the protective systems of the innate immune system, such as the phagocytic cells, may destroy the antigen before it is encountered by B or T cells and induce an adaptive immune response. Very little foreign antigen typically survives the innate immune system's various host defense systems intact. If it does, however, only a very small number of B- or T-cell antigen receptors require engagement to initiate a protective adaptive immune response.

B-cell antigen receptors may interact directly with an invading microbe, but αβ TCRs recognize only "processed" antigenic peptides. In addition, the αβ TCR recognizes foreign antigen only when the antigen is attached to the surface of other cells (antigen-presenting cells [APCs] or target cells; Fig. 10.1).

APCs include macrophages, B cells, and the various dendritic cells (Chapters 2, 12, and 20). Dendritic cells, as discussed later, are APCs par excellence (Box 10.1; see Chapters 12 and 20). These APCs are very efficient at endocytosing extracellular antigen, processing it, and presenting it, usually along with costimulators that complete the immune activation process. Antigen peptides are presented to T cells by APCs in association with MHC class II molecules (Chapter 8).

Target cells are any nucleated cells infected with intracellular pathogen. Malignant cells may also become target cells. Antigen derived from intracellular pathogen or tumor is processed into peptides that are then presented to T cells in association with MHC class I molecules.

Antigen recognition by T lymphocytes is thus said to be *MHC restricted.* The major subsets of T lymphocytes, the T-helper cells (CD4⁺) and the cytotoxic T lymphocytes (CD8⁺), have different MHC restrictions. Thus the CD4⁺ T cell–APC interaction is MHC class II restricted, and the CD8⁺ T cell–target cell interaction is MHC class I restricted (Chapters 7, 8, and 15). The process whereby antigen becomes associated with self MHC molecules for presentation to T cells is called *antigen processing.*

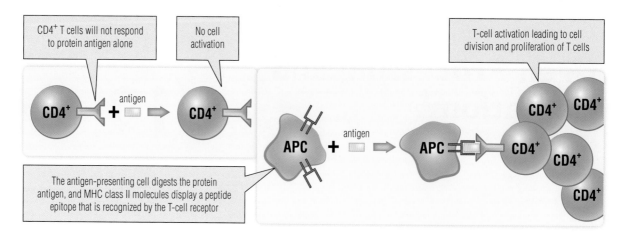

Fig 10.1 Antigen presentation to T cells by antigen-presenting cells (APCs). *MHC,* major histocompatibility complex.

PATHWAYS OF ANTIGEN PROCESSING

Peptide antigens generated in the cytosolic compartment of the cell, such as from viruses and bacteria that replicate in the cytosol, bind to class I MHC molecules for presentation to CD8+ T cells (Chapter 7). Peptide antigens generated in endosomes from the endocytic uptake of extracellular antigens, such as toxins, or from microbes captured in endosomes, such as after the phagocytic uptake of certain bacteria by macrophages, bind to class II MHC molecules for presentation to CD4+ T cells. This means that CD8+ T cells can monitor the intracellular environment, and CD4+ T cells can monitor the extracellular environment for pathogens.

The intracellular pathway traversed by an antigen is the primary factor in determining whether an antigen will be presented on class I or class II MHC molecules, not anything particular about the antigen itself.

MECHANISMS OF ANTIGEN PROCESSING

Extracellular (Exogenous) Antigens

Extracellular, or exogenous, antigens are either extracellular proteins, such as a protein vaccine, or proteins derived from a pathogen in an endosome after uptake. These antigens are processed for eventual presentation on MHC class II molecules to CD4+ T lymphocytes (Fig. 10.2A). First, however, they must be internalized by the APC. Soluble antigen is endocytosed intact. Pathogens are internalized through a specialized process called *phagocytosis* (Chapter 21) by which they enter the endosome pathway. Some organisms have evolved to live inside the endosome, such as *Mycobacterium tuberculosis*. These organisms are located inside the cell but are still extracellular in the sense that they are not present in the cytosol.

In any event, the endosome containing the antigen becomes acidified and fuses with a lysosome (see Fig. 10.2) and is then degraded by cellular proteases, first to peptides of different sizes and ultimately to amino acids. During this process, peptides are

generated in the size range that can bind to class II MHC molecules (9 to 30+ amino acid residues).

The APC also synthesizes new class II MHC molecules in the endoplasmic reticulum. These molecules move out through the Golgi apparatus, eventually becoming part of a vesicle that buds off the Golgi and that may fuse with an endosomal vesicle containing peptides from an extracellular or vesicle-derived antigen. In the pathway from the endoplasmic reticulum through the Golgi, the empty binding site of class II MHC is "protected" from binding other peptides (eg, self peptides) by a molecule known as the *invariant chain*. In the acidic environment of the endosome, this protection is removed by proteolytic action, and the class II binding site is available for occupancy by any appropriate peptide available in the endosome. The endosome containing "occupied" MHC class II molecules is then routed into the exosomal pathway and fuses with the cell surface membrane. In this way, a foreign antigen can be presented to the repertoire of TCRs and can induce the appropriate T cell to proliferate (see Fig. 10.2A).

Intracellular (Endogenous) Antigens

Intracellular, or endogenous, antigens such as viral proteins are processed by "target cells" for eventual presentation on class I MHC molecules to CD8+ T cells (cytotoxic T lymphocytes; see Fig. 10.2B). In this case, peptides that are foreign antigens are generated in the cytoplasmic compartment. These may be derived by proteolysis, via the normal cellular machinery, of viral proteins being synthesized and assembled in the cytoplasm of a virally infected cell. In Figure 10.2B, a viral protein is being synthesized in the cytosol. The cellular degradative machinery, most importantly a complex of proteases known as the *proteasome,* may enzymatically cleave some of the viral protein molecules through various polypeptide and peptide intermediate steps until peptides of 8 to 11 residues are formed; these can bind to class I MHC molecules. Many of the peptides undergo further degradation, making them irrelevant to the immune system. However, some enter the endoplasmic reticulum, where they associate with MHC class I molecules.

Cells contain a variety of proteasomes that are constantly recycling cellular proteins. Components of the proteasome

 T-cell receptor (TCR)

 Immunoglobulin (Ig)

 Antigen

 MCH I

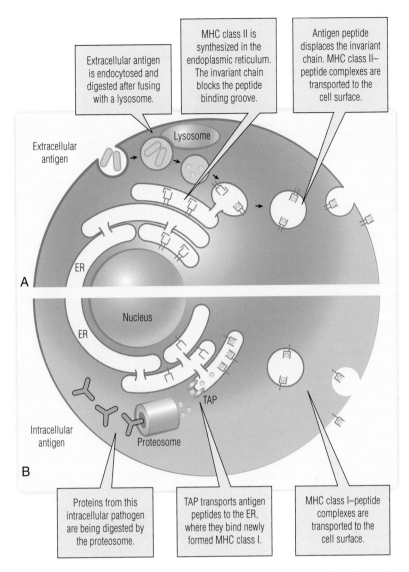

Extracellular antigen is endocytosed and digested after fusing with a lysosome.

MHC class II is synthesized in the endoplasmic reticulum. The invariant chain blocks the peptide binding groove.

Antigen peptide displaces the invariant chain. MHC class II–peptide complexes are transported to the cell surface.

Lysosome

Extracellular antigen

ER

A

Nucleus

ER

TAP

Intracellular antigen

Proteosome

B

Proteins from this intracellular pathogen are being digested by the proteosome.

TAP transports antigen peptides to the ER, where they bind newly formed MHC class I.

MHC class I–peptide complexes are transported to the cell surface.

Fig 10.2 Processing pathways for extracellular antigens (**A**) and intracellular antigens (**B**). *ER,* endoplasmic reticulum; *MCH,* major histocompatibility complex; *TAP,* transporter associated with antigen presentation.

involved in processing proteins derived from pathogens are encoded in the large multifunctional protease (*LMP*) gene situated in the MHC (see Fig. 8.1). During infection, the cytokine interferon γ is released and increases the transcription of *LMP*. Thus during infection, proteolysis of proteins derived from pathogens is increased.

Peptides are carried into the endoplasmic reticulum by a two-chain molecule known as *transporter associated with antigen presentation* (TAP), which permits the peptides to traverse the membrane bilayer of the endoplasmic reticulum and bind in the empty peptide-binding groove of nascent MHC class I molecules being synthesized in the endoplasmic reticulum. Binding of these small peptide antigens is critical for the final stages of assembly of MHC class I molecules. In the absence of peptide, class I molecules are unable to fold correctly and are not found at the cell surface. MHC class I molecules complete their biosynthesis in the Golgi and move out to the surface membrane via the exocytic pathway. After fusion of a Golgi with the surface membrane, foreign antigenic peptides associated with MHC

class I molecules may interact with T lymphocytes bearing receptors capable of binding this MHC-antigen complex (CD8+ or cytotoxic T lymphocytes).

Class I or II Association

It is important to note that the likelihood of an antigen becoming associated with class I or class II MHC is determined solely by the route of trafficking through the cell, not by some special property of the antigen, as illustrated in Figure 10.2. The processing of antigens in this way also explains why polysaccharides, lipids, and nucleic acids are not recognized by αβ T cells; they are not processed to fit into the binding groove of the MHC molecules.

Processing of cytosol- and endosome-derived antigens to result in association with MHC class I or class II molecules, respectively, results in the activation of different subsets of T cells (Fig. 10.3 and Table 10.1). Presentation of extracellular antigen on MHC class II activates CD4+ T cells. CD4+ T cells provide

 MCH II

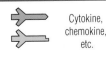 Cytokine, chemokine, etc.

 Complement (C′)

 Signaling molecule

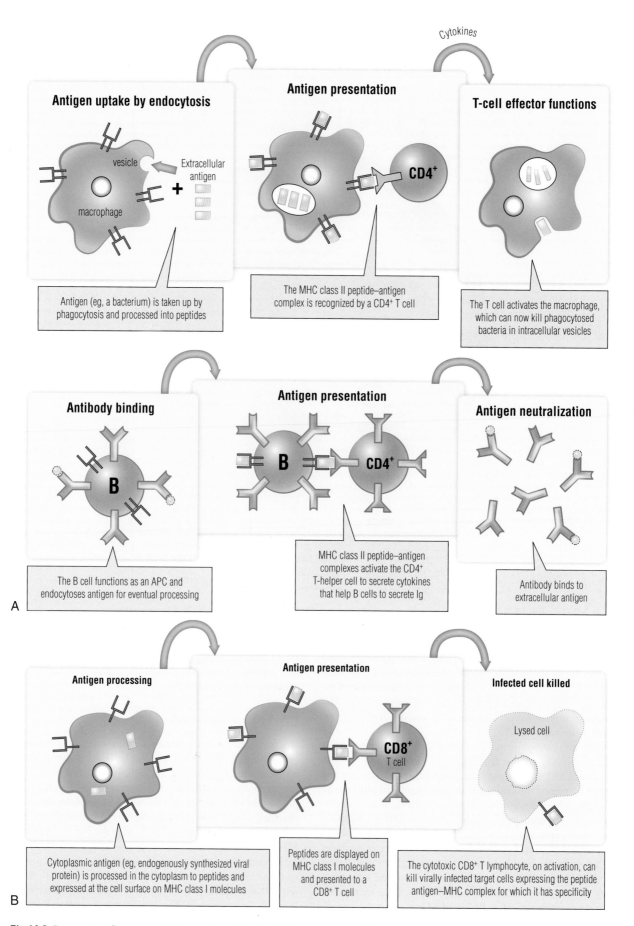

Fig 10.3 Presentation of antigens to different subsets of T cells. **A,** Major histocompatibility complex (MHC) class II–associated extracellular antigen is presented to T-helper cells (CD4+ T cells) either by macrophages or by B cells. **B,** MHC class I–associated cytosolic antigen is presented to cytotoxic T lymphocytes (CD8+ T cells). *APC,* antigen-presenting cell; *Ig,* immunoglobulin.

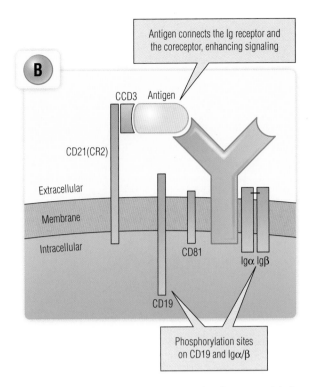

Fig 11.3 The B-cell receptor–coreceptor complex. *Ig*, immunoglobulin.

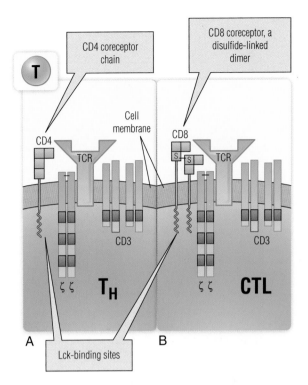

Fig 11.4 The T-cell receptor (TCR)–coreceptor complex. *CTL*, cytotoxic T lymphocyte; *T_H*, T-helper cell.

to CD54 or intercellular adhesion molecule 1 (ICAM-1) on APCs. These adhesion molecules are discussed further in Chapter 13. The T-cell receptor–MHC, coreceptors, and adhesion molecules together form an immunologic synapse between the APC and T cell (see Fig. 7.8).

Coreceptor Molecules in B-Cell Activation

As previously described, the antigen-specific receptors on B and T cells are unable to transduce signals without the help of invariant proteins such as Igα/Igβ and CD3. However, optimal signaling requires even more cell-surface molecules, known as *coreceptor molecules*. The B-cell coreceptor (Fig. 11.3) can cocluster with the BCR and increase the efficiency of signaling by several thousandfold. As shown in Figure 11.3, the B-cell coreceptor consists of three proteins: CD21, also known as *complement receptor 2* (CR2); CD19; and CD81. Protein antigens bound to complement component C3d (see Chapter 20) can bind simultaneously to both CD21 and the BCR. This enables the CD21-CD19-CD81 coreceptor complex to cluster and cross-link with the BCR and induce phosphorylation reactions on the intracellular tail of CD19. This phosphorylation allows PTKs that belong to a family of similar enzymes (the Src family) to bind to the cytoplasmic tail of CD19 and increase the concentration of signaling molecules around the BCR, thereby enhancing the efficiency of signaling (see Fig. 11.3).

Coreceptor Molecules in T-Cell Activation

Optimal signaling through the TCR only occurs when coreceptor molecules are involved. The TCR coreceptor molecules are CD4 and CD8 (Fig. 11.4). As discussed in Chapters 7 and 10,

CD4 binds to MHC class II molecules and CD8 binds to MHC class I molecules. When, for example, the TCR binds to an MHC class II–peptide complex on an APC, CD4 on the T cell binds to the MHC class II molecule (Fig. 11.6). The tyrosine kinase Lck, an Src kinase, is associated with the cytoplasmic domain of CD4 (and CD8). Consequently, Lck is localized with the TCR complex when CD4 binds to MHC class II–peptide complexes or when CD8 binds to MHC class I–peptide complexes.

Lck is integral in the signaling cascade in T cells, and again, coreceptor molecule involvement increases the concentration of these signaling molecules in the vicinity of the TCR. The presence of the CD4 or CD8 coreceptors has been estimated to reduce the number of MHC-peptide complexes required to trigger a T-cell response by about a hundredfold.

■ SIGNALING EVENTS

Intracellular molecules, chiefly PTKs and protein tyrosine phosphatases (PTPs), form the link between receptor activation and activation of biochemical pathways that amplify and transmit the signal. Within seconds of cross-linking the BCR, PTK enzymes of the Src family (Box 11.1) phosphorylate ITAMs in the receptor protein cytoplasmic tails (Fig. 11.5). Phosphorylation of the receptor tails attracts other signaling molecules to the cytoplasmic side of the receptor. In B cells, the critical molecule is another PTK known as Syk, which binds to the phosphorylated ITAM sequences in Igα and Igβ and is then itself activated by phosphorylation. Syk may be phosphorylated by the Src family kinases associated with the BCR, as shown in Figure 11.5, or it may be phosphorylated by another Syk molecule bound to an adjacent BCR chain.

 MCH II

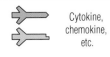 Cytokine, chemokine, etc.

 Complement (C')

 Signaling molecule

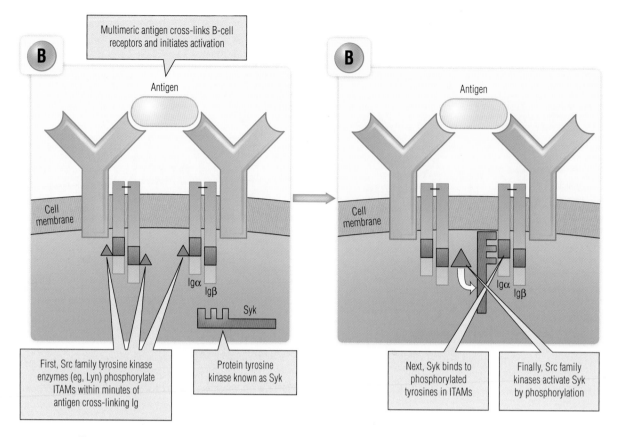

Fig 11.5 Earliest events in activation of B cells. *Ig*, immunoglobulin; *ITAM*, immunoreceptor tyrosine-based activation motif.

A related series of steps occurs in T cells. Clustering of the TCR, CD3, and CD4/CD8 proteins on recognition of peptides displayed by MHC molecules on APCs brings the PTK known as Lck into the receptor complex (see Fig. 11.6). Lck phosphorylates the ITAMs in the cytoplasmic sequences of CD3 and ζ chain. This attracts the PTK ZAP-70, which is unique to T cells and natural killer (NK) cells. ZAP-70 is part of the same PTK family as Syk and binds to the ITAMs of the ζ chains. More than one ZAP-70 molecule may bind to a ζ chain because of the multiple ITAMs per ζ chain (see Fig. 11.6). ZAP-70 is then phosphorylated by Lck, and phosphorylation activates the PTK activity of ZAP-70.

Once a critical number of Syk or ZAP-70 kinases are activated in B or T cells, respectively, the signal is transmitted onward from the membrane and is amplified by activation of several pathways. The important role of PTKs in lymphocyte function is indicated by the occurrence of immunodeficiency in the presence of mutations that affect PTK function (Box 11.2).

■ AMPLIFICATION THROUGH SIGNALING PATHWAYS

For the signal to be propagated from the membrane to the nucleus, where it can have a major impact on a cellular response, several biochemical pathways are used that are similar in B and T cells and that amplify the signal while propagating it.

In both B and T cells, three main signaling pathways are used. The first involves phosphorylation and activation of the enzyme phospholipase Cγ (PLC-γ). This is triggered by Syk or ZAP-70 (Figs 11.7 and 11.8). Activated PLC-γ then stimulates two pathways that involve diacylglycerol (DAG) and protein kinase C and also inositol 1,4,5-trisphosphate (IP$_3$) and the serine-threonine–specific protein phosphatase calcineurin. The third main pathway involves activation by Syk or ZAP-70 of adapter proteins that then activate single-chain guanosine triphosphate (GTP)–binding proteins (eg, Ras). The Ras family of proteins then activates signaling pathways that lead through the mitogen-activated protein (MAP) kinases directly to activation of transcription factors (see Figs 11.7 and 11.8).

Phosphorylation of PLC-γ by Syk in B cells (see Fig. 11.7) and phosphorylation of PLC-γ by ZAP-70 in T cells (see Fig. 11.8) leads to migration of PLC-γ to the cell membrane, where it catalyzes the cleavage of phosphatidylinositol 4,5-bisphosphate to produce DAG and IP$_3$. The latter causes cytoplasmic calcium ion levels to increase, which, among other events, activates several calcium-dependent enzymes, including the serine-threonine–specific protein phosphatase calcineurin, which is responsible for dephosphorylating the nuclear factor of activated T cells (NF-AT) family of transcription factors. Despite its name, NF-AT is required for expression of genes for cytokines in T and B cells. The serine-threonine kinase protein kinase C is activated by interaction with DAG and phosphorylates several

 T-cell receptor (TCR)

 Immunoglobulin (Ig)

Antigen

MCH I

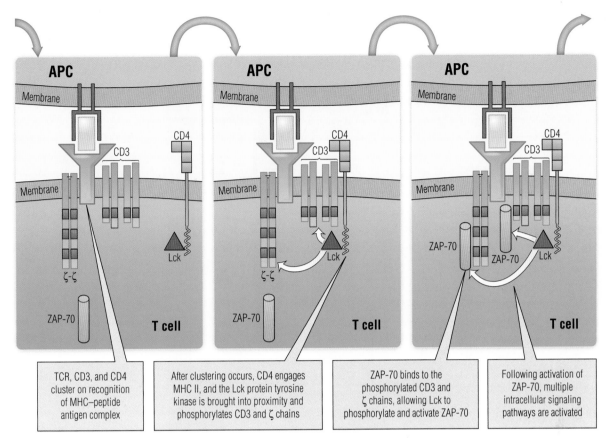

Fig 11.6 Earliest events in activation of T cells. *APC,* antigen-presenting cell.

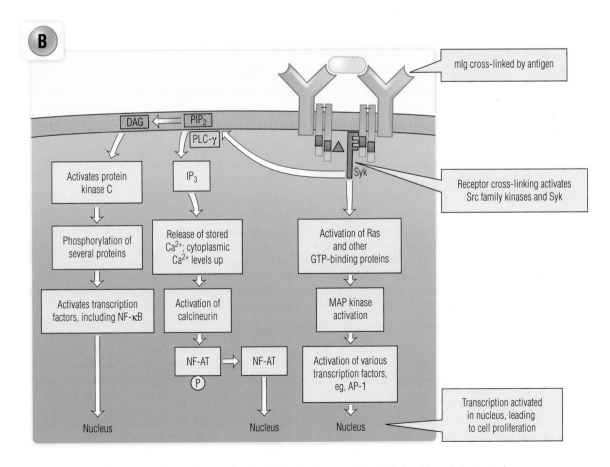

Fig 11.7 Major signaling pathways in B cells. *AP-1,* activation protein 1; *DAG,* diacylglycerol; *IP₃,* inositol
1,4,5-trisphosphate; *MAP kinase,* mitogen-activated protein kinase; *NF-AT,* nuclear factor of activated T cells;
NF-κB, nuclear factor-κB; *PIP₂,* phosphatidylinositol 4,5-bisphosphate; *PLC-γ,* phospholipase Cγ.

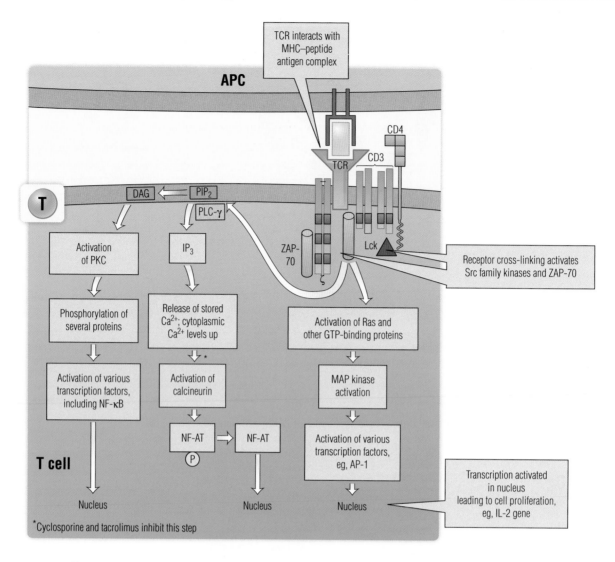

Fig 11.8 Major signaling pathways in T cells. *AP-1*, activation protein 1; *APC*, antigen-presenting cell; *DAG*, diacylglycerol; *GTP*, guanosine triphosphate; *IP₃*, inositol 1,4,5-trisphosphate; *MAP kinase*, mitogen-activated protein kinase; *MHC*, major histocompatibility complex; *NF-AT*, nuclear factor of activated T cells; *NF-κB*, nuclear factor κB; *PIP₂*, phosphatidylinositol 4,5-bisphosphate; *PKC*, protein kinase C; *PLC-γ*, phospholipase Cγ; *TCR*, T-cell receptor.

cellular proteins, eventually leading to the activation of transcription factors that include nuclear factor κB (NF-κB). The third signaling pathway involves activation of the small GTP-binding proteins of the Ras family. These signaling molecules operate through activation of the MAP kinase family of enzymes, which activate several transcription factors, including one called *activation protein 1* (AP-1).

■ RESPONSE

The various transcription factors—including NF-AT, NF-κB, and AP-1—act on several lymphocyte genes to enhance their transcription. This prepares T and B cells for proliferation and differentiation. Cellular proliferation requires the rapid synthesis of nucleotides so that new DNA can be produced. This is a target for immunosuppressive drugs. In B cells, secretion of

immunoglobulin can be a consequence of cellular activation. In T cells, activation leads to enhanced expression of cytokines, such as interleukin 2 (IL-2), which is an essential component of an effective T-cell response, being a growth factor for T cells. Immunosuppressive drugs can modulate this response (Box 11.3).

To preserve homeostasis, a T-cell response must be regulated and eventually terminated, although how this is accomplished is not fully understood. Certainly, as antigen (pathogen) is successfully eliminated, the source of the stimulus is removed and the T-cell response will diminish. Apoptosis, or programmed cell death (see Chapter 17), is a mechanism that may also contribute to termination of a T-cell response in certain circumstances. Also, if T cells fail to receive a costimulatory signal (such as CD28 with CD80; see Chapter 16), they enter a state of functional unresponsiveness known as *anergy*.

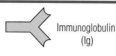 T-cell receptor (TCR)   Immunoglobulin (Ig)   Antigen   MCH I

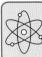

BOX 11.1 Intracellular Signaling: Role of Protein Tyrosine Kinases and Protein Tyrosine Phosphatases

Phosphorylation is a common biochemical mechanism by which cells regulate the activity of proteins. Protein kinases affect protein function by adding phosphate groups to proteins. These phosphate groups are added to tyrosine residues by tyrosine kinases, such as ZAP-70, and to serine or threonine residues by serine-threonine kinases, such as protein kinase C. The phosphate groups can be removed by protein phosphatases. In general, phosphorylation *activates* enzymes, and dephosphorylation *inactivates* enzymes.

Several protein kinases are essential in signal transduction in lymphocytes, and it is important that you recognize some of the most important ones. For example, activation of the receptor-associated tyrosine kinases of the Src ("Sark") family informs the interior of B and T lymphocytes that the antigen receptor is occupied. Two of the major Src family kinases in lymphocytes are designated Lyn and Lck. Another family of tyrosine kinases that is particularly important in lymphocytes is the Syk family. There are two members of this family, Syk and ZAP-70.

Tyrosine kinases, such as Lyn and Lck, tend to be activated early in signaling pathways, whereas serine-threonine kinases, such as protein kinase C and calcineurin, tend to be important in later stages of signaling.

BOX 11.2 Immunodeficiency Diseases and Protein Tyrosine Kinases

A 10-month-old boy presented with recurrent infections. Since the age of 6 months he has had two bouts of pneumonia and recently had meningitis. An older brother and an uncle died of infection. Tests show he has no immunoglobulin and no B cells. Genetic tests show that he has a mutation in the Bruton tyrosine kinase (*BTK*) gene. This type of mutation causes X-linked antibody deficiency. Boys with this mutation present when they are about 6 months old, the age at which immunoglobulin G (IgG) that crossed the placenta during fetal life is used up. Treatment with immunoglobulin can prevent these infections. Figure 11.9 shows a patient with Btk enzyme deficiency receiving immunoglobulin replacement, which is required every 3 weeks when given intravenously. Such replacement helps ensure a healthy life.

The important role of protein tyrosine kinases (PTKs) in lymphocyte function is underlined by the effects of mutations in the gene that encodes these enzymes (*BTK*).

Defective *BTK* leads to a disease known as *X-linked agammaglobulinemia*, in which all the classes of immunoglobulin are severely depleted and no circulating B cells are present. *BTK* is involved in phosphoinositide hydrolysis during B-cell receptor signaling in pre–B cells, and defects in *BTK* result in impaired B-cell development and thereby prevent normal antibody production.

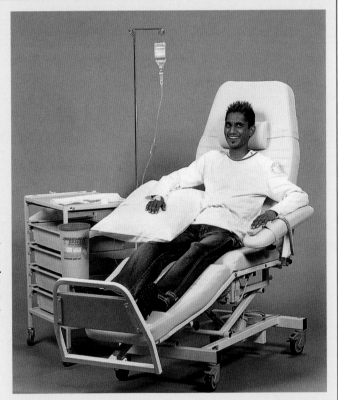

Fig 11.9 Patient with defective *BTK* that led to X-linked agammaglobulinemia. (From Helbert M. *The Flesh and Bones of Immunology.* London: Mosby; 2006.)

 MCH II

 Cytokine, chemokine, etc.

 Complement (C')

Signaling molecule

BOX 11.3 Immunosuppressive Drugs: Mechanism of Action

A 29-year-old woman was diagnosed 7 years ago with cardiomyopathy. There is no specific treatment for her condition, and she has developed worsening heart failure. She has been on the waiting list for a heart transplant for the past 3 months. Once a heart becomes available from a cadaveric donor, she undergoes the transplant procedure. Human leukocyte antigen (HLA) matching (Chapter 34) is not usually practical in this situation because heart transplant recipients cannot wait for a good HLA match and must take what is available. She receives a combination of three immunosuppressive drugs immediately after the transplant and stays on these for the rest of her life.

Several immunosuppressive drugs are used to prevent allograft rejection (Chapter 34). These are remarkable drugs that have revolutionized the field of transplantation surgery. Their availability has saved thousands of lives and has made organ transplantation "doable," even when there is no perfect HLA match available. Over 100,000 people in the United States will take these medications for the duration of their lives. All these drugs prevent graft rejection but have the disadvantage of leaving the patient open to infectious disease because the immune response has been inhibited.

Both cyclosporine and tacrolimus function by preventing T-cell cytokine gene transcription mediated by nuclear factor of activated T cells (NF-AT). They accomplish this by forming a complex with cytoplasmic proteins called *immunophilins*. The drug-immunophilin complex inhibits the action of calcineurin (see Fig. 11.8). Without the dephosphorylation reaction mediated by calcineurin, NF-AT is unable to enter the nucleus to promote gene transcription, such as of the gene for interleukin 2 (IL-2). In the absence of this cytokine, lymphocyte proliferation is inhibited and the immune response is suppressed.

Two other drugs inhibit the action of IL-2 on T cells. This means that even if IL-2 is produced, the opulation of T cells that respond to the graft, in this case the donor heart, cannot grow. Sirolimus (rapamycin) is an oral drug that blocks the effects of IL-2. In contrast, basiliximab is a monoclonal antibody that prevents the receptor for IL-2 from functioning.

T-cell proliferation can also be blocked by drugs that inhibit the synthesis of nucleotides. Azathioprine inhibits the synthesis of purines. Because it is active in a wide range of cell types, it can have side effects. Mycophenolate mofetil is an inhibitor of guanine synthesis. It is mainly active in lymphocytes and so has fewer side effects than azathioprine.

LEARNING POINTS Can You Now …

1. Draw the B- and T-cell receptor complexes and list the molecules involved?
2. Recall that B- and T-cell activation is more optimal with the aid of coreceptor complexes?
3. Describe with a diagram the earliest biochemical events in B- and T-cell activation?
4. List the major signaling pathways triggered in B and T cells by antigen recognition?
5. Recall the mechanism of inhibition of T-cell activation by immunosuppressive drugs such as cyclosporine and tacrolimus?

 T-cell receptor (TCR) 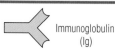 Immunoglobulin (Ig)   Antigen   MCH I

Hematopoiesis

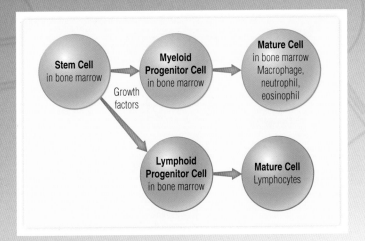

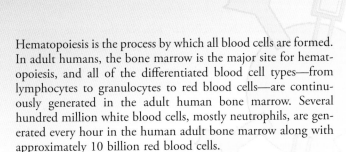

Hematopoiesis is the process by which all blood cells are formed. In adult humans, the bone marrow is the major site for hematopoiesis, and all of the differentiated blood cell types—from lymphocytes to granulocytes to red blood cells—are continuously generated in the adult human bone marrow. Several hundred million white blood cells, mostly neutrophils, are generated every hour in the human adult bone marrow along with approximately 10 billion red blood cells.

The leukocytes, both lymphoid and myeloid cells, were briefly described in Chapter 2. This chapter, as illustrated in the above figure, explains their development from stem cells to progenitor cells to mature cells. Chapter 13 describes the structure and function of the lymphoid organs, where lymphocytes are generated and mature. The process by which lymphocytes move from the organs of lymphoid generation, chiefly the bone marrow and thymus in humans, to the spleen, lymph nodes, skin, mucosa, and so on, where they encounter antigen, is known as *lymphocyte recirculation*, or *lymphocyte trafficking*, and *homing*. Chapter 13 also explains the way that lymphocytes recirculate and home to different tissues as well as the important role of cell adhesion molecules in these processes.

THREE MAJOR STAGES OF HEMATOPOIESIS

Hematopoiesis can be divided into three major parts, and each part involves very different types of cells and includes stem cells, progenitor cells, and mature cells (Fig. 12.1). Hematopoietic stem cells (HSCs) are pluripotent and self-renewing. They give rise to all the blood cell types (lineages). HSCs do not express cell lineage–specific marker proteins, such as CD3 on T cells or CD19 on B cells, but they do express a protein designated as *CD34,* which allows them to be manipulated for use in stem cell transplantation (Box 12.1).

HSCs migrate during embryonic development to the fetal liver and bone marrow. There they are induced to differentiate further by the large number of growth factors found in these tissues. Included among these growth factors are the colony-stimulating factors (CSFs). Specific CSFs induce differentiation of particular cell lineages, which are discussed later.

In the presence of these various growth factors, including the CSFs, the HSCs become progenitor cells (see Fig. 12.1). Progenitor cells are less primitive than HSCs, and they have some commitment to develop along a particular cell lineage.

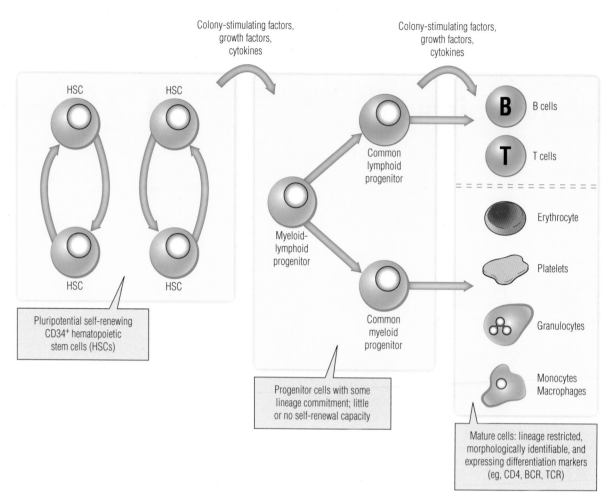

Fig 12.1 The three major stages of hematopoiesis. *BCR*, B-cell receptor; *HSC*, hematopoietic stem cell; *TCR*, T-cell receptor.

Progenitor cells cannot replenish stem cells. Under the influence of growth factors, two separate immune system progenitor cells develop: the common lymphoid and common myeloid progenitor cells. These cells give rise to mature cells, which have fully differentiated, such as T cells (see Fig. 12.1).

LYMPHOID CELLS

Development

Figure 12.2 illustrates the major overall stages in the development of B and T cells from the common lymphoid progenitor (CLP). The initial stages of T-lymphocyte precursor (thymocyte) development, but not human pre–B-cell development, are under the influence of the cytokine interleukin-7 (IL-7), which is produced and released from nonlymphoid stromal cells in the bone marrow. IL-7 is one of several cytokines affected by X-linked severe combined immunodeficiency (X-SCID; Box 12.2). Most T lymphocytes develop in the thymus from thymocyte precursors derived in the bone marrow (Chapters 13 and 15), and much of the B-lymphocyte development takes place in the bone marrow (Chapters 13 and 14). The developmental pathway for natural killer (NK) cells is not

yet well defined. NK cells are part of the innate immune system; their role in viral and tumor immunity is further described in Chapter 34.

Lymphoid Cell Types

Cells

Lymphoid cells produce antibody and express immunoglobulin as an antigen-specific receptor along with several other important molecules, such as major histocompatibility complex (MHC) class II molecules and the coreceptor molecule CD19. Morphologically, lymphoid cells have a large nucleus surrounded by a small rim of cytoplasm. In addition to producing antibody to combat extracellular infections, they can also function as antigen-presenting cells (APCs). They may be stimulated by antigen to form a larger blast cell (plasma cell; see Fig. 2.5B) with more cytoplasm, extensive endoplasmic reticulum, and secretory capacity for antibody.

T Cells

Morphologically, T cells resemble unstimulated B cells (see Fig. 2.5); that is, they are small lymphocytes with a large nucleus and little cytoplasm. They can be stimulated by antigen to become

 T-cell receptor (TCR)

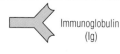 Immunoglobulin (Ig)

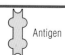 Antigen

 MCH I

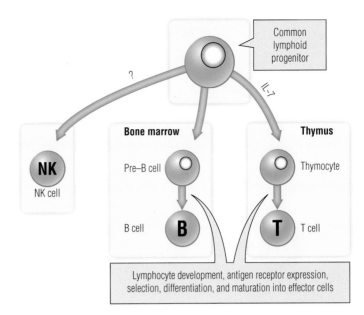

Fig 12.2 Overview of the development of the lymphoid cell lineage. *IL,* interleukin; *NK,* natural killer.

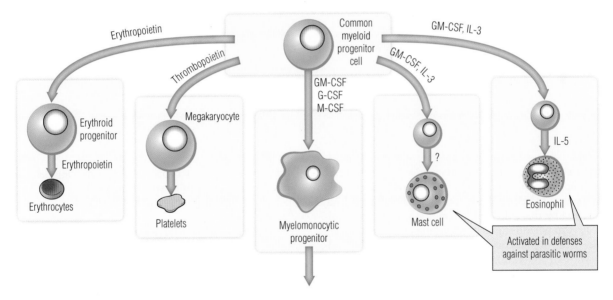

Fig 12.3 Overview of the development of the myeloid cell lineage. *CSF,* colony-stimulating factor; *G,* granulocyte; *GM,* granulocyte-macrophage; *IL,* interleukin; *M,* macrophage.

lymphoblasts with more cytoplasm and organelles. T cells consist of two major subsets: CD4+ helper cells and CD8+ cytotoxic T lymphocytes (Chapter 15). They also express an antigen-specific T-cell receptor and are the major source of antigen-specific protection against viral infection and other intracellular infections.

Natural Killer Cells

NK cells are lymphocytes insofar as they are derived from the common lymphoid precursor, they share growth factor with other lymphocytes (IL-2 and IL-7), and they have a similar appearance under the microscope (see Fig. 2.4). However, unlike T and B cells, NK cells do not rearrange genes for receptors. They are part of the innate immune system, and they kill certain virally infected cells and some tumor cells (Chapter 22). NK cells carry receptors that are specific for molecules expressed on infected cells or cells altered in other ways—for example, those

that express tumor-specific antigens. They have a role in initiating responses of T-helper cells, such as TH1, to intracellular pathogens.

NK cells are closely related to a newly discovered group of cells, the innate lymphoid cells. Like NK cells, these innate lymphoid cells have much in common with conventional lymphocytes but do not have rearranged receptor genes. They also have a role in initiating specific immune responses to different types of pathogens.

■ MYELOID CELLS

Development

Figure 12.3 depicts the main stages in the development of the other major white blood cells, the granulocyte and

 MCH II

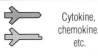 Cytokine, chemokine, etc.

 Complement (C′)

 Signaling molecule

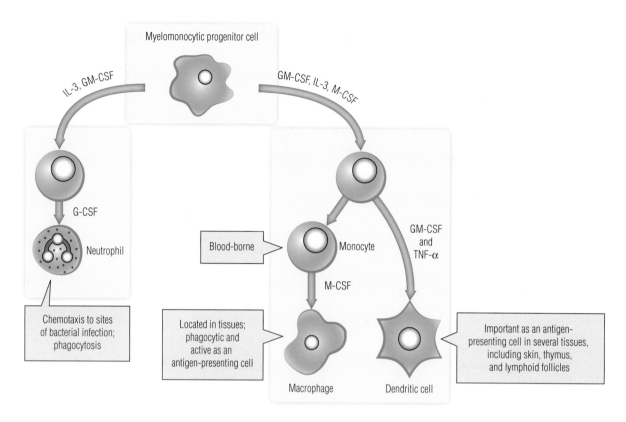

Fig 12.4 Overview of the development of the monocyte-macrophage lineage. *CSF,* colony-stimulating factor; *G,* granulocyte; *GM,* granulocyte-macrophage; *IL,* interleukin; *M,* macrophage; *TNF,* tumor necrosis factor.

monocyte-macrophage lineages. These cells derive from the same common myeloid progenitor (CMP) that gives rise to erythrocytes and platelets. The various differentiation pathways are stimulated by the actions of different growth factor combinations. Erythropoietin stimulates development of erythrocytes, and the CSFs—granulocyte-macrophage CSF (GM-CSF), granulocyte CSF (G-CSF), and monocyte- macrophage CSF (M-CSF)—stimulate development of the myelomonocytic progenitor cells and, ultimately, induce the production of neutrophils, monocytes, macrophages, and dendritic cells (DCs; Fig. 12.4). Various specific CSF-cytokine combinations are necessary for the differentiation of each of the myeloid cell types.

Myeloid Cell Types

Neutrophils

Neutrophils exhibit phagocytic and cytotoxic activities, and they migrate to sites of inflammation and infection in response to chemotactic factors. They are short lived, with a half-life of about 6 hours. Approximately 1011 neutrophils are estimated to be generated every day in the adult human. They contain both primary granules, loaded with lysosomal enzymes that include myeloperoxidase and elastase and secondary granules that contain lysozyme, collagenase, and so on. These cells are often referred to as *polymorphonuclear neutrophils* (PMNs) because they have nuclei with two to five lobes. Their role as a first line of defense in the innate response to bacterial infections is

discussed further in Chapter 21. Their development under the influence of G-CSF is discussed in Box 12.3.

Mast Cells

Mature mast cells have large granules that can be stained purple with dyes. These granules contain heparin and histamine. Mast cells express specific receptors on their surface for the Fc region of certain immunoglobulins (ie, FcRγ and FcRε). These cells have important roles in allergic responses (see Chapter 26), and they are activated through their receptors for immunoglobulin E (IgE) to release the above substances.

Eosinophils

Eosinophils (see Fig. 2.5) are characterized by a nucleus with two or three lobes. They have large, specific granules that contain heparin as well as peroxidase and other hydrolytic enzymes. These cells have phagocytic and cytotoxic activity and express Fc receptors, specifically FcRγ and FcRε. These cells also function to combat certain parasitic infections, particularly worms (Chapter 21).

Monocytes and Macrophages

Monocytes (see Fig 2.5) are the largest blood cells. They contain many granules and have a lobular-shaped nucleus. Monocytes phagocytose, have bacteriocidal activity, and can carry out antibody-dependent cell-mediated cytotoxicity (ADCC; Chapter 21). Monocytes migrate out of the blood into the tissues and become tissue macrophages, such as the Kupffer

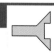 T-cell receptor (TCR)

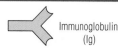 Immunoglobulin (Ig)

 Antigen

 MCH I

cells of the liver. They express the monocyte-macrophage marker protein CD14. Macrophages have a central role at the dividing line between the innate and specific immune response because of their role in antigen processing and presentation.

Dendritic Cells

DCs (see Fig. 2.5) are irregularly shaped cells with many branchlike processes. The two main types of DCs are *conventional DCs* (cDCs) and *plasmacytoid DCs* (pDCs). Both cDCs and pDCs are derived from the same myelomonocytic progenitor cell as macrophages (see Fig 12.4). DCs migrate to the tissues such as the skin, where they take on a sentinel role. These cells are sometimes called *Langerhans cells*. In the presence of infection and under the influence of cytokines, they mature and migrate to lymphoid organs, where they present antigen, activate T cells, and help develop a protective adaptive immune response.

DCs have a special role in presenting antigen to T cells, as described in the box in Chapter 10. The cDCs secrete IL-12, which activates the TH1 subset of T cells, and pDCs secrete the antiviral cytokine interferon-alfa.

BOX 12.1 Autologous Hematopoietic Stem Cell Transplantation

A 56-year-old woman is receiving cytotoxic chemotherapy for leukemia. The chemotherapy is very potent and has damaged her bone marrow stem cells. She has become very anemic and is bleeding because of her low platelet count. She is also contracting serious infections because her neutrophil count is so low. Fortunately, she has autologous stem cells available, which she receives by infusion. She makes a gradual recovery.

Stem cell infusions are used in a variety of settings. Different sources of stem cells are available. Autologous stem cells can be removed from samples and can be stored at very low temperatures that preserve the cells from destruction. These stem cells are returned to the patient via autologous bone marrow transplantation after chemotherapy to help the patient quickly reconstitute immune and blood cells. Because this is the patient's own marrow, there are no complications with regard to transplant rejection. However, the process of obtaining the bone marrow usually involves a relatively painful surgical procedure to aspirate cells from the pelvic bones under general anesthesia.

Large numbers of autologous hematopoietic stem cells (HSCs) can be mobilized into the blood by giving patients granulocyte colony–stimulating factor (G-CSF). The HSCs are then identified by their expression of the CD34 molecule and are harvested from the blood. Peripheral blood harvesting has been found to generate more stem cells than does bone marrow aspiration. It is also less painful for the patient and is becoming the approach of choice in preference to autologous bone marrow transplantation for certain patients.

Stem cells can also be obtained from donor marrow or blood. Donor cord blood from a newborn has the best potential for regeneration, although stem cells derived from donors are a form of allogeneic transplantation and carry the risk of rejection. The general topic of transplantation is discussed in greater detail in Chapter 34.

Induced stem cells may be used in the future. Induced stem cells are derived from normal cells, such as fibroblasts, which are easily obtained from a skin biopsy. They have been reprogrammed so that silenced stem cell genes are reactivated.

BOX 12.2 X-Linked Severe Combined Immunodeficiency

A 7-week-old male infant is suffering from a range of life-threatening infections. Blood testing shows normal levels of B cells but absent T cells. Genetic testing is carried out and confirms the presence of X-linked severe combined immunodeficiency (X-SCID). Fortunately, the boy has an older sister who is able to donate stem cells. He undergoes transplantation and makes a good recovery.

Compare this infant with the baby with X-linked antibody deficiency in Box 11-2. The boy with antibody deficiency did not get sick until he was about 6 months old. Up to that point, he was protected by antibodies from his mother.

Boys affected by X-SCID are born without T cells or natural killer (NK) cells, have nonfunctional B cells, and, if untreated, will rapidly die from infection. Although normal numbers of B cells are present in these patients, they are nonfunctional. This is because of both a lack of T cells to provide help and an inherent B-cell defect. Stem cell transplantation is an effective treatment for these boys; however, in many cases a human leukocyte antigen–matched donor is tragically unavailable.

The mutation on the X chromosome responsible for X-SCID has been identified. The mutation is in the gene for a subunit of several cytokine receptors, including the receptors for interleukins 2, 4, 7, 10, 15, and 21. The cytokine receptor subunit is referred to as the *common cytokine receptor γ-chain*, or the *γc chain*. The B-cell defect in these boys may be related to the lack of a functioning IL-4 receptor due to the mutation in γc.

 MCH II

 Cytokine, chemokine, etc.

 Complement (C′)

 Signaling molecule

BOX 12.3 Administration of Granulocyte Colony–Stimulating Factor for Neutropenia

Because of its important role in hematopoiesis, granulocyte colony-stimulating factor (G-CSF) has become a well-characterized protein. The G-CSF gene has been cloned, and a recombinant form of G-CSF has been produced for use in treatment because it causes an increase in neutrophil production in the bone marrow. Apart from its role in autologous stem cell transplantation, in vivo administration of G-CSF has been approved for the treatment of neutropenias caused by several conditions, including cancer chemotherapy and acute leukemia. The enhanced neutrophil levels produced by G-CSF treatment have been shown to protect these otherwise neutropenic patients from life-threatening bacterial infections (see Box 21.1).

LEARNING POINTS ⚛ Can You Now ...

1. Draw the developmental pathway from stem cell through progenitor cell to mature lymphoid and myeloid cells?

2. Describe the role of colony-stimulating factors and other growth factors in the developmental pathways to lymphoid and myeloid cells?

3. List several important morphologic features and functional activities of B and T lymphocytes, natural killer cells, neutrophils, mast cells, eosinophils, monocytes, macrophages, and dendritic cells?

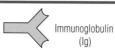 T-cell receptor (TCR)

 Immunoglobulin (Ig)

Antigen

 MCH I

Organs and Tissues of the Immune System

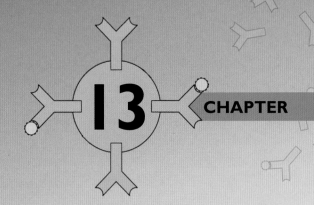

13 CHAPTER

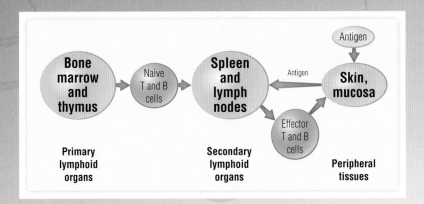

Up to this point, we have primarily discussed the genes, molecules, and cells that function in the immune response. However, host defense responses take place in a whole organism, not in isolated cells or among subcellular components. It is now necessary to consider the immune response in the context of a physiologic system. The above figure depicts the main topics for this chapter: the structure and function of the primary and secondary lymphoid organs and how lymphocytes are produced, expanded, come into contact with antigen, and mature into effector cells capable of a protective immune response.

▩ PRIMARY AND SECONDARY LYMPHOID ORGANS

The immune system is made up of distinct compartments, the organs and tissues, which are interconnected by the blood and lymphatic vessels. This network comprises those organs and tissues in which lymphocytes are produced, *the primary lymphoid organs,* and those in which they come into contact with foreign antigen, are clonally expanded, and mature into effector cells, the *secondary lymphoid organs.*

In the embryonic human, the *primary lymphoid organs*—that is, the place where lymphocytes are generated—are initially the yolk sac, then the fetal liver and spleen, and finally the bone marrow and thymus (Fig. 13.1). By puberty, most lymphopoiesis is B-lymphocyte production in the marrow of the flat bones, such as the sternum, vertebrae, and pelvis.

The human *secondary lymphoid organs* are generally considered to be the spleen and lymph nodes. In addition, specialized mucosa-associated lymphoid tissue (MALT) lines the respiratory, gastrointestinal, and reproductive tracts, and a cutaneous immune system is also present. These organs are distributed as shown in Figure 13.1. Lymphocytes lodge in the secondary lymphoid organs, and they expand clonally on contact with the antigen appropriate for their specific antigen receptors. They also recirculate among these organs via the blood and lymphatic systems. This lymphocyte recirculation, or *trafficking,* connects the various lymphoid compartments to create one system (discussed later).

Lymphocytes are dispersed to almost all tissue sites; therefore almost all the tissues in the human body could be thought of as lymphoid. However, some sites—such as eye, testes, and brain—do not have lymphoid cells and are said to be *immunologically privileged.* The most important sites of lymphocyte dispersal are the spleen, lymph nodes, MALT, and skin. Each of these is described briefly in this chapter to create a context for understanding the physiology of the immune response.

Bone Marrow

As described in Chapter 12, the bone marrow is the major hematopoietic organ in humans. All of the blood cell types are generated in the bone marrow. T- and B-cell generation takes place in these internal cavities; development from B-cell progenitors to immature B cells occurs in a radial direction toward

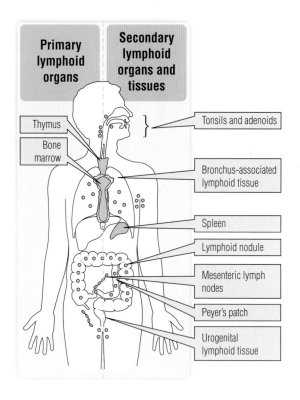

Fig 13.1 Major lymphoid organs in the adult human. (Modified from Roitt I, Brostoff J, Male D. *Immunology*, 6th ed. London: Mosby; 2001.)

the center of the bone. This process is described in more detail in Chapter 14. Immature T cells are produced in the bone marrow but migrate to the thymus to fully mature.

Hematopoiesis is facilitated in the bone marrow by a mixture of cells that provide a source of the growth factors and cytokines essential for the development of the various blood cell types.

Thymus

The thymus is a bilobed organ found in the anterior mediastinum. The thymus forms from epithelial cells from the third pharyngeal pouch, the corresponding brachial clefts, and the pharyngeal arch. The thymus grows until puberty and then undergoes progressive involution. By late adulthood, it is largely adipose tissue with only a small amount of lymphoid tissue remaining. The main role of the thymus is to select T cells that are able to recognize self major histocompatibility complex (MHC), known as *positive selection,* and to destroy T cells that recognize self antigen (Chapter 15) Figure 13.2 shows a schematic drawing of the thymus, which has three main areas:

1. The subcapsular zone contains the earliest progenitor T cells.
2. The cortex is densely packed with developing T cells undergoing selection.
3. The medulla contains fewer, but more mature, T lymphocytes; these have survived the selection processes and are about to be released to the periphery (Chapter 15).

The thymus is the primary site of T-cell development. Most T-cell progenitors (more than 95%) die in the thymus through

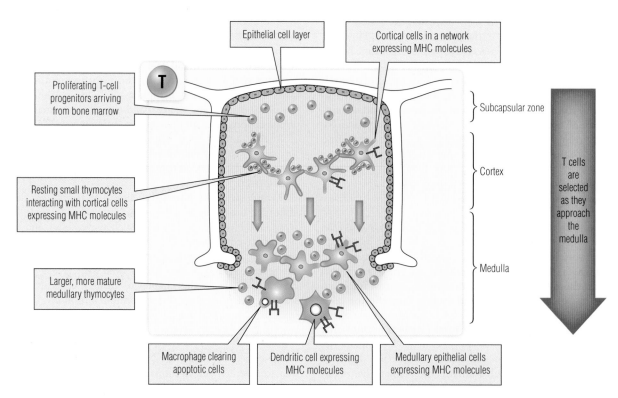

Fig 13.2 A simplified schematic showing the cellular organization of the thymus (T). *MHC,* major histocompatibility complex.

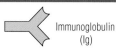 T-cell receptor (TCR)

 Immunoglobulin (Ig)

Antigen

 MCH I

the process of apoptosis. An extensive network of epithelial cells and antigen-presenting cells is involved in the selection process that leads to the development of an appropriate T-cell receptor repertoire. An outline of some of the important cell-cell interactions in T-cell development is found in Figure 13.2, and this topic is developed in more detail in Chapter 15.

Lymph Nodes

Lymph nodes function as the meeting place for antigen and T and B lymphocytes, and they are one site of lymphocyte active proliferation in response to infection. Lymph nodes are bean shaped and are usually found clustered in groups at sites where numerous blood and lymph vessels converge. For example, a large collection of nodes is found in the armpit (axillary nodes). Each lymph node is organized into several areas (Fig. 13.3). The cortex is predominantly the site of B cells and contains a number of spherical follicles of B cells. If B cells become activated and start proliferating, they produce a germinal center. Follicles that contain germinal centers are called *secondary follicles.* The lymph node paracortex is predominantly a CD4+ T-cell area, and the medulla of the node contains a mixture of B cells, T cells, and macrophages.

Circulating lymphocytes enter the node via specialized high endothelial venules (HEVs) in the paracortex; the important role of HEVs in lymphocyte trafficking is discussed later. Antigens arrive in the lymph that flows in from the peripheral tissues. Antigens present in solution or as small particles in suspension are filtered out of the lymph and are presented to B cells in the primary follicles.

Lymph also contains dendritic cells (Chapters 10 and 12) that carry antigen on surface MHC molecules. These dendritic cells enter the paracortex and search out CD4+ T cells able to recognize the antigens they are presenting. If antigen recognition

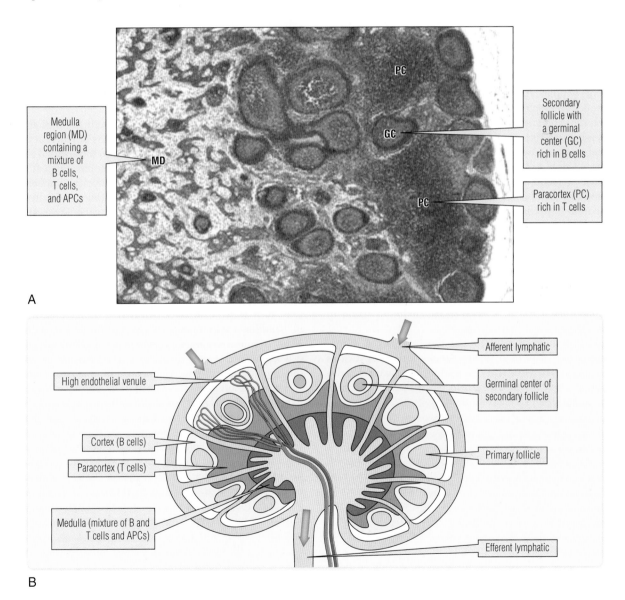

Fig 13.3 Lymph nodes. **A,** Stained section of a node. **B,** A simplified schematic showing the organization of a node. *APC,* antigen-presenting cell. (**A,** From Kerr JB. *Atlas of Functional Histology.* London: Mosby; 2000.)

 MCH II

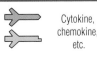 Cytokine, chemokine, etc.

 Complement (C')

 Signaling molecule

takes place, an immunologic synapse is temporarily formed. Otherwise, the dendritic cell will continue to search for T cells capable of recognizing antigen. CD4 T cells that have been stimulated in this way will proliferate, enlarging the paracortex. Some T cells will also migrate into the neighboring germinal center, where they may provide help to B cells responding to antigen.

During lymphocyte activation, fluid and cells are accumulated in the node, which leads to lymph-node enlargement—the "swollen gland" typical of response to infection. After the immune system clears the infectious agent, the node returns to its normal size and can no longer be palpated. The location of the swollen lymph nodes reflects the site of infection. For example, an infected finger leads to swollen axillary nodes. More generalized swollen nodes (*lymphadenopathy*) reflect a generalized infection or tumor.

Spleen

The spleen, a secondary lymphoid organ about the size of a clenched fist, is found in the left upper quadrant of the abdomen. The spleen is a major lymphoid organ and has similar functions to lymph nodes—namely, antigen-lymphocyte interactions and subsequent lymphocyte activation and proliferation. Unlike lymph nodes, the spleen is not connected to the lymphatic system, so cells and antigen arrive and leave through the blood. The spleen has two additional functions. First, it contains a very high number of macrophages, which filter the blood, removing microbes and dead red blood cells. Second, it is the main site for responses to blood-borne antigens and is the source of B cells that respond in the absence of T-cell help to bacterial cell wall polysaccharide antigens (Box 13.1). The spleen contains two main areas: the *red pulp* contains chiefly macrophages and red blood cells in the process of disposal, and the *white pulp* contains dense lymphoid tissue. The spleen has been estimated to store about 25% of the total lymphocytes in the body. The histology of the white pulp is similar to that of lymph nodes and is segregated into B- and T-lymphocyte areas. The T cells are chiefly found around blood vessels, whereas B cells are found mainly in follicles.

Like lymph nodes, the spleen can also be enlarged during some infections. These tend to be systemic infections such as malaria, Epstein Barr virus (EBV) infection, and bacterial endocarditis. The spleen is also enlarged in blood diseases and with some malignancies and liver conditions.

Mucosa-Associated Lymphoid Tissue

The mucosal immune system handles antigen at a contact point between the host and the environment, and it is an important first line of defense. MALT consists of structured lymphoid aggregates, more diffuse populations of mucosal lymphocytes, and the circulation of cells within this system. MALT is not a stand-alone immune system, although cells within MALT do behave in some unique ways.

Lymphoid aggregates include the tonsils in the mucosa of the pharynx. Just like any other lymphoid tissue, after repeated bouts of infection, secondary follicles develop in the tonsils, which then become painful and swollen. Peyer patches are another type of lymphoid aggregate found in the small intestine.

Figure 13.4A shows a stained section through a Peyer patch. There are no villi over the Peyer patch; instead, the follicle-associated epithelium (FAE) contains a specialized cell type (M cells) that takes up antigens that are inhaled or ingested (Fig. 13.4B, C). Antigens are taken up by M cells by the process of *pinocytosis,* the cellular intake of small vacuoles that contain fluid and molecules. By a transcellular transport process called *transcytosis,* the M cells transport antigens into the subepithelial tissues, where they encounter lymphocytes. Underneath the follicle-associated epithelium are lymphoid follicles. If these are actively responding to infection, a germinal center may be present. The B cells within the follicle secrete immunoglobulin A (IgA) across the epithelium (Fig. 13.4D). IgA is initially bound to the poly-Ig receptor, and after transport across the epithelial cell membrane, it retains a piece of this receptor—now known as *secretory component*—that may help protect it from degradation in the gut lumen.

Secretion of IgA, as opposed to other immunoglobulin classes, is stimulated by the cytokine known as *transforming growth factor β* (TGF-β), secreted by epithelial cells. TGF-β also has broadly suppressive effects on T cells. This is thought to be important to ensure tolerance of peptides derived from food proteins (Chapter 18), so-called oral tolerance.

Mucosal Lymphocytes

The mucosal epithelium of the gastrointestinal, respiratory, and reproductive tracts contains large numbers of lymphocytes. The lamina propria lymphocytes are similar to those found elsewhere in the body; intraepithelial lymphocytes are different and are mostly T cells (~90%) and a greater than typical number (maybe as much as 10%–20%) are γδ T cells (Fig. 13.5). In general, intraepithelial lymphocytes act to protect the host against viral and bacterial pathogens encountered in the gut.

Skin: The Cutaneous Immune System

The skin is the major physical barrier to pathogen entry, and it is a very important interface between the immune cells and the external environment. The skin has many lymphoid accessory cells, such as dendritic cells, that have critically important roles in handling environmental antigens that penetrate the skin. Many immune responses are initiated in the skin; consequently, it is reasonable to view the skin as another peripheral organ of the immune system—the cutaneous immune tissue.

Figure 13.6A shows inflamed skin during a delayed-type hypersensitivity (DTH) response. This type of response is described in more detail in Chapters 23 and 31. The lymphoid cells involved in immune reactions in the skin are shown in Figure 13.6B. The epidermal layer of the skin has numerous dendritic cells called *Langerhans cells,* which are very important in antigen processing and presentation (Chapter 10). Langerhans cells have a sentinel role in the skin. When they detect infection, they phagocytose and process antigen. At the same time, they migrate via lymphatics to the regional lymph node to present antigen to T cells.

The T cells found in the epidermal layer, the *intraepidermal T cells,* are chiefly CD8⁺ T cells that carry γδ T-cell receptors (Chapter 7) at a higher frequency than is typical, similar to the situation described earlier for the intraepithelial T cells of the MALT. The T-cell receptors on these intraepidermal T cells also represent a restricted set of specificities, which suggests a focus

 T-cell receptor (TCR)

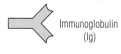 Immunoglobulin (Ig)

 Antigen

 MCH I

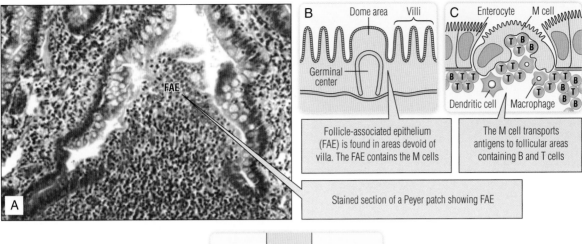

B Dome area | Villi
Germinal center

Follicle-associated epithelium (FAE) is found in areas devoid of villa. The FAE contains the M cells

C Enterocyte | M cell
Dendritic cell | Macrophage

The M cell transports antigens to follicular areas containing B and T cells

Stained section of a Peyer patch showing FAE

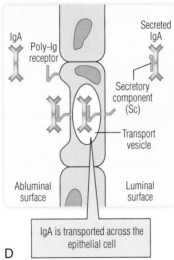

D

IgA | Poly-Ig receptor | Secreted IgA

Secretory component (Sc)

Transport vesicle

Abluminal surface | Luminal surface

IgA is transported across the epithelial cell

Fig 13.4 Mucosa-associated lymphoid tissue (MALT). **A,** Stained section of a Peyer patch (gut-associated lymphoid tissue [GALT]). **B,** The organization of GALT in Peyer patches. **C,** An M cell in the intestinal follicle-associated epithelium (FAE). **D,** Transport of immunoglobulin A (IgA) across epithelium.

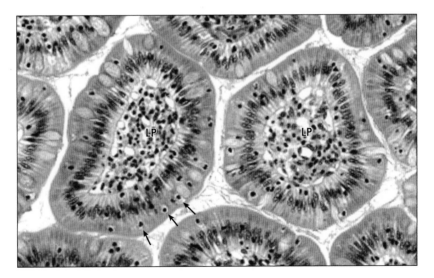

Fig 13.5 Cross section of the small bowel showing the two types of mucosal lymphocytes: lamina propria (LP) and intraepithelial lymphocytes. This section has cut across several villi. At the core of each villus are some lamina propria containing lymphocytes in the connective tissue. Intraepithelial lymphocytes *(arrows)* are also scattered around the epithelium.

 MCH II

 Cytokine, chemokine, etc.

Complement (C′)

 Signaling molecule

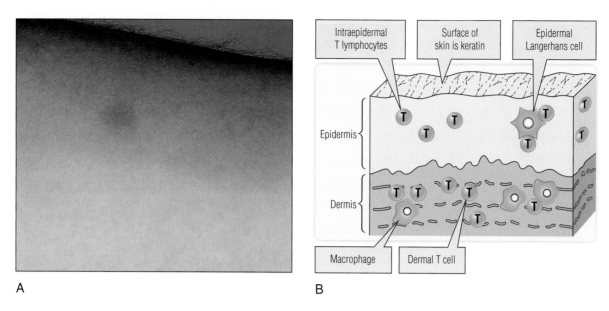

A

B

Fig 13.6 Skin: the cutaneous immune system. **A,** Inflamed skin during a delayed-type hypersensitivity test. **B,** A simplified schematic of skin showing antigen-presenting cells (APCs) and Langerhans cells.

on frequently occurring pathogens that infect through the skin. The underlying dermis is rich in macrophages and T cells (see Fig. 13.6B; see also Fig. 23.8).

■ LYMPHOCYTE TRAFFICKING

Trafficking refers to movement of leukocytes around the body. At this point, the discussion of trafficking is confined to lymphocytes; trafficking of other white blood cells is discussed in Chapter 21. Unlike red cells, which circulate passively with the flow of blood, lymphocytes actively move around the different compartments of the body. The six elements of lymphocyte trafficking are (1) recirculation, (2) homing, (3) extravasation, (4) diapedesis, (5) chemotaxis, and (6) synapse formation.

Lymphocyte Recirculation

Most mature T and B cells are in constant circulation via the bloodstream and lymphatics (Fig. 13.7) and move constantly from tissue to tissue. It has been estimated that a lymphocyte makes a full circuit of the human body—from the blood to the tissues to the lymphatic system and returning to the blood—once or twice a day. This recirculation is important to ensure that the small number of lymphocytes specific for any given antigen have the best chance to find that antigen in any possible body site.

The first recirculation pathway is from blood to lymph node. For example, naïve T lymphocytes—that is, T lymphocytes that have not yet encountered the antigen they have specificity for (their *cognate antigen*; Chapter 15)—constantly circulate among the secondary lymphoid organs until they encounter antigen or die. This circulation through the lymphoid organs maximizes the chance to encounter antigen displayed on a professional antigen-presenting cell: a requirement to activate a naive T cell (Chapter 15). By comparison, effector T cells—so-called *memory T cells,* long-lived cells that retain "memory" of contact with

antigen and respond faster (Chapter 17)—follow two different recirculation pathways. First, effector T cells are attracted into tissues where inflammation is present. Second, effector T cells recirculate again and again to the same type of tissues. After exposure to antigen in the MALT, lymphocytes may leave and home to other mucosal tissues. This trafficking provides a potential target for vaccination, using mucosal vaccines for the initial stimulation (Box 13.3). Other populations of effector T cells recirculate into different tissues, such as the skin. Positioning T cells that have already been primed by contact with antigen in peripheral sites, where they can screen for antigen, enhances the likelihood of effective protection via a secondary immune response (Chapter 17). Figure 13.7 outlines lymphocyte recirculation pathways.

Homing

Homing refers to the differential migration of lymphocytes to specific tissues. Lymphocyte homing is regulated by receptor-ligand interactions between members of the different families of cell adhesion molecules (CAMs). Several extensive families of CAMs exist that include selectins, addressins, and integrins.

Naive T cells recognize HEVs in lymph nodes. To do this, naive T cells express L-selectin, which recognizes and binds GLYCAM1 expressed in the lining of HEVs. GLYCAM1 is a member of the addressin family of molecules. In contrast, integrin $\alpha4/\beta6$ on effector lymphocytes and MADCAM1 on endothelium in mucosa promote homing into the gut, for example. Thus different ligand pairs promote homing of different lymphocytes into different tissues. Some of these are shown in Figure 13.8.

Lymphocyte Extravasation

Figure 13.9 is a simplified representation of the steps involved in lymphocyte extravasation, which are (1) primary adhesion to

 T-cell receptor (TCR)   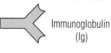 Immunoglobulin (Ig)   Antigen   MCH I

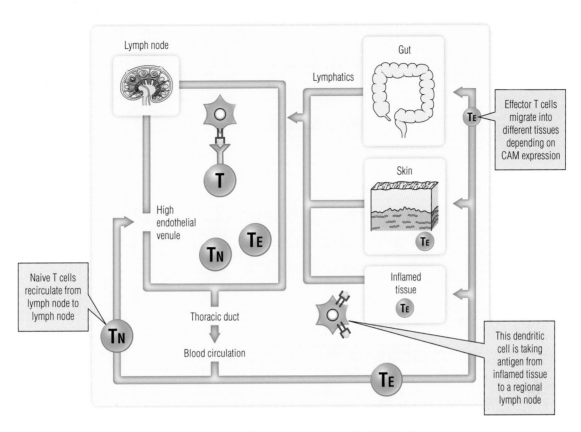

Fig 13.7 Recirculation of lymphocytes. This figure shows how a naive T cell (TN) will continue to recirculate through lymph nodes. If this T cell encounters a dendritic cell that expresses the cognate antigen, the T cell will transform into an effector T cell (TE). Effector T cells circulate into different tissues depending on their cell adhesion molecule (CAM) expression.

endothelium, (2) lymphocyte activation, (3) secondary adhesion (arrest), (4) diapedesis, and (5) return.

Lymphocytes normally flow freely through the blood vessels. Analyses by videomicroscopy show that they can roll along endothelial cells, slowed down by low-affinity interactions between homing receptor molecules on the lymphocyte cell surface and CAMs on the vascular endothelial cell surface (Table 13.1). If the lymphocyte detects signals of inflammation in the tissue—for example, by detecting inflammatory mediators such as chemokines (Chapter 21)—the lymphocyte may be activated to express additional adhesion molecules that can mediate strong, high-affinity interactions.

The secondary adhesion phase is mediated by high-affinity interactions among various families of CAMs found both on the lymphocyte surface and on the endothelial cells in the tissues, such as leukocyte function–associated antigen (LFA-1) and intercellular adhesion molecule 1 (ICAM1), respectively. This primary adhesion, triggering, and expression of new adhesion molecules takes place in a few seconds, and lymphocyte movement is stopped even in the presence of considerable shear forces from the ongoing blood flow.

Lymphocyte arrest is followed by passage (diapedesis or transmigration) through the tight junction between adjacent endothelial cells into the tissues (see Fig. 13.9). It is important to point out that the specificity of the recirculation-homing process is entirely a function of homing receptor–addressin interactions and is independent of antigen. In fact, most lymphocytes recruited to an infected tissue are not specific for the antigen causing the infection. However, an ongoing immune response influences the retention of lymphocytes at a tissue site and causes release of various factors that stimulate expression of adhesion proteins.

Chemotaxis

Chemotaxis is the directed movement of cells in tissues. For example, a B cell arriving in a lymph node will locate itself in a follicle by following a trail of chemokines. Chemotaxis will also lead lymphocytes to the site of an infection. In this case, inflammatory chemokines are released by macrophages at the site of the infection (Chapter 21).

Synapse Formation

When lymphocytes are interacting with other cells, an immunologic synapse forms. Some of the same CAMs mentioned already in trafficking are temporarily expressed to stabilize the synapse. For example, a T cell that recognizes antigen presented by an antigen-presenting cell (APC) will become activated and will start to express LFA-1, which binds to ICAM1 on the APC to form a link across the synapse.

 MCH II   Cytokine, chemokine, etc.   Complement (C′)   Signaling molecule

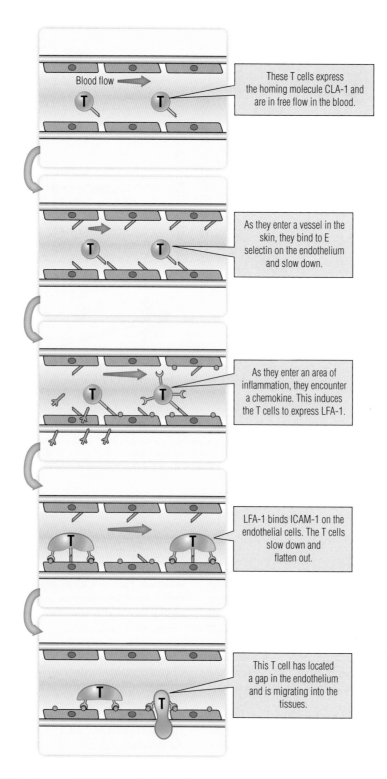

Blood flow

These T cells express the homing molecule CLA-1 and are in free flow in the blood.

As they enter a vessel in the skin, they bind to E selectin on the endothelium and slow down.

As they enter an area of inflammation, they encounter a chemokine. This induces the T cells to express LFA-1.

LFA-1 binds ICAM-1 on the endothelial cells. The T cells slow down and flatten out.

This T cell has located a gap in the endothelium and is migrating into the tissues.

Fig 13.8 How skin-specific T cells respond to local inflammation. The process illustrated would lead to the type of lesion shown in Figure 13.6A. *ICAM1*, intracellular adhesion molecule 1; *CLA-1*, cutaneous lymphocyte antigen 1; *LFA-1*, leukocyte function–associated antigen 1.

 T-cell receptor (TCR) Immunoglobulin (Ig) Antigen MCH I

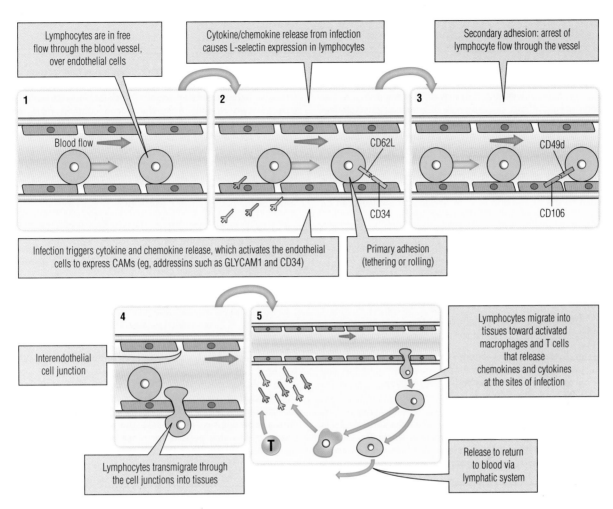

Fig 13.9 Five-step model of leukocyte extravasation. *CAM,* cell adhesion molecule.

TABLE 13.1   Ligands and Cell Adhesion Molecules

Function of Ligand Pair	CAM on Lymphocyte	CAM on Local Tissue
Recirculation of naive T cells to lymph nodes	L selectin on naive T cells	GLYCAM1 on high endothelial blood vessels
Homing of effector T cells into the gut	Integrin α4/β6 on effector lymphocytes	MADCAM1 on mucosal endothelium
Homing of effector T cells into the skin	CLA-1 on effector lymphocytes	E-selectin on skin endothelium
Homing of lymphocytes into inflamed tissue	LFA-1 on T cells activated by chemokines	ICAM1 on inflamed endothelium
Stabilization of immune synapse	LFA-1 on T cells activated by antigen recognition	ICAM1 on antigen-presenting cell

CAM, *cell adhesion molecule;* CLA, *cutaneous lymphocyte antigen;* GLYCAM, *glycosylation-dependent cell adhesion molecule;* ICAM, *intercellular adhesion molecule;* LFA; *leukocyte function–associated antigen;* MADCAM, *mucosal vascular addressin cell adhesion molecule.*

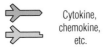 MCH II

Cytokine, chemokine, etc.

 Complement (C′)

 Signaling molecule

BOX 13.1 Risks of Splenectomy

A 28-year-old man presents to the emergency department in shock with low blood pressure and high fever. He underwent an emergency splenectomy 2 years prior but has not been on antibiotics since then. A diagnosis of postsplenectomy invasive sepsis is made. He is resuscitated and started on penicillin and makes a prompt recovery. A day later, pneumococcus is cultured from blood taken in the emergency department, confirming the diagnosis.

The spleen is a soft, spongy organ that bleeds easily following trauma. In certain situations, such as seat-belt–mediated trauma sustained to the midsection in a car accident, the spleen can be ruptured and must be surgically removed.

Several thousand people have undergone splenectomy in the United States. Splenectomized patients are more susceptible to infection by encapsulated bacteria such as pneumococci. This is true for two reasons. First, the spleen contains many of the T-independent B cells that make antibody against the polysaccharide capsule of these bacteria. Second, the spleen contains a large number of macrophages, which phagocytose opsonized bacteria in the blood. Splenectomized patients are significantly at risk for infectious disease and are therefore maintained on life-long prophylactic antibiotics. They also receive vaccines against some of the pathogens for which they are at risk.

BOX 13.2 Lymphadenopathy

A 26-year-old man attends your clinic complaining of lumps in his throat. On further questioning, he has had a sore throat for about 4 days and is very anxious because his father was recently diagnosed with laryngeal cancer. On examination, your patient has some redness of the fauces and tonsils, which are slightly enlarged with two small (approximately 1-cm diameter) lymph nodes in the right anterior triangle. You explain that the patient's symptoms are most consistent with an acute viral infection of the upper respiratory tract and that treatment

is not necessary. To be safe, you take a throat swab to rule out bacterial pathogens.

Lymphadenopathy is usually the consequence of acute infection. Localized lymphadenopathy occurs as a consequence of localized infection, as is the case here, and is usually associated with a localizing sign; in this case, the throat was inflamed. Lymphadenopathy that persists for more than a few days or affects many different sites may indicate other disease processes, such as chronic infection (eg, tuberculosis or HIV) or malignancy.

BOX 13.3 Mucosal Vaccines

Many pathogens, both bacterial and viral, invade the host via mucosal tissue. For example, HIV is primarily sexually transmitted; influenza invades through the respiratory mucosa; and *Shigella* and *Escherichia coli* cause enteric infections and diarrhea. For this reason, it would be very desirable to be able to vaccinate and induce a mucosal immune response that would prevent entry of such pathogens. Notably, vaccination at one mucosal site can confer immunity at other mucosal sites because of lymphocyte migration to other mucosal tissues.

For mucosal vaccines to work, they have to overcome the generally immunosuppressive environment of the gut. To do this,

biotechnologists are developing substances called *adjuvants* to overcome oral tolerance. Given that the mucosal tissues are major sites of interaction with pathogens, it is very important that we continue to learn more about mucosal immunology. It is likely that our rapidly developing understanding of the mucosal immune system will lead to effective mucosal vaccines that will confer long-term protection against pathogens such as HIV, influenza, rotaviruses, and enteropathogenic bacteria. The impact worldwide of such mucosal vaccines would be enormous.

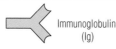 T-cell receptor (TCR)   Immunoglobulin (Ig)   Antigen   MCH I

LEARNING POINTS Can You Now…

1. Describe the immune response in terms of a systemic physiologic response?
2. Describe the role of the bone marrow in lymphocyte generation and B-cell maturation?
3. Draw the cellular organization of the thymus and describe the role of the thymus in T-lymphocyte generation and maturation?
4. Draw the structure of the spleen and describe its role as a major site of responses to blood-borne antigens? As a "filter" for the blood? As a site of T-independent antibody synthesis?
5. Draw the structure of a lymph node and describe its role as a filter for the lymph and as a major site for responses to lymph-borne antigens?
6. Describe the role of the various mucosa-associated lymphoid tissue (MALT) as a first line of defense?
7. Describe the important role of the skin as a part of the immune system?
8. Draw the major recirculation pathways of lymphocytes around the organs and tissues of the immune system?
9. Draw the five-step model of lymphocyte extravasation?

 MCH II

 Cytokine, chemokine, etc.

Complement (C')

 Signaling molecule

14 B-Cell Development

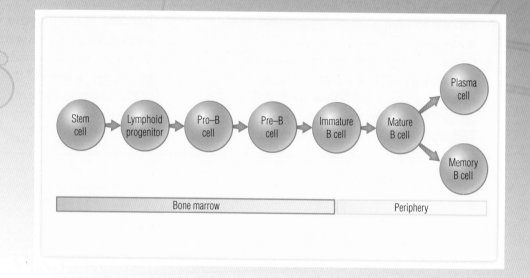

As discussed in Chapters 6 and 11, membrane-bound antibody molecules on the surface of B cells comprise a key part of the B-cell receptor (BCR) responsible for recognizing antigen. A series of developmental stages results in expression of the antigen-specific BCR. B lymphocytes that express a diverse repertoire of BCRs, as yet unselected, are continually generated in the bone marrow. Before reaching maturity, the developing B cells undergo a selection process, referred to as *negative selection,* in an attempt to ensure that their antigen receptor does not recognize self antigen; otherwise, antiself reactivity may result in autoimmunity (Chapter 28). Those B cells that survive negative selection disperse to the peripheral lymphoid organs (Chapter 13), where they may encounter the foreign antigen they have specificity for, become activated, and ultimately terminally differentiate into antibody-producing cells. Those cells that do *not* encounter the appropriate antigen die over a few weeks. This chapter and the figure above illustrate the developmental stages of the B cell, from hematopoietic stem cell to conventional mature B cell. At the end of the chapter, two unconventional B-cell populations are described, the T-independent and B1 B cells.

■ EARLY B-LYMPHOCYTE DEVELOPMENT

Stem Cell to Immature B Cell

The B-cell lineage is derived from lymphoid progenitor cells that differentiate from hematopoietic stem cells (Chapter 12). B cells are produced throughout life, but differentiation first occurs in the fetal liver and then shifts to the bone marrow soon after birth (Chapters 12 and 13). In the adult bone marrow, B-cell development follows a radially organized maturation pathway in which the least developed cells are close to the endosteal (inner) surface of the bone, and the more mature cells are concentrated in the central marrow space. Immature B cells exit the bone marrow via the sinusoids and migrate to the periphery, typically to the spleen or lymph nodes. Their development in the bone marrow depends on a variety of growth factors contributed by bone marrow stromal cells (Chapter 12).

From the earliest cell progenitor, the hematopoietic stem cell, the B-cell differentiation pathway can be subdivided into several developmental stages. These stages are defined by the rearrangement status of the immunoglobulin (Ig) heavy and light chain genes and the expression of differentiation-specific molecules on the cell surface as shown in Table 14.1.

The earliest committed B-lineage cell is called the *pro–B cell*. This cell is recognized by the appearance of surface markers characteristic of the B lineage, such as CD19, a part of the coreceptor complex (Chapter 11). The recombination activation genes (RAGs) are active in pro–B cells and Ig heavy chain diversity (DH), joining (JH) and variable region (VH) gene segments are rearranged in attempts to produce a heavy chain. Terminal deoxynucleotidyl transferase (TdT) is also active in these cells and increases junctional diversity.

The cell becomes a *pre–B cell* once a μ heavy chain is expressed (see Chapter 6). The μ heavy chain (μ_H) is expressed on the cell surface in association with ψL and μ_H chains (Chapter 11) to form a receptor complex called the *pre–B-cell receptor* (pre-BCR). The pre-BCR plays an important role in transducing signals that lead to proliferation of the pre–B cells and thereby facilitates their further development. Proliferation promotes further development and progression toward the next main stage—the late pre–B cell.

During the pre–B-cell stage, the V(D)J recombinase machinery initiates light chain gene rearrangement. The cell will first attempt to recombine a κ light chain, and if this is unsuccessful, it will then attempt to produce a λ light chain. The appearance of paired light and heavy chain polypeptides on the cell surface as a complete IgM molecule, the BCR, constitutes the transition to an immature B cell. Transcription of the RAG and TdT enzymes is now switched off for the remainder of the cell's life (Fig. 14.1).

TABLE 14.1 Differentiation-Specific Molecules

	Stem Cell	Lymphoid Progenitor	Pro–B Cell	Pre–B Cell	Immature B Cell
CD19 expressed on cell surface	No	Yes	Yes	Yes	Yes
RAG and TdT activity	No	Yes	Yes	Yes	No
μ Heavy chain expressed on cell surface	No	No	No	Yes	Yes
Pre-BCR expressed on cell surface	No	No	No	Yes	Yes
Light chain expressed on cell surface	No	No	No	No	Yes
IgM BCR expressed on cell surface	No	No	No	No	Yes

BCR, B-cell receptor; IgM, immunoglobulin M; RAG, recombination activating gene; TdT, terminal deoxynucleotidyl transferase.

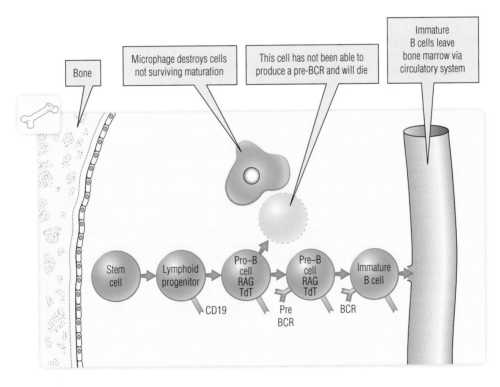

Fig 14.1 In the bone marrow, immature B cells expressing BCRs are produced. *BCR*, B-cell receptor; *RAG*, recombination activation genes; *TdT*, terminal deoxynucleotidyl transferase.

 MCH II

  Cytokine, chemokine, etc.

 Complement (C')

 Signaling molecule

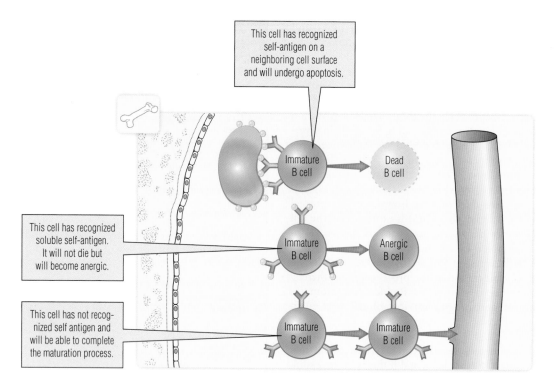

This cell has recognized self-antigen on a neighboring cell surface and will undergo apoptosis.

This cell has recognized soluble self-antigen. It will not die but will become anergic.

This cell has not recognized self antigen and will be able to complete the maturation process.

Immature B cell → Dead B cell

Immature B cell → Anergic B cell

Immature B cell → Immature B cell

Fig 14.2 Negative selection ensures that only immature B cells that do not recognize self antigen are permitted to leave the bone marrow.

At the same time as cells are undergoing the maturational processes described, they are dividing and proliferating. A net result is that high numbers of B cells can be produced. On the other hand, recombination that does *not* result in the successful expression of a pre-BCR or BCR is fatal for cells. This ensures that only B cells with intact BCRs survive the maturation process.

The recombination processes involved in B-cell development that give rise to extensive receptor diversity necessarily generate some antigen receptors that possess self-reactivity. Just by chance, it is likely that some B-cell receptors will recognize some self antigens, and cells that express these receptors will need to either be killed or switched off. This process is referred to as *negative selection*. This selection process results in a pool of immature B cells that do *not* become activated when challenged with self antigen, a condition called *tolerance*. *Self antigen* in this context means macromolecules present in the bone marrow that could be bound by the BCR. These could be either molecules present on the surface of healthy cells or those present in solution in the extracellular matrix.

Self antigens that are abundant on the cell surface and that can extensively cross-link immature BCRs (multivalent antigens) induce apoptosis, leading to an outcome called *clonal deletion*. Immature B cells respond differently to small, soluble proteins that cannot effectively cross-link the immature BCR. When immature B cells are exposed to high doses of such a soluble antigen, responding B cells downregulate expression of IgM and are rendered incapable of becoming activated upon subsequent antigenic challenge, a condition called *anergy*. These B cells are not killed and can in fact be rescued from anergy in some circumstances. B cells that have survived negative selection express increased levels of IgM and begin to express membrane-bound IgD (Fig. 14.2).

IgD is expressed after alternative splicing of heavy chain transcripts (Chapter 6). After B cells progress through this stage, they become mature B cells that express surface IgM and surface IgD. Once the B cell completes the early maturation stages in the bone marrow, it begins to migrate to peripheral lymphoid organs to complete its development. B cells that have fully rearranged Ig genes but have not yet encountered nonself antigen are known as *naive B cells*.

■ THE MATURE B CELL

Additional Tolerance Induction

Because not all self antigens are present in the bone marrow, mechanisms have evolved to ensure that the mature B-cell pool is rendered tolerant to self antigens encountered in the periphery. T-cell help is generally required for the mature B cell to produce antibody. If the mature B cell engages an antigen, and no T cell specific for the antigen responds to provide the necessary signals (Chapters 11 and 16) for the B cell to become fully activated, the cell will undergo clonal deletion or will become anergic. As with immature B cells, the outcome of receptor engagement depends on the antigen encountered. Multivalent antigens generally cause clonal deletion, and univalent antigens induce anergy (Fig. 14.3). However, a population of B cells has evolved to respond specifically to multivalent polysaccharide antigen without T-cell help; these thymus-independent (*T-independent*) B cells are discussed later in this chapter.

 T-cell receptor (TCR)

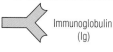 Immunoglobulin (Ig)

 Antigen

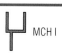 MCH I

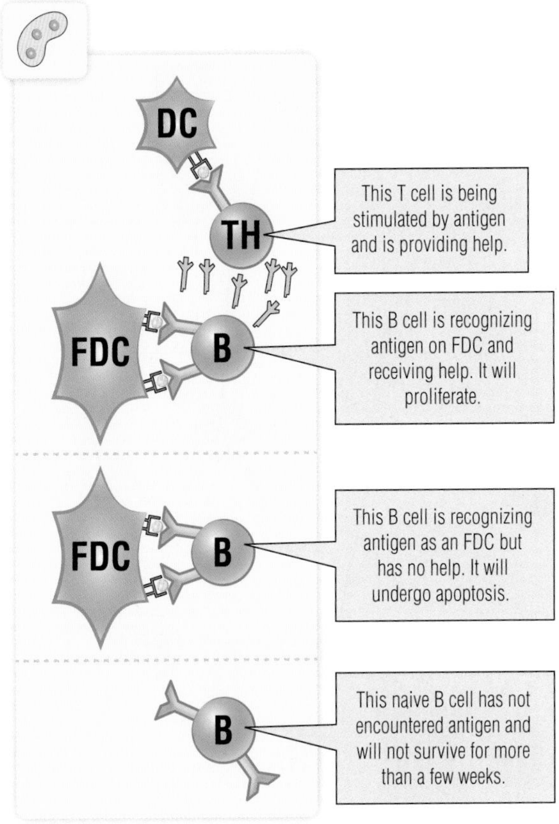
DC
TH
This T cell is being stimulated by antigen and is providing help.
FDC
B
This B cell is recognizing antigen on FDC and receiving help. It will proliferate.
FDC
B
This B cell is recognizing antigen as an FDC but has no help. It will undergo apoptosis.
B
This naive B cell has not encountered antigen and will not survive for more than a few weeks.

Fig 14.3 In a germinal center, a naive B cell has the opportunity to recognize antigen and receive help from a T cell. Only then will it become stimulated and proliferate. *DC,* dendritic cell; *FDC,* follicular dendritic cell; *TH,* T-helper cell.

Activation and Antibody Production

To respond to a specific antigen, B cells usually require T-cell help and presentation of antigen by specialized cells called *follicular dendritic cells* (FDCs). As you read in Chapter 13, follicles in the secondary lymphoid organs provide an environment in which antigen is concentrated and displayed to incoming naive B cells and in which naive B cells, FDCs, and T cells can interact. Each type of secondary lymphoid tissue traps antigen from different sources: the spleen collects blood-borne antigens, antigens in the afferent lymphatic system are trapped in lymph nodes, and mucosa-associated lymphoid tissue (MALT), such as Peyer patches in the gut and tonsils/adenoids in the nasopharynx, acquires antigen from the surrounding mucosal epithelia. After leaving the bone marrow, naive mature B cells continuously recirculate through the blood to follicles in the different secondary lymphoid organs until they encounter their specific antigen. In the absence of its target antigen, the naive B cell traverses this region and eventually reenters the circulation.

FDCs are a specialized type of antigen-presenting cell (APC) found only in lymphoid follicles. They do not express class II major histocompatibility complex (MHC) molecules but instead retain antigen-antibody complexes on their surface attached to Fc receptors or complement receptors. These cells are morphologically similar to other dendritic cells (DCs), with long processes that create networks within the lymphoid follicles, but they may have a different origin from that of the bone marrow–derived MHC class II–expressing DCs described earlier.

As a general rule, naive B cells cannot be activated by antigen alone. A second accessory signal is required to initiate full activation of the B cell (Chapter 16). In the case of protein antigens, the second signal is delivered by an activated T cell with an antigen receptor (T-cell receptor [TCR]) that recognizes the peptide–MHC class II complex displayed by a neighboring APC. Antigens that require this form of B cell–T cell collaboration to initiate an immune response are called *thymus dependent.*

If the B cell encounters its target antigen, antigen engagement by the BCR triggers the B cell to internalize the BCR-antigen complex. Then the antigen is degraded, and in the case of protein antigens, it is processed into peptide–MHC class II complexes, which are subsequently displayed on the cell surface (Chapter 10). Thus B cells can present antigen to T cells, which then reciprocate by providing neighboring B cells with help.

SOMATIC MUTATION AND CLASS SWITCHING IN GERMINAL CENTERS

Driven by antigenic stimulation and the help provided by T cells, activated B cells begin to proliferate rapidly, dividing about once every 6 hours to create a *germinal center,* a lightly stained region within the follicles (see Fig. 13.3A and B) made up of FDCs. During this period, point mutations are introduced at a high rate into the immunoglobulin genes and are not corrected. This unique process is referred to as *somatic hypermutation* and is not permitted to take place without correction in any other cell type. Somatic mutations usually consist of single nucleotide substitutions focused in and around the rearranged variable region exon. Both heavy and light chain variable region exons may be targets of somatic mutation. The introduced mutations may or may not affect how well the BCR binds antigen. Those B cells whose BCRs bind antigen with high affinity (Fig. 14.4) receive survival signals (*positive selection*) from FDCs and germinal center T cells, whereas those that fail to bind antigen soon die by apoptosis. This competition for antigen becomes more important as levels of antigen begin to fall once an infection is brought under control. Positively selected B cells may undergo additional rounds of proliferation, somatic mutation, and antigenic selection. The consequence will be the survival of B cells that produce the highest affinity antibody. The resulting *affinity maturation* is one of the reasons the quality of antibody improves over time. For example, Clinical Box 2.1 shows how antibody levels improve following vaccination. This is in part because more B cells are producing antibody but also largely because the antibody produced increases in affinity over time. Both the quantity of immunoglobulin and the quality of antibody binding (affinity) contribute to the antibody levels.

A second important development that occurs in the germinal center is Ig class switching. Up to this stage in the maturation process, the B cell expresses surface IgM and IgD but secretes only IgM. In many situations it is important for other classes of antibody to be produced. For example, in response to mucosal infection, production of IgA is helpful. T cells are required to provide specific types of help for Ig class switching (Chapters 6 and 16).

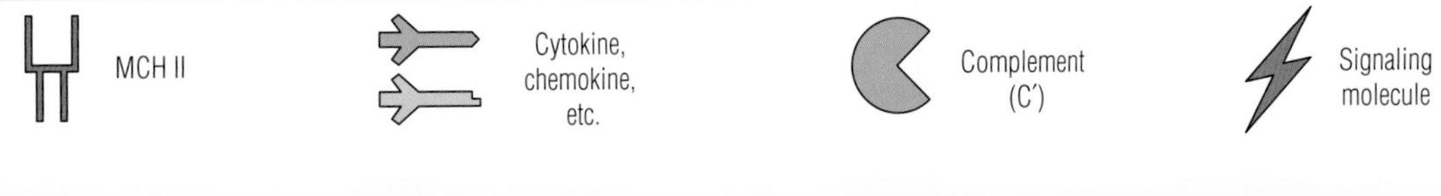
MCH II
Cytokine, chemokine, etc.
Complement (C′)
Signaling molecule

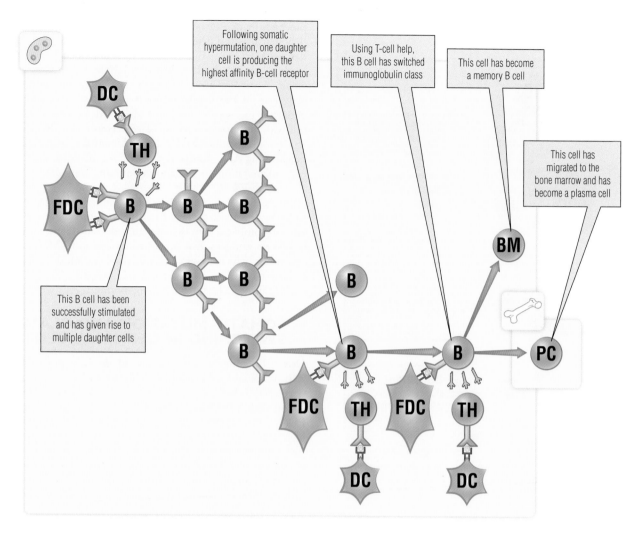

Fig 14.4 Several different fates are possible for developing B cells. They may become class switching or memory B cells (BMs), or they may become plasma cells (PCs). *DC,* dendritic cell; *FDC,* follicular dendritic cell; *TH,* T-helper cell.

At any stage in these maturation processes, B cells may leave the germinal center to terminally differentiate into a plasma cell or become a recirculating memory B cell. Both of these steps require B-cell help. Plasma cells home to the bone marrow where they may secrete large amounts of antibody for a period of at least several weeks.

Memory B cells do not secrete antibody but can be rapidly reactivated upon subsequent antigenic challenge. Look again at Figure 2.4. After the second and particularly the third hepatitis B booster vaccinations, the antibody levels rise rapidly. This is typical of a memory B-cell response.

■ THYMUS-INDEPENDENT ANTIGENS

As described earlier, B cells that respond to polypeptide antigens require two signals to become fully activated: cross-linking with the BCR and help from T cells. However, some antigens are able to activate B cells directly in the absence of T-cell help; hence they are called *thymus-independent* (TI) antigens. Many TI B cells are located in the spleen. TI B cells do not fully develop

until late childhood, which is one reason children are prone to recurrent bacterial infection. TI antigens include repeating polymers, such as bacterial polysaccharides, and certain bacterial cell wall components, such as lipopolysaccharides. These antigens all have multiple repeat motifs and engage several BCRs and in this way overcome the need for a second signal (Fig. 14.5).

TI antigens are often of bacterial origin, and TI responses provide a means to generate an early and specific antibody response against bacterial pathogens that can proliferate quickly and overwhelm the immune system. However, because T cells are not usually mobilized, the antibody repertoire generated during TI responses is limited because T-cell–dependent events that promote affinity maturation, Ig class switching, and B-cell memory are not induced.

TI B cells have two important implications. The first is that it is important to develop vaccines that can induce protection against bacteria that use polysaccharide capsules, such as *Haemophilus* and pneumococcus (*Streptococcus pneumoniae*). These bacteria otherwise cause significant numbers of deaths in

 T-cell receptor (TCR)   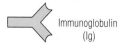 Immunoglobulin (Ig)   Antigen   MCH I

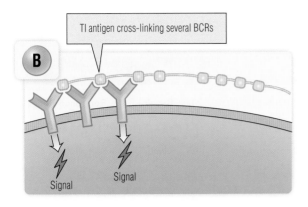

Fig 14.5 T-independent (TI) antigens overcome the need for T-cell help by engaging multiple B-cell receptors (BCRs).

TABLE 14.2 Types of B Cells

	Conventional	T-Independent	B1
Location	Lymph node, spleen, mucosa	Mainly spleen	Peritoneum
Gene rearrangement	Yes	Limited	Limited
Affinity maturation and class switching	Yes	No	No
Spontaneous antibody secretion	No	No	Yes
Antibodies against self antigens	Rare	No	Common

children. However, vaccines based solely on TI antigen polysaccharides do not stimulate T-cell help because they contain no proteins that can be broken down into peptides. Because they do not induce T-cell help, when used as vaccines, polysaccharides induce only low-affinity IgM antibodies with poor immunologic memory. Protein-conjugated polysaccharide vaccines have been developed that have successfully overcome this problem (Chapter 16).

People who have undergone splenectomy are at high risk of invasive infection. As described in Chapter 13, this is partly because these patients have lost a large number of splenic macrophages, which filter the blood. The second reason for the high risk of infection is the loss of TI B cells. This can be overcome by lifelong antibiotics and conjugated polysaccharide vaccines.

▉ B1 B CELLS AND NATURAL ANTIBODIES

B1 cells develop from immature B-cell precursors, but they differ from conventional B cells in several important ways. First, the B1 B cells reside in unusual sites, such as the peritoneum, rather than in conventional lymphoid organs. Second, B1 B cells express different cell surface markers. For example, many, but not all, B1 cells express a surface marker called *CD5* that is not found on conventional B cells.

Unlike conventional B cells, which are constantly being renewed from bone marrow precursors, B1 cells in the adult replenish themselves by continuing division of cells carrying surface IgM (sIgM$^+$) in peripheral tissues, thereby ensuring a persistent B1 population long after their generation has ceased. This property likely contributes to the tendency of B1 cells, particularly the CD5$^+$ cells, to be a frequent source for a relatively common B-cell neoplasm called *chronic lymphocytic leukemia* (Chapter 35).

The B1 cell receptor repertoire is very restricted as a result of preferential use of a few VH genes and limited if any insertional diversity, caused by a lack of TdT expression in these cells. The BCRs expressed on B1 cells are often reactive toward bacterial antigens, such as polysaccharides, and they frequently display polyspecificity—the ability to cross-react with multiple antigens. Hence, B1 cells provide an important protective function against bacterial pathogens early in life until the adult repertoire develops. In this way B1 B cells are similar to TI B cells (Table 14.2).

However, B1 B cells produce antibody without any stimulation from antigen, and the antibodies often cross-react with self antigen. Spontaneously produced, self-reactive antibodies are called *natural antibodies* and may sometimes give rise to autoimmunity, as described further in Chapter 28.

Finally, because B1 B cells only use limited gene rearrangement, do not refine their response over time (by affinity maturation or class switching), and do not develop immunologic memory, they may be viewed as having more in common with the innate immune system than with the adaptive immune system.

 MCH II

 Cytokine, chemokine, etc.

 Complement (C′)

 Signaling molecule

BOX 14.1 Acute Lymphoblastic Leukemia

A 7-year-old girl has a 3-week history of very low energy and weight loss. On examination, she is very pale with lymphadenopathy and some petechiae on her legs. Her physician does a complete blood cell count, which shows low hemoglobin and platelet counts (Table 14.3), which explain the pallor and petechiae, respectively. Her white cell count is raised, and nearly all the white cells are blasts—very immature leukocytes. After looking at the cells, a hematologist thinks they are probably immature lymphocytes and carries out flow cytometry to make sure (Table 14.4). Because they are CD19 positive, flow cytometry is able to show that the abnormal cells are B cells and that they are very immature because they express the enzyme terminal deoxynucleotidyl transferase (TdT). This is very suggestive of a diagnosis of acute lymphoblastic leukemia (ALL). The diagnosis is confirmed by examination of a bone marrow sample.

ALL is the most common childhood cancer in most developed countries, and 80% of children with ALL can be cured. The malignant cells arise from primitive B cells, which probably correspond to pro–B cells (see Fig. 14.1). Although exposure to radiation is a known risk factor for developing ALL, most children with ALL do not appear to have any risk factors operating.

TABLE 14.3 Complete Blood Cell Count

	Test Result	Reference Range
Hemoglobin	8.1 g/dL	11.5-15.5 g/dL
White cell count	23 ×10^6/mL	5-14 ×10^6/mL
Neutrophils	6%	32%-54%
Blasts	93%	0%
Platelet count	36 ×10^6/mL	150-450 ×10^6/mL

TABLE 14.4 Flow Cytometry

CD3	3%
CD4	2%
CD8	1%
CD19	97%
TdT	97%

CD, *cluster of differentiation*; TdT, *terminal deoxynucleotidyl transferase.*

LEARNING POINTS Can You Now…

1. List the different cell types in the B-cell development pathway?
2. Recall the time-dependent changes in cell surface molecules during the B-cell development pathway?
3. Draw the order of rearrangement and expression of immunoglobulin heavy chain and light chain genes during B-cell development?
4. Compare T-dependent and T-independent B-cell activation?
5. Explain antigen-induced tolerance in immature and mature B-cell populations?
6. Describe affinity maturation in terms of B-cell antigen receptor improvement?
7. Describe T-independent B cells and B1 B cells?

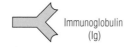 T-cell receptor (TCR)

 Immunoglobulin (Ig)

Antigen

MCH I

T-Cell Development

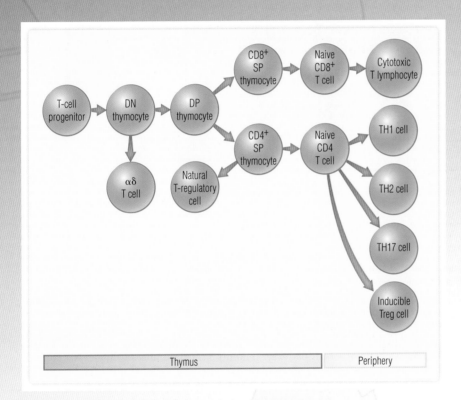

| Thymus | Periphery |

To protect the host from infection, the T-cell population must contain a diverse array of antigen-specific receptors. Each individual T cell expresses a unique receptor capable of recognizing foreign peptide antigen displayed by a self major histocompatibility complex (MHC) molecule. The main topic for this chapter, as shown in the above figure, is how a diverse population of mature T lymphocytes with different antigenic specificities is generated to accomplish several different protective functions for the host.

T lymphocytes are generated in the thymus. T-cell development in the thymus is a multistep process with several built-in checkpoints to ensure that the appropriate differentiation has taken place. As a result of selection, only a small proportion of progenitor T cells, known as *thymocytes,* actually exits the thymus to the periphery as mature T cells; most (>98%) die during the selection processes that establish the T-lymphocyte repertoire.

These thymic selection processes enable the host to develop a T-cell repertoire that is self-tolerant but self-restricted (Chapter 8). This means that the mature T cells that are selected to develop are capable of recognizing nonself antigenic peptides bound to self MHC molecules, but in general will not recognize self peptides.

Different subsets of mature T cells carry out the functions of cell-mediated immunity, including killing virally infected cells and tumor cells (CD8+ T cells) and providing help for and regulating components of the immune system (CD4+ T cells).

■ THE THYMUS

The architecture of the thymus was described in Chapter 13. You should recall that the thymus is organized into three major areas: the subcapsular zone, the cortex, and the medulla (Fig. 15.1).

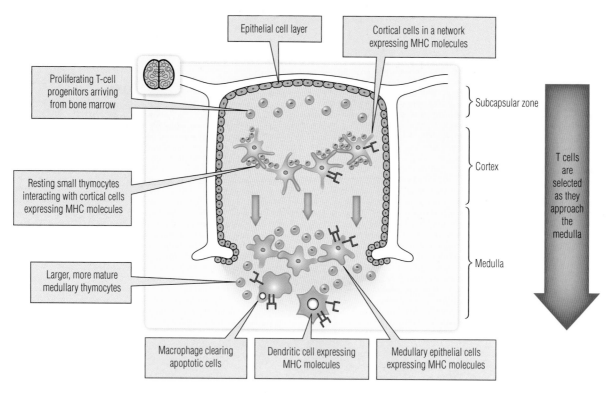

Fig 15.1 Simplified schematic of thymic organization. *MHC,* major histocompatibility complex.

Different populations of stromal cells and thymocytes are found in each of these structurally and functionally distinct regions. The critical role of the thymus in T-cell development is illustrated by the observation that individuals who never develop a thymus (complete Di George syndrome) have minimal numbers of mature peripheral T cells (Box 15.1). Despite the critical nature of the fetal thymus in establishing a T-cell population, after birth the thymus is no longer necessary to maintain mature antigen-specific T cells. After birth, when the maintenance of the pool of peripheral T cells is accomplished by mature T-cell division under the influence of interleukin 7 (IL-7), thymectomy has little impact on T-cell responses in humans.

Overview of the Transition From Thymocyte to Mature T Cell

Thymocyte development takes place over several stages in separate parts of the thymus (Fig. 15-2). An overview of these stages is given here before proceeding to a more detailed discussion.

Upon migrating to the thymus and locating in the subcapsular zone, bone marrow–derived thymocytes do not express, and are said to be *negative for,* the CD4 and CD8 costimulatory molecules characteristic of T cells. They are referred to as *double-negative* (DN) cells (see Fig. 15.2). At this stage, the T-cell receptor (TCR) genes are in the germline (unrearranged) configuration.

As shown in Figure 15.2, the DN thymocyte subpopulation undergoes several important differentiation events. The DN cells become committed to the T-cell lineage as TCR gene rearrangements begin to occur (described later). An important choice

made at this stage is commitment to either the αβ or γδ T-cell lineage. Notably, both these T-cell lineages derive from a common progenitor cell, with commitment to one lineage or the other being a competitive process based on which TCR genes productively rearrange first (compare this with the process of immunoglobulin [Ig] light chain gene expression in B cells; Chapter 14). The majority of thymocytes commit to the αβ TCR pathway, and only a small number of thymocytes commit to the γδ pathway. Because γδ T cells are not MHC restricted, they are not subject to the other thymic developmental processes and leave the thymus at this stage.

The next major step in the T-cell development pathway is the *double-positive* (DP) stage. DP cells express both CD4 and CD8, and such cells are not found outside the thymic cortex. The DP stage is the point at which cells are positively selected (retained) if they express a TCR that can recognize self MHC. At the next step in the T-cell development pathway, the cells migrate to the thymic medulla, where they are negatively selected (deleted) if they express receptors that recognize self peptide antigens with self MHC molecules with high affinity. At this point, depending on whether the TCR interacts appropriately with a class I or class II MHC molecule, the cells become *single positive* (SP): either CD4⁻ CD8⁺ or CD4⁺ CD8⁻. This is known as *lineage commitment.* Some CD4⁺ cells commit to develop into natural T-regulatory cells (nTregs) at this stage.

Order of T-Cell Receptor Gene Rearrangements

Rearrangement of TCR genes begins at the DN stage. The β, γ, and δ genes all attempt to rearrange at this stage. This involves activation of recombination activating genes (RAGs) and

 T-cell receptor (TCR)

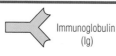 Immunoglobulin (Ig)

 Antigen

 MCH I

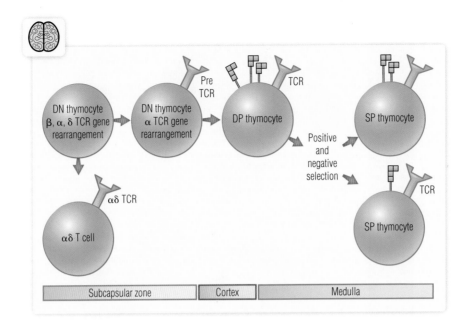

Fig 15.2 Overview of the different pathways of thymocyte maturation. *DN,* double negative; *DP,* double positive; *SP,* single positive; *TCR,* T-cell receptor.

terminal deoxynucleotidyl transferase (TdT), as described in Chapter 7, in addition to multiple gene rearrangements. If a functional γδ receptor is produced, a γδ TCR-expressing T cell results. Those cells with γδ TCRs establish the γδ lineage.

However, the majority of DN cells express a TCR β-chain. Once a functional TCR β-chain is expressed at the cell surface, it complexes with an invariant pre-T α-chain and the CD3 molecule (Chapters 7 and 11) to form a pre-TCR complex. Expression of the pre-TCR allows signal transduction (Chapter 11), and signals from the pre-TCR halt further β-chain rearrangements and allow proliferation of the DP T cells. Proliferation promotes TCR α-chain rearrangement after recombinase expression. Therefore similar to the role of the pre–B-cell receptor ([BCR]; Chapter 14), expression of the pre-TCR is a critical step in the pathway to assembly of an αβ TCR and formation of the αβ T-cell population.

Major Histocompatibility Complex Self Peptide Expression in the Thymus

During their development, immature T cells encounter various populations of cells that express MHC and self peptide. Immature T cells first encounter cortical thymic epithelia, which are involved in positive selection. As the immature T cells migrate into the medulla, they encounter a mixture of dendritic cells, epithelial cells, and macrophages, which are involved in negative selection. All these populations of cells are actively presenting antigenic peptide to the immature T cells.

In the absence of infection, antigen-presenting cells (APCs) process and present self peptide through the pathways described in Chapter 10. This means that normal cytoplasmic proteins are digested by proteasomes and are presented on MHC class I. On the other hand, extracellular proteins are digested in endosomes and are presented on MHC class II.

The cells in the thymic medulla have evolved to express proteins typically expressed in other organs. For example, the only cells normally considered capable of secreting insulin are β-cells of the pancreatic islets. However, thymic medullary cells also secrete some insulin, which is processed into peptides that are presented on MHC class II. A special transcription factor, the autoimmune regulator *AIRE,* enables the thymic medullary cells to express proteins normally only expressed in other organs. *AIRE* gene mutations lead to multiple autoimmune problems, as in the autoimmune polyendocrinopathy candidiasis ectodermal dysplasia (APECED) syndrome (Box 15.2).

Positive Selection: Establishment of Self-Restriction

To continue along the developmental process, the DP cell must first make a successful interaction with MHC molecules on thymic cortical epithelial cells. Most DP cells die in the cortex through apoptosis because they lack TCRs capable of interacting appropriately with self MHC. Only DP cells that have TCRs that recognize self MHC with medium affinity will survive. These cells have been positively selected for being self MHC restricted.

Negative Selection: Establishment of Central Self-Tolerance

The pool of cells generated by positive selection in the thymus is self MHC restricted, but it also includes some self-reactive cells, which could recognize self peptide plus MHC. These self-reactive cells must be eliminated or the host risks autoimmune disease. Elimination of self-reactive cells involves a process called *negative selection* (Fig. 15.3).

This takes place in the thymic medulla, where the developing DP T cells are exposed to a range of peptides that present proteins expressed throughout the body. During negative selection, DP cells that are very strongly reactive (high affinity) with

 MCH II   Cytokine, chemokine, etc.    Complement (C′)    Signaling molecule

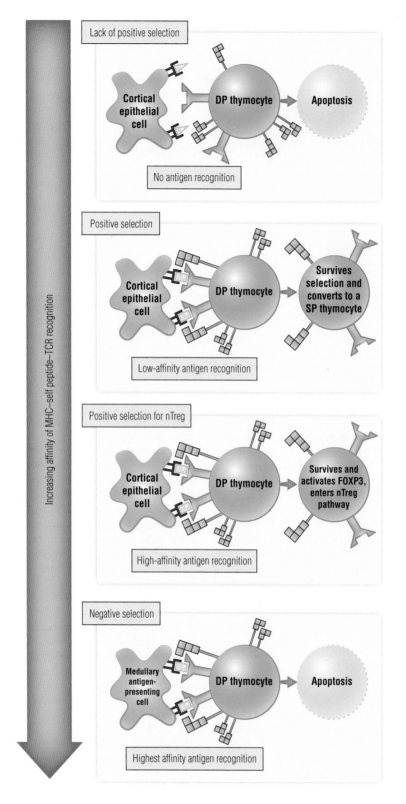

Fig 15.3 The different possible outcomes when a double-positive (DP) thymocyte interacts with thymic antigen-presenting cells. The affinity of the recognition of the major histocompatibility complex (MHC)–self peptide complex by T-cell receptor (TCR) determines the outcome. *DP*, double positive; *nTreg*, natural T-regulatory cell; *SP*, single positive.

 T-cell receptor (TCR)

 Immunoglobulin (Ig)

Antigen

MCH I

self peptides are eliminated, and a state of self-tolerance is established.

The next step depends on whether the DP cell recognizes self antigen presented on MHC class I or class II molecules. Remember that the CD8 molecule recognizes MHC class I and CD4 recognizes MHC class II. DP cells that recognize cell self antigen on MHC class I stop expressing CD4 and become single-positive (SP) CD8⁺ cells. In contrast, DP cells that recognize cell self antigen on MHC class II stop expressing CD8 and become SP CD4⁺ cells.

Within the SP CD4⁺ cells, the 10% of cells with the highest affinity for MHC class II self antigen activate a transcription factor called FOXP3, which commits these cells to a different differentiation pathway, and they eventually mature as natural regulatory cells.

Negative selection is mediated by signal transduction through the TCR, which leads to induction of apoptosis. Apoptotic cells are disposed of by thymic macrophages.

It has been estimated that two-thirds of the cells that survive positive selection in the cortex are subsequently deleted by negative selection in the medulla. Consequently, a very small number of the original thymocytes emerge into the periphery as mature, but still antigen-naive, T cells. The term *naive* refers to the fact that these cells have not yet encountered the foreign, nonself antigen that specifically "fits" their TCR.

T-Cell Receptor Signaling in Positive and Negative Selection

The same molecular interaction—that is, TCR binding to the MHC–peptide antigen complex) mediates both positive and negative selection (see Fig. 15.3).

How can very different outcomes result from the same type of receptor-ligand interaction? It has been suggested that different affinities of interaction between TCRs and MHC-peptide complexes generate different intracellular signals. These signals might be quantitatively or qualitatively different. Investigations are underway to determine the nature of these signals and to establish an answer to this paradox. Currently, one simplified interpretation of the available data would be that high-affinity interactions between the TCR and the appropriate MHC molecule expressed on an appropriate thymic cell lead to negative selection (deletion) of the cell that expresses that TCR, whereas lower-affinity interactions, but not too low—perhaps best described as "intermediate affinity" interactions—between the TCR and the MHC molecule lead to positive selection and continued maturation. Note that a similar phenomenon is seen during B-cell development. B cells that recognize an abundant membrane self antigen during development in the bone marrow also undergo apoptosis in an analogous negative selection process.

■ THE PERIPHERY: NAIVE T-CELL ACTIVATION BY ANTIGEN

The mature T cells that leave the thymus have not yet encountered the antigen that they have specificity for, sometimes referred to as their *cognate antigen*. At this stage, they are said to be *naive mature T cells*. These cells recirculate from the bloodstream to the central lymphoid organs (eg, spleen, lymph nodes, Peyer patches) for years before they die or encounter antigen.

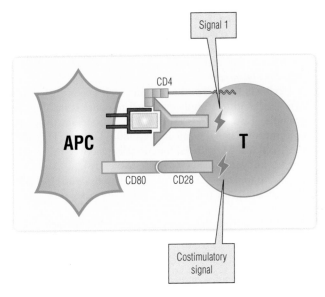

Fig 15.4 Activation of naive T cells. In this example, a CD4⁺ T cell is being activated by an antigen-presenting cell (APC) presenting antigen on major histocompatibility complex class I.

Antigen is usually encountered on a professional APC in a secondary lymphoid organ (Chapter 13). If the TCR recognizes antigen displayed on MHC molecules (first signal) and also receives a second costimulatory signal (Chapter 16), the T cell is activated (Fig. 15.4; Chapter 11). The activated cells then proliferate and undergo clonal expansion and differentiation into effector cells, most of which are short lived. These effector cells are often said to be *antigen primed*, and this process is referred to as *priming the T cells*. These primed *effector cells* undergo several changes, including expression of new cell surface molecules such as CD154 (CD40 ligand) and various adhesion molecules (Chapters 13 and 16). The effector T cells can move into peripheral tissues and other organs to handle pathogen infection directly, or they can migrate to germinal centers to provide help, such as to activate B cells with specificity for the same antigen to secrete antibody.

The end result is a vigorous T-cell response and destruction of the pathogen. Most of the activated T cells then die by apoptosis, restoring homeostasis to the T-cell pool. A few effector cells mature into memory T cells, which can respond faster and more effectively upon reencountering antigen (Chapter 17).

Peripheral T-Cell Tolerance

As described earlier, negative selection is used to help generate a self-tolerant, mature T-cell population. Negative selection taking place in the thymus is referred to as inducing *central tolerance*. However, because not all self antigens are encountered in the thymus, some self-reactive cells may "escape" from the thymus and appear in the periphery. Several mechanisms act in the periphery to ensure that potentially self-reactive T-cell clones that have escaped there are controlled and rendered harmless. For example:

1. Antigen is hidden in immune-privileged sites, such as the brain, eye, or testes.

 MCH II

  Cytokine, chemokine, etc.

 Complement (C′)

 Signaling molecule

2. Paradoxically, if a T cell is specific for a common peripheral antigen and is repeatedly stimulated by encountering high levels of this antigen, the T cell will undergo apoptosis and be deleted. This mechanism is known as *deletion-induced* or *high zone tolerance.*

3. A T cell will not respond to an antigen if one of the components required to stimulate a T-cell response is missing. For example, if no MHC is expressed in the relevant tissue or a costimulatory signal is missing (CD80/CD28; see Fig. 15.3), the T cell will be rendered functionally inactive. This mechanism is known as *clonal anergy* (Chapter 18).

4. Finally, populations of regulatory T cells with specificity for self antigen "police" the periphery and prevent any self-reactivity.

These mechanisms that take place outside the thymus are said to induce *peripheral tolerance* and are discussed in detail in Chapter 18.

Mature T-Cell Responses and Functions

After the naive mature T cell has encountered its cognate MHC-antigen complex and has received a costimulatory signal from a professional APC, it proliferates and differentiates into an effector cell. The CD8+ and CD4+ T-cell subsets can then develop with different effector functions.

By virtue of the different specificities of CD4+ and CD8+ effector T cells, the immune response can monitor extracellular pathogens such as bacteria and intracellular pathogens such as viruses, respectively. CD4+ T cells monitor MHC class II molecules, which display peptides generated in endosomes (eg, from extracellular pathogens taken up by phagocytosis), and CD8+ T cells monitor MHC class I molecules, which display peptides generated in the cytoplasm (eg, from intracellular pathogens such as viruses replicating in the cytoplasm).

CD4+ T Cells

CD4+ T cells recognize antigen displayed on MHC class II molecules. As is discussed in more detail in Chapter 16, CD4+ T cells may differentiate into one of a series of subsets. These include helper subsets, which promote specific types of T-helper (TH) response (by TH1, TH2, and TH17) and Tregs. Which pathway a naive T cell follows depends on the environment in which it is primed and on any danger signals produced by the innate immune system. For example, if a danger signal is present, such as IL-12 in response to an infection, a responding T cell is likely to develop into a TH1 cell. nTregs develop as a result of high-affinity interactions between the TCR and MHC class II self peptide—but not high enough to cause negative selection. A second set of Tregs are *inducible Tregs* (iTregs). These are derived from naive CD4+ T cells in the appropriate environment. Tregs are discussed fully in Chapter 18.

CD8+ T Cells: Cytotoxic T Lymphocytes

Naive CD8+ T cells emerge from the thymus. They require further activation and differentiation to become the effector T cells that recognize virally infected target cells and tumor cells (see Box 15.3). CD8+ T cells recognize antigen displayed on MHC class I molecules. Because MHC class I molecules are found on essentially all nucleated cells of the body, CD8+ T cells can monitor all cells for signs of infection. CD8+ T cells are activated to become effector T cells either by encountering antigen on a professional APC and receiving activation signals from both MHC class I and costimulatory molecules (eg, CD80) or by encountering antigen on a non-APC target cell and receiving a "second signal" from cytokines released by CD4+ T-helper cells.

CD8+ T cells use a variety of mechanisms to suppress intracellular infection and induce apoptosis in infected cells.

The γδ T-Cell Subset

As described earlier in this chapter, γδ TCR–expressing T cells are a minor population (<5%) of all T cells and represent a separate lineage from the αβ T cell. The γδ TCR recognizes antigen very differently from the γδ TCR in that it recognizes certain peptide and nonpeptide antigens without processing and in the absence of MHC class I or II molecules.

The γδ T cell acts as a part of the first line of defense, recognizing microbial invaders in the skin and gut mucosa predominantly. They appear to recognize commonly occurring microbial pathogens.

Their unique ability to recognize some common microbial protein and nonprotein antigens, such as bacterial cell wall phospholipids, without processing and presentation distinguishes them from αβ T cells, which enables them to have a unique protective role in the first line of defense against invading microbes.

 T-cell receptor (TCR)

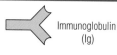 Immunoglobulin (Ig)

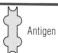 Antigen

 MCH I

BOX 15.1 Partial Di George Syndrome

As a neonatologist, you are called to the pediatric surgical unit to see an infant who has been diagnosed as having a fistula between the esophagus and trachea and who is having a series of convulsions due to low calcium levels. An incidental finding is the subtly unusual facial appearance and, on chest radiography, it has been noted that the thymus is absent. This combination is seen in Di George syndrome, where structures derived from the third and fourth pharyngeal pouches do not develop, including the thymus and parathyroid glands, which control blood calcium levels. Fortunately, the infant does not have any cardiac defects, the other major anomaly associated with Di George syndrome. Further testing shows part of chromosome 22 has been deleted, confirming the diagnosis.

This infant continues to develop fairly normally, although she is observed to have a decreased number of CD3$^+$ T cells (Fig. 15.5). However, her immunoglobulin levels are normal. She handles normal childhood infections well, and she is not provided any special immunologic treatment. By early adulthood, she leads a normal life (Fig. 15.6).

Children with *partial Di George syndrome* tend to develop fairly normally, as in our example, provided they do not have other associated problems such as heart defects. However, patients with *complete Di George syndrome* suffer from opportunistic infections, such as from fungi and viruses, in much the same way as do those with severe combined immunodeficiency disease (SCID; Chapter 32).

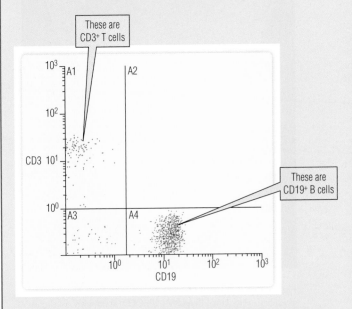

Fig 15.5 Flow cytometric analysis of lymphocytes from a female infant with Di George syndrome. This infant survived despite low T-cell numbers. (Courtesy John Hewitt, Manchester Royal Infirmary, United Kingdom.)

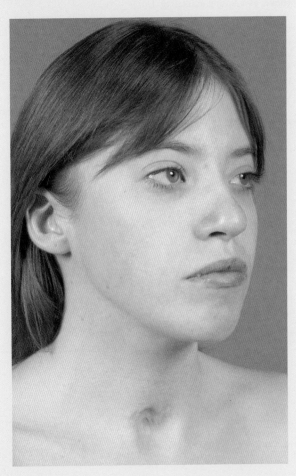

Fig 15.6 A patient with Di George syndrome showing the subtle "elfin-like" appearance of individuals with this syndrome. The scar is from surgery on the trachea. (Courtesy Manchester Royal Infirmary, United Kingdom.)

MCH II   Cytokine, chemokine, etc.   Complement (C′)   Signaling molecule

BOX 15.2 Autoimmune Polyendocrinopathy Candidiasis Ectodermal Dystrophy (APECED)

A 4-year-old boy has become unwell and experiences diarrhea, weight loss, low blood pressure, and difficulties at preschool. He is diagnosed with celiac disease (Chapter 28), but even after he goes on a gluten-free diet, he does not improve. Subsequently, his doctors note that he has adrenal failure and hypothyroidism, and they also note that he has *Candida* infection of the mouth. His brother also has thyroid disease. These features are suggestive of autoimmune polyendocrinopathy candidiasis ectodermal dystrophy (APECED) syndrome. He has genetic testing, and homozygous mutations in the *AIRE* gene are found, which confirms APECED. The hypothyroidism and adrenal failure are treated with hormone replacement, and his *Candida* infection is treated. As a final complication, our patient develops alopecia totalis as a young adult (Fig. 15.7).

APECED is caused by mutations in the *AIRE* gene. As a consequence, thymic cells are unable to express proteins that represent organs such as the thyroid. Because of this defect, thymocytes that recognize peptides derived from these proteins are not deleted, which allows autoreactive T cells to leave the thyroid and cause autoimmune disease. The reason for the *Candida* infection is explained in Chapter 16.

APECED is a rare cause of autoimmune disease. However, it does illustrate the consequences of failure of central tolerance.

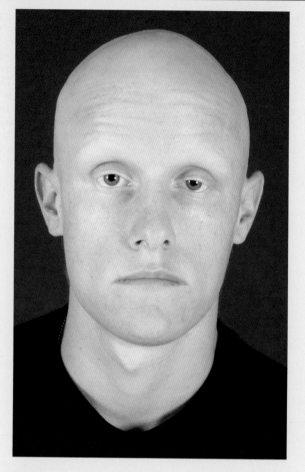

Fig 15.7 Patient with autoimmune polyendocrinopathy candidiasis ectodermal dysplasia (APECED) syndrome. As a result of autoimmunity, he has celiac disease, thyroid disease, adrenal disease, and alopecia totalis.

 T-cell receptor (TCR) Immunoglobulin (Ig)   Antigen MCH I

BOX 15.3 Acute Epstein-Barr Virus Infection

Most people have been infected with Epstein-Barr virus (EBV). In the developing world infection takes place in early childhood, but it is usually asymptomatic. In the developed world, infection is usually delayed until adulthood; 70% of people who become infected develop infectious mononucleosis (IM), also known as *glandular fever*. Symptoms of IM include a sore throat, malaise, lymphadenopathy, and possibly an enlarged spleen. EBV infects its target cell, the B cell, for life, and thus it establishes a latent infection. Infected B cells proliferate, although very little free virus is produced. EBV increases are associated with malignancy: infection leads to a fivefold increase in the risk of B-cell lymphoma, a complication discussed in Chapter 35. EBV also increases the risk of autoimmunity; for example, it doubles the risk of multiple sclerosis.

From the point of view of the host response, acute EBV is characterized by a massive increase in the number of CD8+ T cells in the peripheral blood. The increase appears to be of EBV antigen–specific T cells (Fig. 15.8). It has been suggested that the enormous expansion of T cells during acute EBV infection may be a result of the expansion of a few dominant clones of CD8+ T cells with specificity for EBV antigens—a so-called *oligoclonal expansion*.

The original EBV-specific CD8+ T cells are generated in the thymus through random T-cell receptor (TCR) gene rearrangement and lineage commitment to the CD8+ cell lineage.

A few EBV-specific CD8+ T cells are clonally expanded on contact with EBV antigens in the periphery. Help from CD4+ T cells is required at this stage. When these CD8+ T cells mature, they become EBV-specific cytotoxic T lymphocytes (CTLs). However, there is also an increase in the number of T cells without the appropriate TCR, which cannot recognize EBV. These bystander cells are increased in number because of the secretion of growth factors by the immune system during acute EBV. CD4+ T cells respond to acute EBV infection and produce high levels of cytokines such as interleukin 6 (IL-6), interferon (IFN) γ, and tumor necrosis factor (TNF). These cytokines contribute to the fever and fatigue observed in these patients.

An antibody response, mostly immunoglobulin M (IgM), is also mounted during acute EBV. After a few months, Ig class switching takes place, and most of the antibodies against EBV become IgG. The antibody response is not as useful as the CTL response in limiting this infection. However, the combination of antibody and CD8+ CTLs reduces but does not eliminate the infection. This infection is a good example of how the immune system may not always be able to accomplish "sterilizing immunity" but sometimes has to settle for limiting infection. The CTL and antibody responses to EBV must be maintained for the rest of the infected individual's life. This also requires "help" from CD4+ T cells—the subject of Chapter 16.

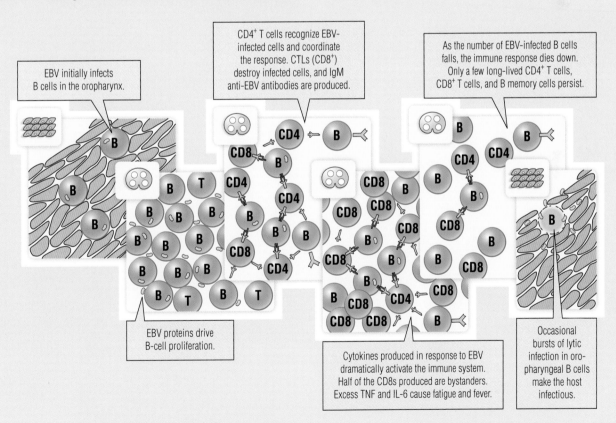

Fig 15.8 Infection with Epstein-Barr virus (EBV) and immune responses. *CTL,* cytotoxic T lymphocyte; *IL,* interleukin; *TNF,* tumor necrosis factor.

 MCH II

 Cytokine, chemokine, etc.

Complement (C')

 Signaling molecule

LEARNING POINTS Can You Now ...

1. Recall the role of the thymus in establishing the T-cell repertoire?
2. Draw the major steps in the pathway of T-cell development and indicate the cell surface molecules expressed at different stages?
3. Describe special features of antigen presentation in the thymus?
4. Compare positive and negative selection?
5. Draw the events involved in naive T-cell activation?
6. Recall the mechanisms used to generate central and peripheral tolerance in T cells?
7. List the functional properties of different T-cell subsets?
8. Compare and contrast the roles of $\gamma\delta$ and $\alpha\beta$ T cells?

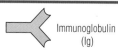 T-cell receptor (TCR)

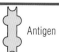 Immunoglobulin (Ig)

 Antigen

MCH I

T-Cell Interactions and
T-Cell Help

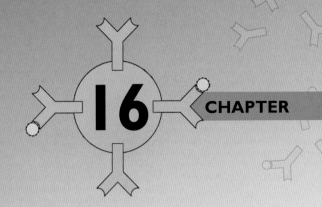

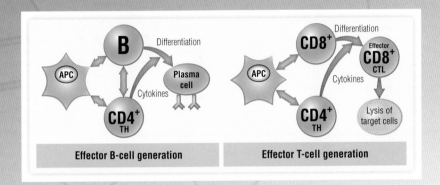

Effector B-cell generation   **Effector T-cell generation**

Some of the basic concepts of cell-cell interaction and cooperation in immune responses were introduced in Chapter 2. Chapters 7 and 8 explained how T-cell receptors (TCRs) recognize antigen only when it is presented by major histocompatibility complex (MHC) molecules on antigen-presenting cells (APCs), an example of the requirement for cell-cell interaction in generating an immune response. In addition, the need for costimulatory signals provided by interaction with other cells for the full activation of B and T lymphocytes was introduced as a concept in Chapter 11 and was discussed further in Chapter 15. At this point, it is appropriate to bring these concepts together and, as illustrated in the above figure, to explain the critical role of cell-cell interaction in generating the signals required to produce effector B cells (plasma cells) and effector T cells (T-helper cells and cytotoxic T lymphocytes [CTLs]). This chapter also discusses how specific immune responses are tailored to combat different types of pathogens.

■ GENERATION OF STIMULATED, OR PRIMED, B AND T CELLS

Foreign soluble antigen produced by pathogens in tissues passes through lymphatics to lymphoid organs, such as the spleen and lymph nodes (Chapter 13). Antigen is also collected at sites of infection and is brought to secondary lymphoid organs by dendritic cells (DCs). This process brings B and T cells into proximity with soluble antigen and APCs bearing foreign antigen and stops their migration. B cells with a B-cell receptor (BCR) specific for available antigen then takes up the antigen via

receptor-mediated endocytosis. Antigen processing takes place with the eventual display of antigenic peptides on the B-cell surface in association with MHC class II molecules (Chapter 10; Fig. 16.1).

In this regard, B cells can function as APCs for T cells, which constantly scan for APCs that display appropriate MHC–antigenic peptide complexes; when they are detected, a cell-cell interaction takes place between the T cell and the APC. Contact with an MHC–foreign peptide antigen complex results in signaling through the TCR (Chapter 11) that, in addition to activating biochemical pathways in the cell, strengthens the adhesive bond between the cells by inducing expression of cell adhesion molecules (CAMs). Some of the most important receptor-ligand pairs involved in the T cell–APC interaction are illustrated in Figure 16.2.

After antigen recognition, a redistribution of molecules occurs in the membranes of the respective cells. The cell's cytoskeleton proteins are actively involved in redistribution of transmembrane proteins in the lipid bilayer of the cell surface membrane so that receptor-ligand pairs migrate into the area of close contact between the cells to form the immunologic synapse. Among the molecules that form the synapse are those shown in Figures 16.2 and 16.3—for example, TCR, CD4 or CD8, lymphocyte function–associated antigen 1 (LFA-1), CD28, CD154 on the T cell and MHC, intercellular adhesion molecule 1 (ICAM-1), CD80, and CD40 on the APC.

At this point, we have reached the stage where activated B and T cells specific for the same antigen are present in the same zone of a lymph node.

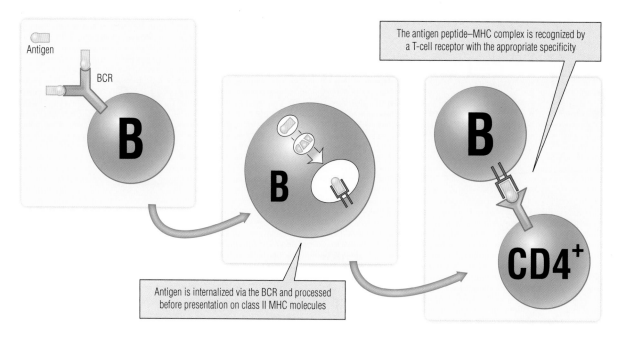

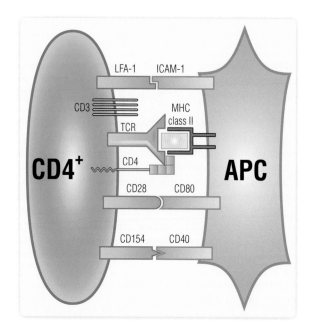

Fig 16.1 B-cell presentation of antigen to T-helper cells. *BCR*, B-cell receptor; *MHC*, major histocompatibility complex.

Fig 16.2 The major cell-surface molecules involved in the interaction of T cells with antigen-presenting cells (APCs). *ICAM-1*, intercellular adhesion molecule 1; *LFA-1*, leukocyte function–associated antigen 1; *MHC*, major histocompatibility complex; *TCR*, T-cell receptor.

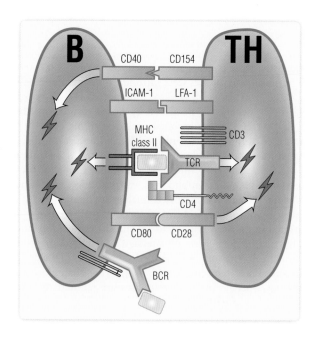

Fig 16.3 Formation of a B cell–T cell conjugate. *BCR*, B-cell receptor; *ICAM-1*, intercellular adhesion molecule 1; *LFA-1*, leukocyte function–associated antigen 1; *MHC*, major histocompatibility complex; *TH*, T-helper cell; *TCR*, T-cell receptor.

 T-cell receptor (TCR)   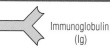 Immunoglobulin (Ig)   Antigen   MCH I

GENERATION OF EFFECTOR CELLS

The immune system adapts its responses for different types of infection. For example, although immunoglobulin G (IgG) is produced in response to many different types of infection, IgE is most appropriate for combating worm infections. T-helper (TH) cells release cytokines, which drive the immune response in one direction or another in response to infection. In this example, TH1 cells promote production of IgG, whereas TH2 cells promote IgE.

CD4+ T-Helper Interaction With B Cells

B cells that express MHC class II antigenic peptide complexes can be recognized by CD4+ TH cells and a B cell–T cell conjugate (see Fig. 16.3). Next, a release of cytokines from the T cell and delivery of costimulatory signals from membrane-bound receptor-ligand pairs occurs. These signals, plus signals from the BCR, cause some B cells to differentiate into plasma cells that secrete IgM (a primary response).

As discussed previously, some of the activated B cells do not differentiate into plasma cells but instead initiate formation of a germinal center in the lymphoid follicles (see Fig. 14.4). In the germinal center, B cells receive help, which enables two important processes to take place. First, the germinal center B cells are subject to rapid somatic mutation in their variable region gene segments, and they undergo selection to retain those cells that have a higher-affinity immunoglobulin (affinity maturation; Chapter 14). The second process that takes place in the germinal center is Ig class switching. As a result of class switching, the μ heavy chain is no longer transcribed and is replaced by the γ, ε, or α heavy chain to produce IgG, IgE, or IgA, respectively.

In the germinal center, a TH cell first recognizes antigen presented by an antigen-presenting cell. Two pairs of costimulatory molecules are next expressed, CD28/CD80 and CD40/CD154. Formation of these pairs of molecules stimulates differentiation in both the T cell and the B cells. A mutation in the human gene that encodes CD154 causes the X-linked hyper-IgM syndrome (see Box 16.2). This disease demonstrates the critical role of the CD40-CD154 interaction in the response to T-dependent antigens.

When B cells switch immunoglobulin class in the presence of TH1 cells, they switch to IgG production. This class switch is mediated by the TH1 cytokine interferon gamma (IFN-γ). However, if the immune system is responding to worm or arthropod infection, interleukin 4 (IL-4) is produced by TH2 cells. This stimulates class switching to IgE. As discussed in Chapter 22, IgE has a special role in helping clear these infections. In contrast, in the mucosal immune system, B cells class switch to produce IgA. This is driven by a different cytokine, transforming growth factor beta (TGF-β), which is secreted by dendritic cells (Fig. 16.4).

A few of the activated germinal center B cells become long-lived quiescent memory B cells, as described in Chapter 17. Similarly, some of the activated T cells also become memory T cells. Subsequent encounter with antigen by these memory cells leads to a more rapid and more effective secondary, tertiary, or subsequent immune response.

CD4+ T-Helper Interaction With CD8+ T Cells

CD8+ CTLs kill cells infected with intracellular pathogens, usually viruses. CTLs can also kill tumor cells. CD8+ T cells require activation signals before they can differentiate into effector CTLs with the full range of cytotoxic granule proteins, perforin, and other molecules required to kill a target cell by inducing apoptosis (Chapter 22). The required activation signals are recognition of antigen (ie, MHC–antigenic peptide complexes) and costimulatory signals from antigen-specific CD4+ TH cells. This is another example of the requirement for cell-cell interaction to generate an immune response, in this case, a cell-mediated immune response. As shown in Figure 16.5, CD4+ TH cells recognize viral antigen displayed on APCs; activation of the CD4+ TH cell causes release of IL-2, which stimulates viral antigen-specific CD8+ T cells. TCR recognition of viral antigen, plus a second signal via the IL-2 receptor (IL-2R; see Fig. 16.5), stimulates differentiation of the CD8+ T cell into an effector CTL, capable of cell killing upon encountering a virally infected target cell. For the most effective killing, CTLs need to be stimulated with IFN-γ secreted by a TH1 cell (see below).

PROVIDING THE MOST APPROPRIATE IMMUNE RESPONSE FOR A GIVEN PATHOGEN

The immune system makes different types of response to different pathogens. Three different T-helper cell types—TH1, TH2, and TH17—coordinate responses to different types of pathogens through their interaction with other cell types. These are summarized in Table 16-1 and Figure 16.6.

Some of the simplest types of pathogen are those that live in the extracellular space. Examples of these include many different types of fungi and bacteria. The fungus *Candida albicans* is a well-studied example of an extracellular pathogen. Extracellular pathogens such as *Candida* are first recognized by innate immune system cells using their pattern recognition molecules. These cells, including dendritic cells, secrete the cytokine IL-23, which stimulates the development of the TH17 subset of T-helper cells. Thus CD4+ T cells able to recognize antigen from *Candida* costimulated with IL-23 will develop into TH17 cells.

TH17 cells secrete IL-17, which attracts neutrophils to the site of infection. Neutrophils kill extracellular pathogens such as *Candida* either through phagocytosis or through extracellular "traps" (Chapter 21). IL-17 also stimulates epithelial cells to secrete antimicrobial peptides, which help kill the pathogens.

The transcription factor RORγt is responsible for IL-17 secretion. In TH17 cells, the genes for RORγt and IL-17 are epigenetically modified to enhance transcription. These modifications are retained in individual cells and are passed on to daughter cells. This ensures immunologic memory is specific both for the *Candida* antigen and the TH17 response. Thus an important role for TH17 cells is to rapidly activate the appropriate mechanisms to kill the fungi when *Candida* invades again.

Many organisms have evolved to live inside cells. Intracellular pathogens include mycobacteria, which have evolved to live inside phagosomes, and all viruses that need to live inside the cytoplasm to survive. Note that for part of their life cycle,

 MCH II Cytokine, chemokine, etc.   Complement (C') Signaling molecule

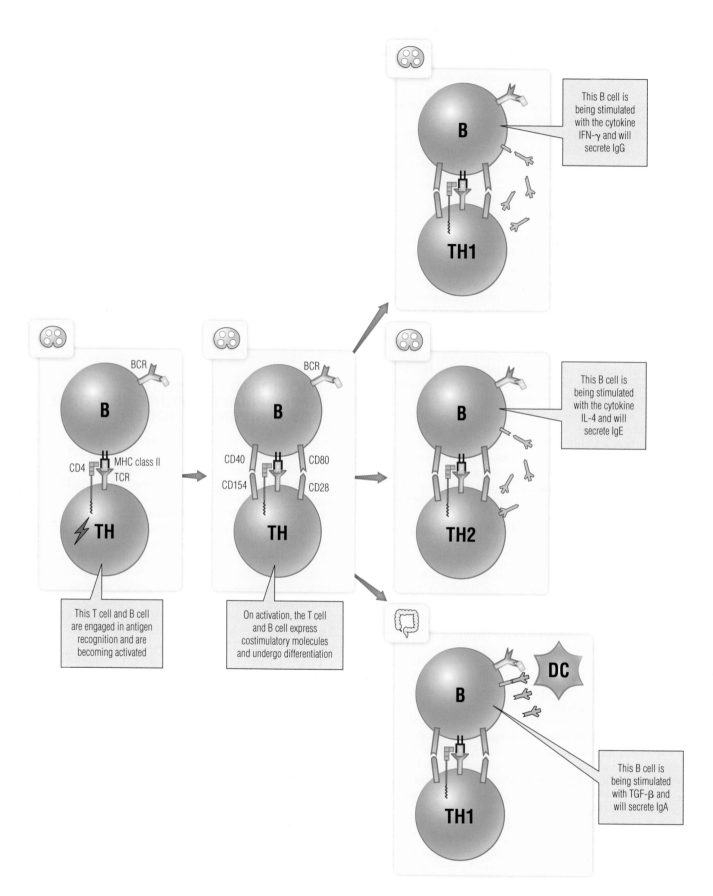

Fig 16.4 B cells secrete immunoglobulin M (IgM) until they undergo Ig class switching, which is regulated by cytokines secreted from T-helper (TH) or dendritic cells. *BCR,* B-cell receptor; *DC,* dendritic cell; *IFN,* interferon; *IL,* interleukin; *MHC,* major histocompatibility complex; *TCR,* T-cell receptor; *TGF,* transforming growth factor.

BOX 16.1 Epigenetics and T-Helper Cells—cont'd

In these circumstances, it would be helpful to manipulate clones of T-helper cells to alter their phenotype. The "epigenetic landscape" (Fig. 16.8) illustrates the problems that this approach needs to overcome. By the time a pluripotent stem cell has developed into a lymphoid progenitor cell, it has already acquired many epigenetic modifications. In the bone marrow, it will mature into either a B or T cell, acquiring more modifications. In the thymus it acquires even more modifications to become either a CD4⁺ or CD8⁺ cell and, finally, in the periphery, it acquires the modifications to become either a TH1, TH2, or TH17 cell.

In the epigenetic landscape, cells travel down valleys during their maturation processes and acquire epigenetic modifications as they go along (Fig. 16.8A). The ridges in between valleys indicate the epigenetic obstacles that would need to be overcome to alter one population to make it more like another. For example, so far it has proven impossible to travel back "uphill" and produce

a stem cell from a differentiated lymphocyte. However, in some circumstances, TH1 cells switch to a TH17 phenotype, and vice versa (Fig. 16.8B). Using prolonged immunotherapy, it is also possible to alter an immune response from a TH2 pattern to a TH1 pattern (Chapter 27). Immunotherapy is routinely used to treat severe allergies. However, in immunotherapy, it is not clear whether individual cells or clones of cells are having their phenotype altered epigenetically or whether TH2 cells are being killed or made inactive and being replaced with separate TH1 cells.

Immunotherapy takes a long time and is not free from risks. Epigenetic modifications are subject to investigation for simpler and safer drug treatments. For example, drugs that boost the TH1 response may be helpful in cancer, whereas in autoimmune disease, drugs that reduce TH1 responses would have more potential.

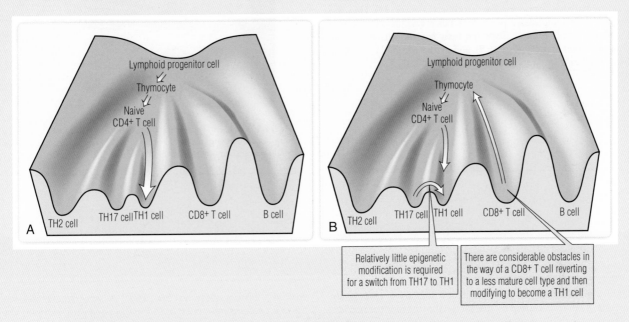

Fig 16.8 A T-helper (TH) cell's journey through the "epigenetic landscape." **A,** The route taken by a cell or population of cells maturing into TH1 cells. **B,** The obstacles in the way of a CD8⁺ T cell developing into a TH1 cell and how it may be relatively simple for a TH17 cell to change to a TH1 phenotype.

 MCH II   Cytokine, chemokine, etc.   Complement (C')   Signaling molecule

BOX 16.2 B Cell–T Cell Interaction: CD40/CD154 and X-Linked Hyper-Immunoglobulin M Syndrome

A 10-month-old child has had a series of bacterial chest and sinus infections since about 6 months of age. He was found to have low immunoglobulin G (IgG) and low IgA but high IgM. These abnormalities are consistent with the hyper-IgM syndrome, and the diagnosis was confirmed when his T cells were shown not to express CD154 (CD40 ligand). He can produce only IgM because his T cells are unable to offer appropriate help to induce B cells to switch Ig class. He was started on Ig replacement and responded well, with a decreased frequency of chest and sinus infections. Hyper-IgM syndrome also affects T-cell function; because CD154 is absent, T cells cannot communicate normally with antigen-presenting cells.

Boys with hyper-IgM syndrome are especially vulnerable to protozoal infections of the liver and gastrointestinal tract. At the age of 8 years, this child showed evidence of infection with *Cryptosporidium*. Fortunately, he has a sister with an identical human leukocyte antigen (HLA) type, and she was able to act as a bone marrow donor for her brother (Chapter 34). This is a prolonged and unpleasant procedure, but it was his only hope of improving T-cell function. Over the next few months, his condition improved steadily (Fig. 16.9), and at the age of 11 years, he was competing in national skiing championships!

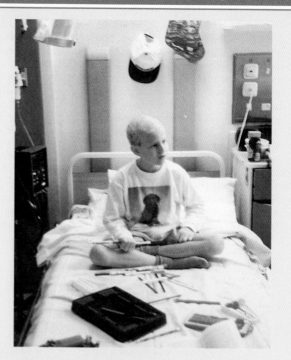

Fig 16.9 A boy with hyper-immunoglobulin M syndrome recovering from bone marrow transplant. His hair loss is a consequence of the conditioning chemotherapy required for bone marrow transplant.

BOX 16.3 Exploiting Our Knowledge of B-T Cooperation to Prevent Bacterial Meningitis With a Conjugate Vaccine

Until the advent of national vaccination that used a conjugate vaccine, meningitis caused by the bacterial pathogen *Haemophilus influenzae B* (HIB) was a serious concern. The disease peaks in infants age 10 to 11 months because until about the age of 18 to 24 months, children are unable to mount the effective T-independent response required for protection against the bacterial pathogen. In severe cases, HIB may cause neurologic damage or even death. The original vaccine was a purified capsular polysaccharide, a T-independent antigen that did not function well in infants younger than about 20 months. In addition, T-independent B cells do not develop immunologic memory and are not effective at immunoglobulin class switching or affinity maturation. Knowledge of T-dependent immune responses and B cell–T cell cooperation in immune responses led to the development of a vaccine in which the bacterial polysaccharide was coupled covalently to a protein. This conjugate vaccine induced far better responses than the unconjugated vaccine, even in very young children. Several proteins have been used for the conjugate, including the protein component of tetanus vaccine. In countries where this conjugate *Haemophilus* vaccine is being used, the incidence of meningitis has dramatically declined. Since 1993, the incidence of HIB-mediated meningitis has declined by 95% in U.S. children younger than 5 years.

B cells with immunoglobulin receptors for the bacterial capsular polysaccharide component of the vaccine take up the conjugate by receptor-mediated endocytosis. The protein component of the conjugate can then be processed and presented on the surface of the B cell associated with MHC class II molecules. The MHC class II–vaccine peptide complex can then be recognized by a T-helper cell of the appropriate specificity. The T-helper cell then activates the B cell to make antibody against the bacterial polysaccharide. The general principle is as illustrated in Figure 16.10.

 T-cell receptor (TCR)

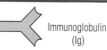 Immunoglobulin (Ig)

 Antigen

 MCH I

BOX 16.3 Exploiting Our Knowledge of B-T Cooperation to Prevent Bacterial Meningitis With a Conjugate Vaccine—cont'd

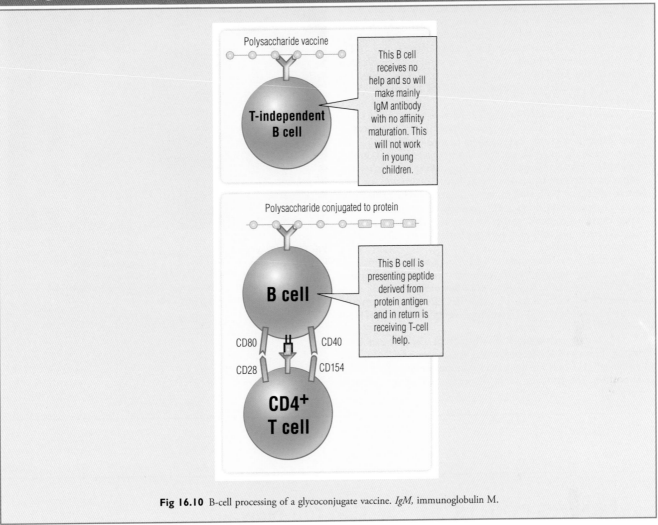

Fig 16.10 B-cell processing of a glycoconjugate vaccine. *IgM*, immunoglobulin M.

 MCH II   Cytokine, chemokine, etc.   Complement (C')   Signaling molecule

BOX 16.4 Oral Candidiasis

A 43-year-old woman presents with a sore mouth and some difficulty swallowing. She has had these symptoms for 2 weeks and is otherwise well, not taking any medications, and not pregnant. Her family doctor recognizes *Candida* infection (Fig. 16.11), and the patient responds promptly to antifungal medication. However, the *Candida* returns 2 weeks later. This leaves the doctor with problem of figuring out why the patient has developed *recurrent* candidiasis.

Candida is a common problem at all ages and in both sexes. For example, many people who take antibiotics develop *Candida*. This happens because the bacteria normally competing for resources in the mouth are killed off, and *Candida* can take over. *Candida* is also seen frequently in people taking corticosteroids, either as tablets or as inhalers, for asthma. Corticosteroids have broad effects on both antigen-presenting cells and T cells. Cytotoxic chemotherapy drugs also frequently cause *Candida*. These drugs cause neutropenia, so that the very cells that defend against *Candida* are unavailable. However, our patient is on none of these common medications.

Another very rare cause of recurrent *Candida* is the autoimmune polyendocrinopathy candidiasis ectodermal dysplasia (APECED) syndrome (see Box 15.2), but our patient has none of the other features of this. In APECED, patients produce autoantibodies against IL-17, which prevents T-helper 17 (TH17) cells from functioning normally.

Her doctor remembers that recurrent *Candida* can be a feature of early HIV infection, which causes loss of CD4⁺ T cells, including TH17 cells. He does an HIV antibody test and the result is positive. The patients starts antiretroviral therapy and does very well.

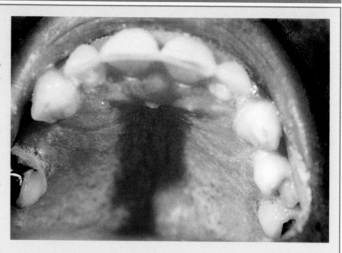

Fig 16.11 The white lesions on this man's palate are oral candidiasis, which is a marker of mild immunodeficiency. It is often the first opportunistic infection to manifest in patients with HIV. Oral candidiasis is also often seen in other mild secondary immunodeficiencies. (Courtesy St. Bartholomew's Hospital, London, United Kingdom.)

LEARNING POINTS Can You Now...

1. Describe how naive B and T cells are primed by cell-cell interactions with antigen-presenting cells?

2. Outline the differences between TH1, TH2, and TH17 responses?

3. Define *epigenetics* and give an example of epigenetic modification of T-helper cells?

4. Describe how a glycoconjugate vaccine induces a protective response?

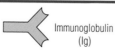 T-cell receptor (TCR)   Immunoglobulin (Ig) Antigen   MCH I

Immunologic Memory and Homeostasis

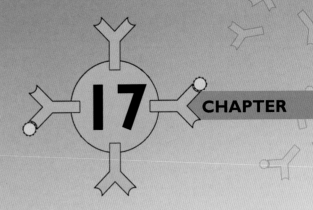

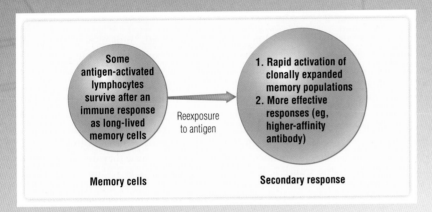

Some antigen-activated lymphocytes survive after an immune response as long-lived memory cells

Reexposure to antigen

1. Rapid activation of clonally expanded memory populations
2. More effective responses (eg, higher-affinity antibody)

Memory cells   **Secondary response**

One of the hallmarks of the adaptive immune system is that it "remembers" previous encounters with antigen (Chapter 2). As shown in the above figure, this chapter describes how memory cells are established and how the memory response is generated, and it explains the advantages of immunologic memory to the individual who reencounters a pathogen. Immune memory is very important in protection from infectious agents, and it allows the host to initiate the secondary immune response on subsequent encounters with a pathogen. This secondary immune response was initially discussed in Chapter 2 and is characterized by being:

- Faster (hours instead of days)
- More vigorous, producing more antibody and higher-affinity specific antibody (Fig. 2.7)
- More specific; for example, T-helper 1 (TH1) or TH2 in the case of T-cell help or immunoglobulin G (IgG) or IgE in the case of immunoglobulin

As described in Chapters 2 and 4 (see also Chapter 25), vaccination takes advantage of immunologic memory. Vaccines against infectious diseases such as smallpox and poliomyelitis have been some of the most important achievements of medical science. Along with improved hygiene and sanitation, vaccines have saved countless lives, and they have been responsible for dramatically improving the quality of life for millions of people throughout the world. However, although great successes have come from taking advantage of the existence of immunologic memory, we still have much to understand about how immunologic memory is established and maintained. This chapter

presents a summary of what is most important about long-term immunologic memory.

LONG-TERM IMMUNOLOGIC MEMORY

Long-term immunologic memory refers to the capacity to generate an enhanced and more effective immune response to an antigen that was last encountered in the distant past. Long-term memory is thought to result from the presence of clonally expanded, antigen-specific B and T lymphocytes that persist in a resting state for many years and, in some cases, for a lifetime. For example, vaccinia virus–specific T cells have been demonstrated in individuals vaccinated with this 50 years prior to prevent smallpox (variola; Box 25.1). Studies of human populations living in isolated island communities have shown antibody-mediated protection against measles virus that persisted for more than 65 years.

B-Cell Memory

Naive B cells activated by antigen differentiate into effector B cells (plasma cells) that secrete antibody (Chapter 14). In a primary response, the plasma cells secrete a relatively low-affinity antibody, whereas in a secondary response a higher-affinity antibody is secreted.

After an initial exposure to an antigen, antibody may be secreted by plasma cells for many months. This is helpful because

TABLE 17.1 Antibody Responses		
	Primary Response	**Secondary Response**
Time period to response	5-10 days	1-3 days
Antibody class	Mainly IgM	IgG, IgA, or IgE
Affinity for antigen	Low	High

Ig, immunoglobulin.

TABLE 17.2 Features of T Cells		
	Naive T Cell	**Memory T Cell**
Speed of response	Slow (responders based in lymph nodes)	Faster (responders may be based in tissues and are epigenetically modified)
Strength of response	Low (low frequency of responders)	High (frequency of responders is high)
Specificity of response	None	May have specified T-helper phenotype or tissue distribution

it means that antibody is present the moment a pathogen enters the body (Box 17.1).

Somatic hypermutation takes place during the secondary response to generate a higher-affinity binding site for antigen (Chapters 6 and 14). Immunoglobulin (Ig) class switching can take place during a primary response, but typically a primary antibody response is mostly IgM, whereas a secondary antibody response can be IgG, IgA, or IgE (Table 17.1).

Over time antibody levels fall, and memory B cells are required to secrete new antibodies on reexposure to the pathogen. It is likely that the memory B cell is derived from an activated B cell that has undergone genetic changes (somatic hypermutation) in variable region gene segment DNA to create a more effective antibody (Fig. 17.1).

The memory B cell preserves the higher-affinity antigen receptor that has been derived by sequential somatic genetic changes. On subsequent exposure to antigen, it is this memory cell that responds, not another naive cell. Evidence that this is true comes from the observation that individuals exposed to a pathogen early in life, such as measles virus, respond to the same epitopes on the pathogen when reexposed later in life, and they do not respond to new epitopes present on the pathogen even though they are antigenic. This observation is consistent with secondary and subsequent exposure to antigen activating preexisting memory cells rather than inducing the differentiation of new naive cells. The advantage to the host is that a secondary response, a more rapid and higher-affinity response, is generated; this allows the infection to be eliminated sooner than if a new primary response were generated.

T-Cell Memory

Memory T cells are produced during primary responses to infection. It is not clear whether they are produced from activated T cells before they become effector T cells or whether they are produced from effector T cells or both. In acquiring the memory phenotype, T cells undergo significant epigenetic modification so that they express very specific patterns. During proliferation, these gene expression patterns are passed to daughter cells. Chapter 16 explained how these epigenetic modifications are acquired.

The cardinal features of T-cell memory are faster, more vigorous, and more specific responses to infection (Table 17.2). Memory T cells are able to respond faster to infection than naive T cells for several reasons. First, naive T cells express L-selectin, which commits them to recirculating to lymph nodes (Chapter 13) rather than other tissues. This places naive T cells in the

perfect position for interacting with antigen-presenting cells (APCs) such as dendritic cells. In contrast, much like effector T cells, memory T cells express a range of cellular adhesion molecules, which permits them to enter a variety of tissues. This can place memory T cells at the front line when an infection occurs. In addition, the epigenetic changes that have taken place mean that genes are more rapidly transcribed. For example, cytokine genes may be more loosely arranged around histone, making them more open to transcription. Because they may be placed in the frontline tissues and because their genes are epigenetically modified, memory T cells respond faster to infection.

The memory T-cell response is more vigorous than the primary T-cell response because there are more T cells with a receptor specific for antigen in the pool of memory T cells. In the thymus, the T-cell receptor genes are rearranged randomly. After positive and negative selection, the chances that any given T cell will recognize any given peptide antigen are very low (on the order of 1:10,000 to 1:100,000). In the primary T-cell response, specific T cells proliferate. At the peak of a primary response, the number of specific T cells may increase by 10,000. Although many of these cells will die through apoptosis (see Fig. 17.1), the frequency of surviving specific T cells that contribute to long-term memory may be on the order of 1:100 to 1:1000.

The memory T-cell response is more specific than the primary response. This applies mainly to CD4$^+$ T-helper (TH) cells, which will acquire TH1, TH2, TH17, and possibly other phenotypes when they become memory cells. These specific phenotypes, along with restricted recirculation patterns, lead to very specific patterns of response. For example, TH1 memory cells specific for influenza tend to be enriched in the lung, exactly where they are required.

As you read in the previous chapter, T-independent B-cell memory does not mature until late infancy. For this reason, individuals experience the highest rate of infection in the first 2 years of life. From age 2 until about 20, T- and B-cell memory is being built progressively, and individuals experience infections at an intermediate level. It is only from about age 20 onward that people stop experiencing numerous infections. T-cell memory can last for at least 50 years, probably through the survival of clones of T cells and their daughter cells rather than individual memory cells (see immunity after smallpox vaccine in Chapter 25). Unfortunately, after about 60 years, immune senescence develops (Chapter 33), and the rate of infection increases again.

 T-cell receptor (TCR) 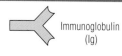 Immunoglobulin (Ig)  Antigen MCH I

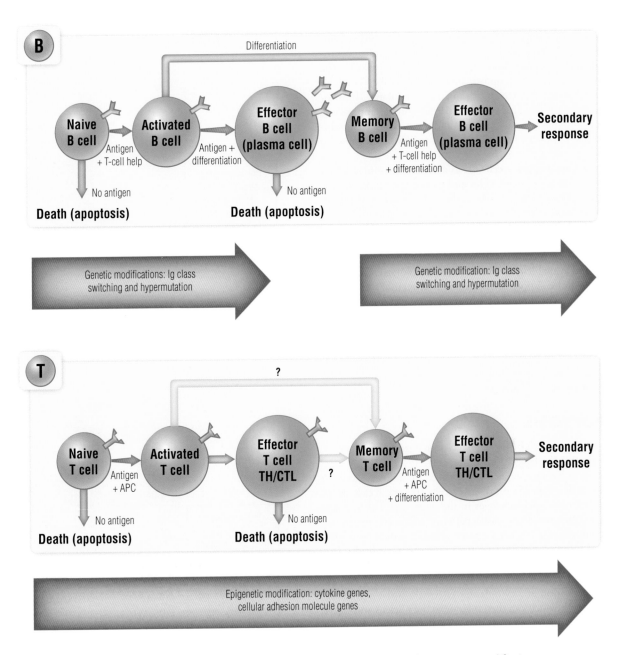

Fig 17.1 Differentiation pathway of memory cells. During B-cell differentiation, there are genetic modifications, but during T-cell differentiation, after the naive T-cell stage, there are only epigenetic modifications. *APC*, antigen-presenting cell; *CTL*, cytotoxic T lymphocyte; *Ig*, immunoglobulin; *TH*, T helper cell.

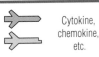 MCH II

 Cytokine, chemokine, etc.

Complement (C′)

 Signaling molecule

■ LYMPHOCYTE HOMEOSTASIS

Given that it is possible for us to retain immunologic memory of every foreign antigen encounter we have ever had, even if the number of memory cells generated in each immune response were small (and it is usually substantial), there would eventually be an issue of availability of appropriate body sites to maintain these cells. However, the blood and lymphoid tissues have space for only a finite number of cells, Fortunately, like other lymphocytes, most effector and memory cells appear to die eventually, probably by programmed cell death (apoptosis). The mechanisms involved in apoptosis are further described later and in detail in Chapter 22. Cell death maintains a balance (homeostasis) between the need for vast clonal expansion of lymphocytes in primary responses to new antigens and the need for maintaining memory cells with the limited number of suitable sites for lymphocytes.

Most activated effector cells die as antigen is eliminated and levels of costimulatory molecules and interleukin 2 (IL-2), the T-cell growth factor, fall. Without these, the level of proapoptotic proteins increases (see Box 17.2), and the cell undergoes apoptosis and dies.

Clones of antigen-specific memory cells survive for longer periods. For these memory cells to survive, they need to compete for space and available growth factors (eg, cytokines). Given that these are in finite supply, it is possible that memory cells from some antigenic encounters do not survive long term. Conceivably, some memory cells are better adapted for survival under these conditions. For example, they have a reduced need for cytokines and growth factors; therefore they are more competitive in terms of ability to survive. This could mean that immunologic memory of some antigens may be more stable than memory of some other antigens.

■ APOPTOSIS

Apoptosis is triggered through receptor-ligand interactions, mainly the Fas–Fas ligand interaction (Fig. 17.2).

Binding of Fas ligand, such as expressed on a killer T cell, to Fas, such as is expressed on a target cell, triggers a cascade of intracellular biochemical changes in the target cell. Fas interacts with several proteins in the "death pathway" eventually to activate a proteolytic enzyme known as *caspase,* which is critical in activating several more proteolytic enzymes in the caspase cascade. This proteolytic cascade is somewhat analogous to the kinase cascade of cell activation (Chapter 11). The critical step of the caspase cascade is activation of a cytoplasmic enzyme, caspase-activatable DNAse (CAD), which can then migrate to the nucleus and cleave DNA into the small fragments that are a characteristic end point of apoptosis (see Table 17-3 and Chapter 22).

Several genes have been found to promote cell death, and several genes also inhibit cell death (see Box 17.2). The family of death-inhibiting genes includes the *BCL* genes. A gene initially detected in B-cell lymphomas (Chapter 35), *BCL2* is typical of the death-inhibiting or antiapoptotic genes. One explanation that has been proposed for the survival of long-term memory cells is that they have a higher than usual level of expression of the Bcl family of proteins. This characteristic protects them from antigen-induced cell death and facilitates their long-term survival.

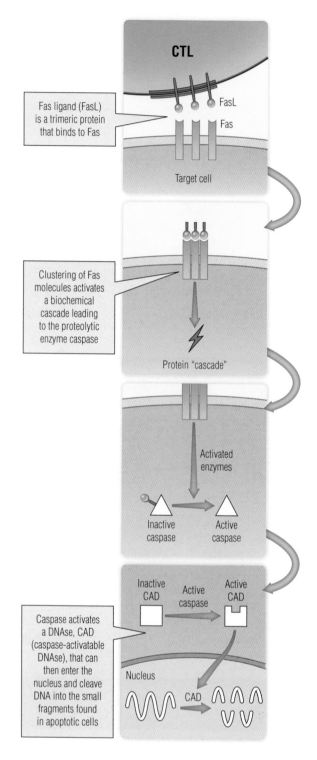

Fig 17.2 Cell death pathway. The role of receptor-ligand interactions (Fas–Fas L) to activate caspase and, finally, caspase-activatable DNAase (CAD), which degrades DNA. *CTL,* cytotoxic T lymphocyte.

 T-cell receptor (TCR)

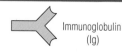 Immunoglobulin (Ig)

 Antigen

 MCH I

BOX 17.1 Entry to Medical School: Immunologic Memory

Annie and Belinda have both been accepted to medical school. To be able to start school, they must have hepatitis B antibody levels of over 100 mIU/mL (rules vary in different countries). Annie completed her initial vaccination of three injections 6 weeks previously (see Fig. 2.7). A blood test shows her antibody levels are 135 mIU/mL, so she can start school.

Belinda was vaccinated against hepatitis B 4 years previously when she worked one summer as a laboratory assistant. At that time she had a blood test that showed antibody levels of 180 mIU/mL. However, when she is tested again at her medical school screening, her antibody levels have fallen to 43 mIU/mL. She has

a booster vaccine, and 2 weeks later her levels have increased to 380 mIU/mL, so she is allowed to start school.

To protect against hepatitis B from a needle-stick injury, antibody needs to be present in the blood at a high level (deemed to be more than 100 mIU/mL in this case). A course of three hepatitis B vaccine injections achieves this in most people, although antibody levels may fall over time. A booster vaccine induces memory B cells to mature into plasma cells and to start secreting antibody again. Because this is a memory response, higher levels of antibody are achieved—faster than in the primary response.

BOX 17.2 Apoptosis: Programmed Cell Death

Apoptosis is a mechanism for the elimination of excess or damaged cells. It is an evolutionarily conserved process initiated by the dying cell, and it represents a form of controlled cellular destruction. Several genes have been identified that either promote or inhibit apoptosis (Table 17-3). Antiapoptotic genes could confer characteristics such as longer than usual survival. The most important of the antiapoptotic genes appears to be *BCL2*. Antiapoptotic genes of the *BCL2* type appear to work by raising the so-called *apoptotic threshold* of a cell; that is, the dose of apoptosis initiator required for a cell expressing the Bcl-2 protein is greater than in the absence of Bcl-2.

The gene *BCL2* was originally detected as a mammalian oncogene involved in a human chromosomal translocation between chromosomes 14 and 18, detected in more than 70% of lymphomas. The chromosomal translocation results in increased expression of Bcl-2, which imparts a relative resistance to apoptosis on the resulting B tumor cells (Chapter 35).

TABLE 17-3 Death-Inhibiting and Death-Promoting Genes

Antiapoptotic (Death-Inhibiting) Genes	Proapoptotic (Death-Promoting) Genes
BCL2	BAX
bcl-X_L	BAK1
BCL2L2	BCL2L11

LEARNING POINTS Can You Now ...

1. Recall examples of the major medical triumphs that resulted from artificial induction (by vaccination) of immunologic memory?

2. List the major differences between a primary and a secondary immune response?

3. Draw a model for the differentiation pathway of memory lymphocytes?

4. List the qualitative and quantitative changes that distinguish memory from naive lymphocytes?

5. Draw the principal features of the apoptotic pathway?

6. List the characteristics of memory cells that help to ensure their survival?

 MCH II   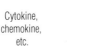 Cytokine, chemokine, etc.   Complement (C′)   Signaling molecule

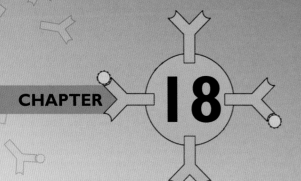

Regulation of the Immune System

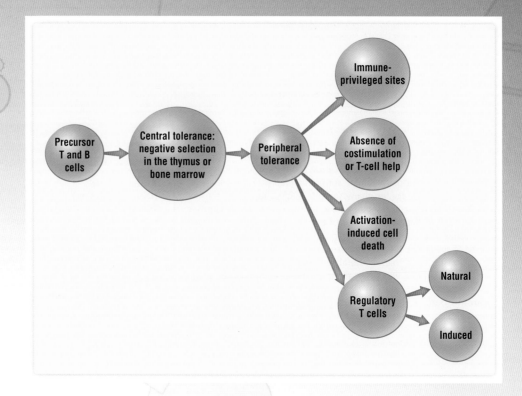

The immune system is capable of preventing and eradicating serious infections. As discussed in Chapter 35, it can also combat tumors. To achieve these goals, the immune system has developed potent effector mechanisms. When the immune system is unregulated, it can cause considerable damage, and unregulated immune responses to self can cause autoimmune disease. For example, common autoimmune diseases such as type 1 diabetes and rheumatoid arthritis both cause a 10-year reduction in life expectancy and also cause considerable symptoms during life. In addition, immune responses to harmless environmental substances can lead to allergies. The most severe type of allergic response, anaphylaxis, causes several hundred deaths per year in the United States. These examples illustrate what can go wrong when the immune response is not regulated. The rest of this chapter describes immune-regulation mechanisms.

■ TOLERANCE

The immune system is tolerant of self antigens and harmless environmental antigens. *Tolerance* can be defined as a state of unresponsiveness to molecules the immune system has the capacity to recognize and attack. In other words, although the receptors for self or harmless environmental antigens are produced during receptor gene rearrangement, cells that express these receptors are actively killed or are kept from functioning.

We have involved multiple "checkpoints" to prevent the devastating effects of autoimmunity or allergy. These are outlined in the above figure. Tolerance to self antigen is achieved through *central tolerance* in the thymus and bone marrow and *peripheral tolerance* in all other tissues. Peripheral tolerance involves a variety of different mechanisms, some of which were mentioned briefly in Chapter 15. Harmless environmental antigens are not

TABLE 18.1 Key Features of B- and T-Cell Tolerance

	B Cells	T Cells
Central tolerance	Bone marrow: B cells that recognize self antigen undergo apoptosis	Thymus; failure to recognize self MHC (no positive selection) causes cells to die through apoptosis Thymus; recognizes self peptide plus self MHC at high affinity; cells die through apoptosis or become Tregs
Peripheral tolerance	Absence of T-cell help (for protein antigens) induces anergy	Immune-privileged sites Absence of costimulation induces anergy Repeated or high-dose exposure to antigen induces activation-induced cell death Tregs

MHC, *major histocompatibility complex*; Tregs, *T-regulatory cells*.

expressed in the thymus or bone marrow, so tolerance to these is achieved through peripheral mechanisms.

Tolerance mechanisms are slightly different for B cells and T cells. The mechanisms of tolerance are summarized in Table 18.1. Mechanisms are not 100% effective by any means. The observation that autoimmune diseases, such as diabetes or rheumatoid arthritis, and allergies are common indicate how often central and peripheral tolerance mechanisms break down. Understanding these mechanisms will help you understand treatments for these conditions. This chapter reviews central tolerance and discusses peripheral tolerance mechanisms.

Central Tolerance

Immature B cells that recognize self antigen in the bone marrow undergo negative selection and die through apoptosis. For T cells, the process in the thymus is more complicated. Thymocytes that do not recognize self major histocompatibility complex (MHC) do not succeed in being positively selected and die through apoptosis. However, most thymocytes that recognize self peptide plus self MHC at high very affinity also die through apoptosis (negative selection). Some CD4+ thymocytes that recognize self peptide plus self MHC become T-regulatory cells (Tregs) (see Fig. 15.3). Through these mechanisms, 95% to 99% of thymocytes die during the selection processes in the thymus. Those that leave the thymus do not recognize self peptide plus self MHC at high affinity unless they are regulatory T cells. Naive T cells that leave the thymus are subject to a second checkpoint: peripheral tolerance.

Peripheral Tolerance

Immune-Privileged Sites

Immune-privileged sites are those that tolerate the presence of antigen without an immune response. T cells do not circulate

through immune-privileged tissues. In addition, immunoglobulin (Ig) may also not be able to diffuse into these tissues at significant levels. Examples of immune-privileged tissues include the central nervous system, the eye, and the reproductive organs—tissues that have some physical barriers against the immune system. For example, it is difficult for Ig molecules to diffuse across the blood-brain barrier, so IgG levels in the cerebrospinal fluid (CSF) are less than one-hundredth of those in the blood. In addition, levels of costimulatory molecules is low in these tissues, so T-cell activation cannot take place. Finally, Fas ligand (FasL) is expressed in some immune-privileged sites, and FasL induces apoptosis in T cells that gain entry into these tissues.

Immune privilege operates only in homeostasis. If any of these organs is damaged by trauma, or if infection triggers inflammation, resident macrophages will transport antigen from the tissue to the local lymph nodes, provoking a potential immune response. In addition, inflammation triggered by the innate immune system will affect cellular adhesion molecule (CAM) expression so that T cells will begin to recirculate through these tissues.

The placenta and fetus are a special type of immune-privileged tissue. In this example, T cells are prevented from functioning if they enter the placenta. On the other hand, IgG antibodies are actively pumped across the placenta into the developing fetus.

Absence of Costimulation or T-Cell Help. As explained in Chapter 16, T cells require costimulation to become activated. Costimulation is normally provided by the antigen-presenting cell (APC) or other cells in the vicinity that respond to the infection. If a T cell recognizes antigen presented on an MHC molecule without costimulation, the T cell will not respond and will enter a state of dormancy referred to as *anergy* (Fig. 18.1A).

Anergic T cells are not dead and survive for some time. If the costimulation is provided at some point in the future, anergy can be reversed and the T cell can complete activation. This observation has important implications for vaccines. Those that contain only a protein antigen are not very effective. This is because although the protein is processed by APCs and the peptides may be recognized by CD4+ T cells, no costimulation is available and an immune response will not take place. To overcome this, an adjuvant is added to the vaccine. The adjuvant is a substance that will stimulate the innate immune system to provide costimulation. Adjuvants are described as improving the "immunogenicity" of a vaccine. Many vaccines use very mild adjuvants. For example, aluminum hydroxide (alum) is used in hepatitis B vaccine. In the future, more potent adjuvants will be developed to make more immunogenic vaccines (Chapter 25).

T-independent B cells can respond to polysaccharide without T-cell help (Chapter 14). However, most B cells that respond to protein antigens will become anergic if they do not receive T-cell help (Fig. 18.1B). So if a T-helper cell is no longer able to provide help because of a tolerance mechanism, any B cells involved in the same immune response will also become anergic.

Activation-Induced Cell Death

Activation-induced cell death (AICD) occurs in T cells that have been exposed repeatedly to the same antigen. These T cells begin

 MCH II

 Cytokine, chemokine, etc.

 Complement (C')

 Signaling molecule

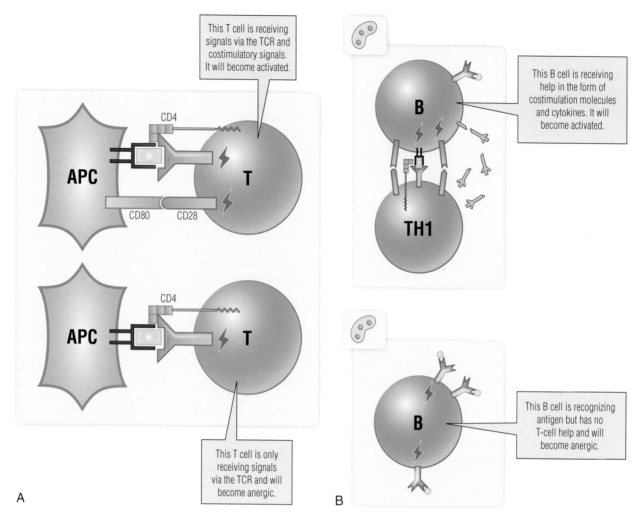

Fig 18.1 The lack of T cells (**A**) and B cells (**B**) can cause cells to become anergic as a result of lack of costimulation or T-cell help, respectively. *APC,* antigen-presenting cell; *TH1,* T-helper 1.

to express both Fas and FasL and either kill themselves or are killed by neighboring cells. These T cells are irreversibly lost from the T-cell repertoire (Fig. 18.2). Eventually, clones of responding T cells are permanently deleted.

Regulatory T Cells

Tregs exert peripheral tolerance in an antigen-specific manner. Like other CD4⁺ T cells, they have antigen receptors that are specific for MHC class II and antigenic peptides. Tregs can have specificity for self antigens and harmless environmental antigens and so have a role in preventing autoimmunity and allergy, respectively.

The two different types of Tregs are shown in Figure 18.3. *Natural Tregs* (nTregs) are produced during T-cell maturation in the thymus. They can be produced if a thymocyte recognizes self antigen plus MHC class II at high affinity (see Fig. 15.3). In these circumstances, the master transcription factor FOXP3 may be activated. This transcription factor regulates genes that steer the cell down the Treg differentiation pathway. Although nTregs

develop in the thymus, they participate in tolerance in the periphery.

Induced Tregs (iTregs) develop from naive T cells in the periphery under specific conditions. For example, in the gastrointestinal tract, the cytokine transforming growth factor beta (TGF-β) is secreted by epithelial cells and dendritic cells. If a naive T cell in a mesenteric lymph node is exposed to TGF-β during antigen stimulation, it may mature into an iTreg. This process is referred to as *oral tolerance* (see Box 18.2). The evolutionary benefits of this are that peptides derived from food or from harmless gut bacteria do not trigger an immune response. Also, iTregs can be induced when antigen exposure is repeated. In other instances, immunosuppressive drugs "force" naive T cells recognizing antigen for the first time to become iTregs. This is of considerable benefit in transplantation and also has implications for other branches of medicine in which it would be desirable to suppress the immune response. This is why the study of iTregs is an area of rapid development, and you may read elsewhere about T-helper 3 (TH3) and Tr1 cells, which are probably subsets of regulatory T cells, although they are not describe here in detail.

 T-cell receptor (TCR)

 Immunoglobulin (Ig)

Antigen

 MCH I

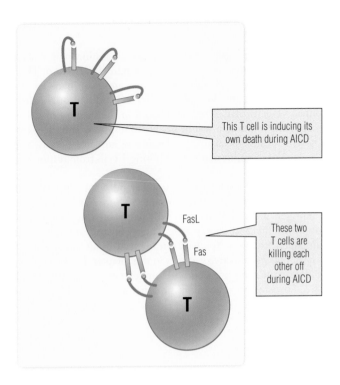

Fig 18.2 Activation-induced cell death (AICD) drives T cells to kill themselves or one another using Fas and Fas ligand (FasL).

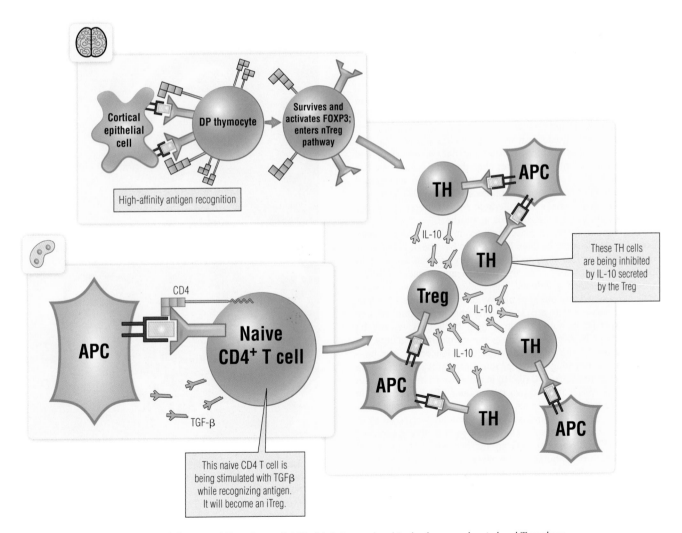

Fig 18.3 *Top left,* A natural T-regulator cell (nTreg) is being produced in the thymus and an induced T-regulator cell (iTreg) is being produced in the mesenteric lymph nodes. *Right,* A Treg is inhibiting neighboring T-helper (TH) cells by secreting interleukin 10 (IL-10). *APC,* antigen-presenting cell; *DP,* double positive; *TGF,* transforming growth factor.

When they recognize antigen, Tregs can inhibit neighboring T cells by secreting the cytokines interleukin 10 (IL-10) or TGF-β. It is likely that other mechanisms are also involved; for example, nTregs are also able to inhibit T cells through direct contact. T cells that recognize antigen in the vicinity of a Treg recognizing *its* antigen will be unable to respond. Thus Tregs are a potent means for ensuring tolerance of antigens because one Treg is able to inhibit many neighboring T cells from responding to antigen.

You should now be able to understand what types of antigenic stimulation trigger an immune response and what types of antigen are tolerated. This will help you understand how autoimmunity and allergy arise when you read about these in subsequent chapters. You have already read about how adjuvants help in making effective vaccines in this chapter. Boxes 18.1 and 18.2 describe some more clinical implications of tolerance. Table 18.2 shows factors that will favor either an immune response or tolerance.

TABLE 18.2   Factors That Favor Immune Tolerance or Immune Response

Factor	Favors Tolerance	Favors an Immune Response
Dose	High dose induces negative selection in the thymus or bone marrow	Medium dose
Exposure frequency	Multiple exposures over a prolonged period induce AICD	Few exposures
Route	Oral	Intramuscular, subcutaneous
Costimulation	None	Costimulation induced by adjuvant

AICD, *activation-induced cell death.*

BOX 18.1

A 50-year-old man took on beekeeping as a new hobby 5 years ago. He keeps two beehives at the back of his garden (Fig. 18.4). Sometimes he forgets to wear his bee suit, and each summer he is stung about 20 times by his bees. Most of the stings he experiences are painful, but he doesn't have a reaction to them. However, his partner has been stung once each year since the hives arrived. Last summer the partner was stung and developed a widespread rash within 5 minutes of the sting. This year, after having been stung again, the partner felt very dizzy and then lost consciousness 5 minutes after the sting. An allergist has confirmed that the partner has developed bee venom allergy, and this most recent attack was anaphylaxis (Chapter 27). Why is it that the frequent stings are tolerated by one person, but the infrequent stings cause anaphylaxis in another?

Bee venom allergy is most likely to develop in people who are infrequently stung by bees. People who have been stung many times are much less likely to develop allergy to bee venom. This observation illustrates how the dose of an antigen can affect whether tolerance is induced. The beekeeper's partner, who is only exposed to low doses of bee venom, has produced T-helper 2 (TH2) cells, which are stimulating the production of bee venom–specific immunoglobulin E (IgE) by B cells. As will be discussed in Chapter 27, IgE causes the symptoms of allergy. On the other hand, the repeated stings experienced by our beekeeper are stimulating him to produce regulatory T cells. These cells secrete interleukin 10 (IL-10) in response to bee venom and inhibit TH2 cells, cutting down the amount of IgE produced. In addition to immune tolerance, repeated stings drive a predominantly TH2 to a TH1 response. This is sometimes referred to as *immune deviation.* As a result of interferon gamma (IFN-γ) secreted during the TH1 response, IgG against bee venom is produced instead, which contributes to the allergy effects.

Repeated antigenic stimulation leads to immune tolerance and immune deviation, protecting our beekeeper. Similar processes are used clinically in allergen immunotherapy, as described in Chapter 27.

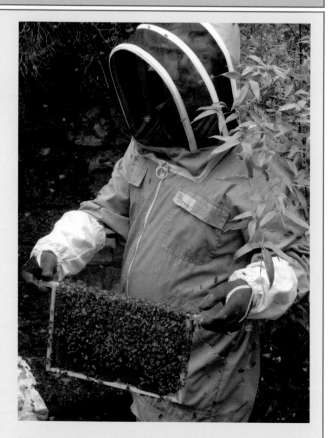

Fig 18.4 This beekeeper is stung repeatedly over the summer but does not have reactions. His partner is stung much less frequently but has had severe reactions.

 T-cell receptor (TCR)   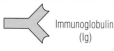 Immunoglobulin (Ig)   Antigen   MCH I

BOX 18.2 Oral Tolerance

Oral tolerance can be defined as the specific suppression of an immune response by prior administration of the antigen by the oral route. The human gut is bombarded by proteins every day. These include proteins in the diet as well as proteins derived from the trillions of commensal bacteria that live harmlessly in the gut. Many of these proteins are not completely digested to amino acids in the gut lumen, and they can be absorbed as either protein or peptides. It is important for the immune system to tolerate these harmless potential antigens.

Gut-associated lymphoid tissues (GALT) behave differently from lymphoid tissues elsewhere in the body. Gut epithelium secretes the cytokine transforming growth factor beta (TGF-β) in response to contact with harmless gut bacteria. TGF-β has two important roles in the gut. Naive T cells being primed by antigen in the gut or mesenteric lymph nodes in the presence of TGF-β will mature into induced T-regulatory cells (iTregs). This suppresses any possible T-cell reaction to the antigen.

On the other hand, if an immature B cell is producing antibody in response to antigen in the gut in the presence of TGF-β, it will class switch to immunoglobulin A (IgA) secretion. As you learned in Chapter 13, IgA has an important role in protecting the mucosal surfaces from infection. The majority of pathogens enter the body through the gut, and IgA acts as a barrier against these. Unlike other classes of antibody, IgA prevents pathogens from invading the body, but it does so without triggering much of a systemic immune response. Thus GALT responds to antigen by producing iTregs and IgA and not by stimulating a potentially dangerous systemic reaction. This is the basis of oral tolerance.

Because of its safety, ease of administration, and specificity for antigen, oral tolerance has been extensively investigated as a means of inducing tolerance in a range of clinical settings. For example, it would be very helpful to switch off responses to self antigen in autoimmune disease or environmental antigens in allergy. It would also help to induce tolerance to proteins used for treatment (for example, factor VIII used to treat people with hemophilia).

Experiments with animals have shown some promise in a wide range of settings. However, numerous clinical trials in humans have so far shown very limited benefits. For example, hay fever (T-helper 2 [TH2]–mediated allergy to grass pollen) can be switched off when grass pollen is administered under the tongue (sublingual immunotherapy; see Chapter 27). This is in part mediated by iTregs and in part by switching TH2 responses to TH1 (immune deviation). Another example of oral tolerance in humans is giving oral insulin to individuals with very early type 1 (insulin-dependent) diabetes (Chapter 28). In a clinical trial of oral insulin, some patients showed evidence of delayed progression of the diabetes. These observations need to be confirmed in other clinical trials.

LEARNING POINTS Can You Now...

1. Outline how central and peripheral tolerance are developed?
2. List what type of antigenic stimulation favors an immune response and what type favors tolerance?
3. Describe one mechanism used to make vaccines more immunogenic?
4. Describe an experimental approach used to improve tolerance of antigens?

 MCH II   Cytokine, chemokine, etc.   Complement (C′)   Signaling molecule

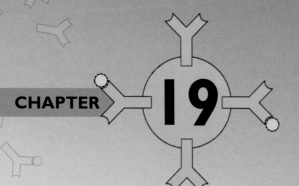

CHAPTER **19** Brief Review of Immune Physiology

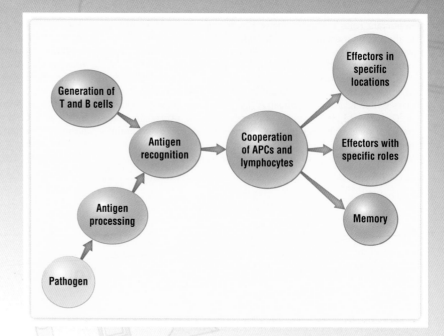

After a discussion of the genes and molecules involved in antigen recognition in Section II, Section III progressed to a discussion of cells, tissues, and organs and a more integrated view of the adaptive immune response as a physiologic system.

At this point, you should have gained a good understanding of the following important topics (also illustrated in the above figure):

- How a repertoire of antigen receptors is developed using gene rearrangement
- How antigen-presenting cells (APCs) process and display antigens for recognition by T cells
- How naive B and T lymphocytes recognize antigen and are then activated to differentiate into effector cells
- How APCs and B and T lymphocytes interact and cooperate in an adaptive immune response
- How lymphocytes recirculate to lymphoid and peripheral tissues
- How specific responses are generated; for example, immunoglobulins (Igs) such as IgG, IgA, or IgE or T-helper 1 (TH1), TH2, or TH17 responses

- How memory of a previous response is maintained to allow a more rapid and effective response on reencountering a pathogen

We established in Chapter 10 that antigen associates with the αβ T-cell receptor (TCR) only after handling by specialized APCs. Most importantly, the route of antigen processing (cytosolic vs. vesicle bound) determines whether an antigen is presented by major histocompatibility complex (MHC) class II molecules to a TCR on a CD4$^+$ T-helper cell or by MHC class I molecules to a TCR on a CD8$^+$ cytotoxic T lymphocyte.

Chapters 11 and 16 described:

- The structure and function of the B-cell receptor (BCR) and the TCR
- The role of coreceptor and costimulatory molecules in optimizing the function of the antigen receptors
- The connection between the antigen receptors and the signal-transduction machinery of B and T lymphocytes

This should have given you an understanding of how lymphocytes become effector cells and the processes involved in lymphocyte activation.

In Chapters 14 and 15, we discussed how the repertoire of B- and T-cell specificities is developed. We learned that orderly processes of gene rearrangement take place in different cell types during B- and T-cell development in the bone marrow and thymus, respectively. How thymocytes and B-cell precursors mature into T- and B-effector cells, respectively, with an appropriate repertoire of antigen receptors was also described. Many similarities are evident in the development of B and T lymphocytes and their respective repertoires of antigen-specific receptors. The greatest difference between the two lineages is that the BCR is subject to continued improvements after exposure to antigen. Thus the processes of affinity maturation and class switching are used to generate a higher-affinity, more effective antibody molecule during the immune response. Although the TCR does not change in structure during an immune response, clonally expanded memory T cells are better able to mount a faster and more effective response when they encounter antigen as a result of epigenetic modification (Chapter 17).

Studies of the adaptive immune response have shown that not only must the lymphoid cells cooperate to mount an effective immune response (Chapter 16), but also that any immune response takes place in a physiologic system of organs and tissues connected by the lymph and blood (Chapters 12 and 13). Lymphocytes recirculate throughout the body, homing to particular lymphoid organs and moving out of the blood into sites of infection as they respond to cytokines and other molecules released from or expressed on the cell surface of activated lymphoid and other cells, particularly APCs. Cell adhesion molecules (CAMs; Chapter 13) are especially important in the trafficking of lymphocytes—the constant patrolling, particularly of naive T lymphocytes, in search of antigen.

It is important to recall the following topics from these chapters:
- The roles of growth factors and colony-stimulating factors in developmental pathways
- The characteristics of the major lymphoid and myeloid cell types
- The cellular organization and major functions of the lymphoid organs
- The cell-cell interactions involved in generating effector B and T cells

Chapter 17 described immunologic memory and also pointed out the existence of mechanisms that maintain lymphocyte homeostasis. Unless there is a response to antigen, such as during an infection, the number of lymphocytes in a human is maintained within a relatively narrow range. Ordered pathways exist with which to generate new lymphocytes when they are required (see Chapters 12, 14, and 15), and pathways for lymphocyte death are ordered and regulated. Chapter 17 briefly describes the process of programmed cell death (apoptosis) and explains how this may be balanced by antiapoptotic molecules encoded by the so-called *death-inhibiting* family of *BCL* genes. This topic will be expanded on in Chapter 22. You should also recall the major differences between a primary and a secondary immune response and the changes that distinguish memory from naive lymphocytes.

Finally, it is important to understand the damage an unregulated immune system can do if it starts reacting to self antigens (causing autoimmunity) or environmental substances (causing allergy). Central and peripheral tolerance reduce the risk of reacting to self, and peripheral tolerance reduces the risk of reacting to harmless substances. Be sure you understand these three things: (1) the mechanisms of tolerance induction in B- and T-cell populations, (2) positive and negative selection mechanisms, and (3) central and peripheral tolerance.

■ INTEGRATED IMMUNE SYSTEM: CONNECTIONS BETWEEN ADAPTIVE AND INNATE RESPONSES

This chapter is a bridge between consideration of the adaptive response and the innate response, and it falls between a section of the book that is chiefly concerned with molecules and a section that presents a more system-wide treatment of immunology. The remainder of this chapter is designed to help the reader bridge that chasm.

The topic of connections between different aspects of the immune system is also central to the next section of the book, Section IV, which otherwise predominantly describes *innate immunity.*

As is developed more fully in the next section, an excellent example of the connection between the innate and adaptive systems is the role played by pattern recognition receptors (PRRs), such as the Toll-like receptors (TLRs; see Box 19.1), of the innate system. The concept of PRRs was introduced in Chapter 2 in connection with mannan-binding lectin (MBL) and the lectin pathway of complement activation. PRRs can bind to molecules that are shared among infectious microbes but are not found in vertebrates—for example, the complex carbohydrates called *mannans* found in the cell walls of yeasts and the lipopolysaccharide (LPS) cell wall components of gram-negative bacteria. LPS is an activator of the innate immune response through stimulation of macrophages (see Box 19.1). Targets such as LPS and mannan are typically found on several different species or even on several unrelated organisms. They are referred to as *pathogen-associated molecular patterns* (PAMPs). PRRs can also recognize other harmful processes not caused by infections, such as burns or other injuries. In these instances, PRRs recognize damage-associated molecular patterns (DAMPs).

Mammals use several PRRs for innate host defense reactions (Fig. 19.1). These can be located in the cell membrane or in the cytoplasm, or they can be in solution in the plasma. PRRs stimulate cells to undergo phagocytosis (Chapter 21) or to secrete antimicrobial peptides. When complement is activated, it can attack microbes directly and does not always need the help of other cells (Chapter 20). Polymorphisms in some pattern recognition molecules are thought to cause disease (see Box 19.2).

Cells of the innate immune system use PRRs to detect the presence of pathogens very soon after invasion. Innate immune system cells take action against the invading pathogen, such as by phagocytosing them or secreting antimicrobial peptides. In addition, when PRRs recognize infection, they also alert the adaptive immune system by sending a danger signal. The danger signal could be a cytokine—for example, interleukins (ILs) 12 or 17—or increased expression of a costimulatory or cellular adhesion molecule. These signals are critical for initiating the adaptive immune response because the adaptive immune system will not begin to respond to infection without a danger signal. This is one form of peripheral tolerance, and it is the coordinated action of the innate and adaptive immune responses that counters attacks by pathogens. The next section of the book describes the innate response in more detail.

  MCH II   Cytokine, chemokine, etc.   Complement (C′)   Signaling molecule

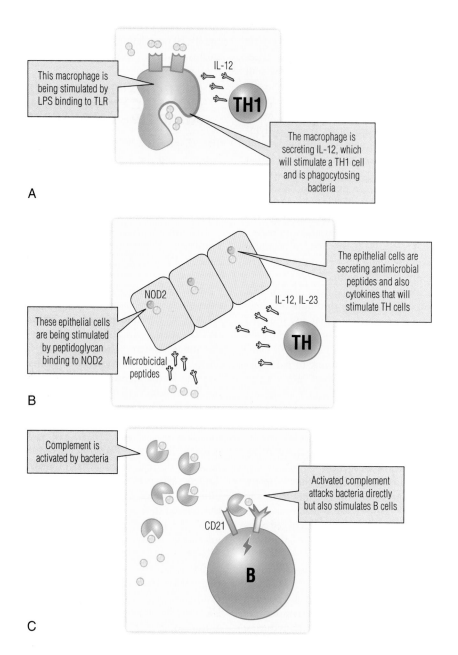

Fig 19.1 Pattern recognition molecules trigger actions from the innate immune system and also activate the adaptive immune system. These include Toll-like receptors (TLRs) (**A**), NOD2 (**B**), and complement (**C**) in solution in the plasma. *IL,* interleukin; *LPS,* lipopolysaccharide; *TH1,* T-helper 1.

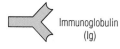 T-cell receptor (TCR)

Immunoglobulin (Ig)

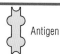 Antigen

 MCH I

BOX 19.1 Role of Toll-Like Receptors as a Link Between Innate and Adaptive Immune Systems

Certain pattern recognition receptors (PRRs) found on antigen-presenting cells (APCs) function as receptors for pathogen-associated molecular patterns (PAMPs) such as lipopolysaccharide (LPS) and transduce activation signals on binding these molecules (Fig. 19.2). LPS is a constituent of many bacterial cell walls. The activated APCs then send danger signals, such as via cytokines, that alert and activate lymphocytes. The PRRs that do this were identified as cell surface receptors after a search for mammalian equivalents of molecules called *Toll receptors,* which have critical roles in the immune systems of insects (Chapter 21). The fruit fly *Drosophila melanogaster* and other insects have well-characterized innate immune systems that confer resistance to microbial infections. A major aspect of host defense in *Drosophila* is the release of antimicrobial peptides. Humans possess molecules that are homologs of Toll: the family of molecules referred to as *Toll-like receptors* (TLRs). There are several different TLRs, each of which recognizes different PAMPs. Many human cell types express members of the family of TLRs. They function as PRRs and bind entities such as LPS. This LPS binding triggers the TLR, whereupon the cytoplasmic domain of the TLR initiates a signaling cascade that leads to activities such as phagocytosis (Chapter 21). The signaling also activates the transcription factor nuclear factor kappa B (NF-κB), which increases production of cytokines such as tumor necrosis factor alpha (TNF-α) interleukins (ILs) 1, 6, and 12; chemokines such as IL-8; and costimulatory molecules (see Fig. 19.1). The cytokines attract antigen-specific lymphocytes and bring the adaptive immune response into play.

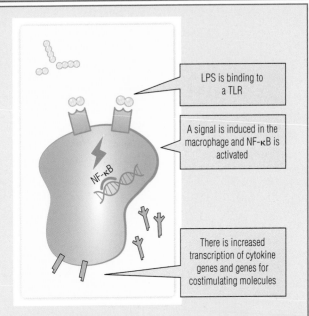

Fig 19.2 Toll-like receptors (TLRs) in activation of antigen-presenting cells (APCs) by microbes. *LPS,* lipopolysaccharide; *NF-κB,* nuclear factor kappa B.

Annotations in figure:
- LPS is binding to a TLR
- A signal is induced in the macrophage and NF-κB is activated
- There is increased transcription of cytokine genes and genes for costimulating molecules

BOX 19.2 Crohn Disease and *NOD2* Polymorphisms

A 27-year-old woman has a 1-year history of diarrhea, abdominal pain, and weight loss and has had some blood and mucus in her feces. Her brother was diagnosed with Crohn disease (CD) 2 years earlier. A colonoscopy is carried out, the results of which show some patchy ulceration in her colon and more extensive ulceration in the terminal ileum as far as the colonoscope can reach. A biopsy shows inflammation affecting the full thickness of the bowel suggestive of CD.

CD is a type of inflammatory bowel disease in which chronic inflammation in the bowel leads to ulceration. Evidence suggests that both T-helper 1 (TH1) and TH17 cells drive the inflammation.

Siblings of people with CD are 30 times more likely to develop CD themselves. The genetic basis appears to be due to the inheritance of polymorphisms in the *NOD2* gene. A polymorphism is a genetic variation that can be found in healthy people. The polymorphisms found in people with CD are found in healthy people but are much more common in people with CD.

In addition, not everyone with CD has inherited the polymorphisms, so they can only be one of several contributory factors to the development of CD.

NOD2 is a pattern recognition receptor (PRR) present in the cytoplasm of many different cell types, including gut epithelial cells. The ligand for NOD2 is peptidoglycan, which is found in many different bacterial cell walls. When NOD2 recognizes peptidoglycan, the cell is stimulated to secret antimicrobial peptides and cytokines, including interleukins (ILs) 23 and 12.

People who have inherited the *NOD2* polymorphisms seen in CD produce a NOD2 molecule that is less effective at binding peptidoglycan. This has led to the theory that individuals who inherit these *NOD2* polymorphisms are prone to bacterial infection of the gut, which then triggers CD. So far, it has not been possible to find evidence to support this theory. It remains just as likely that the abnormal NOD2 molecule triggers chronic inflammation through other means.

 MCH II

 Cytokine, chemokine, etc.

Complement (C')

 Signaling molecule

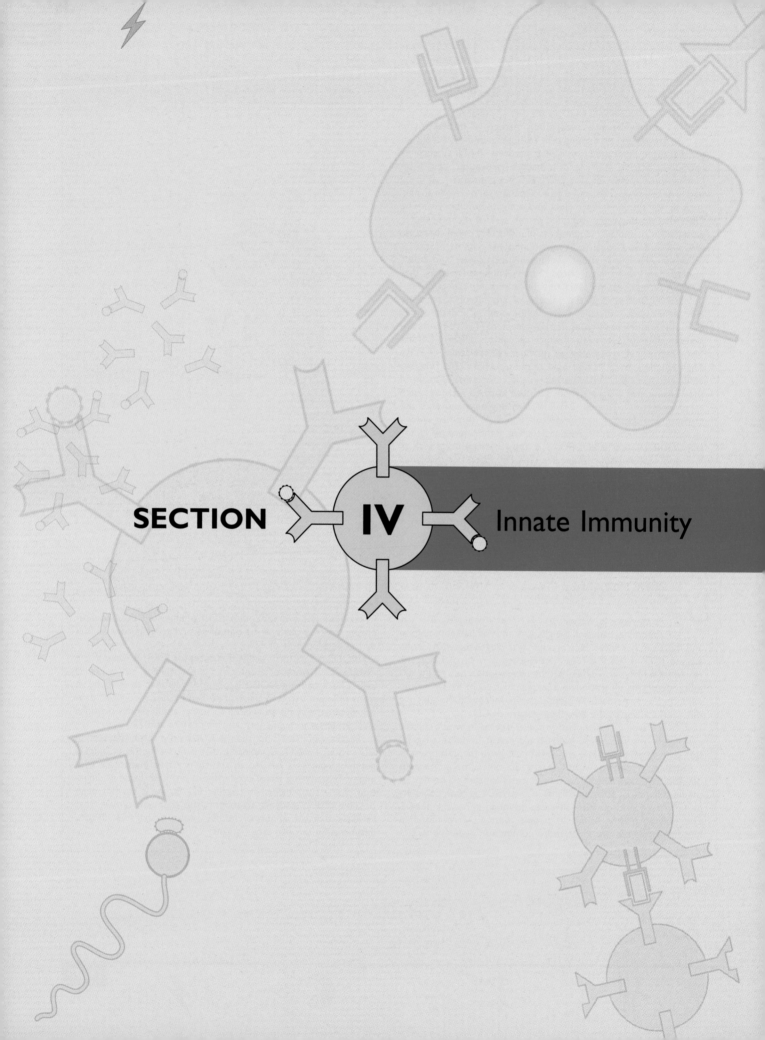

SECTION IV Innate Immunity

Constitutive Defenses Including Complement

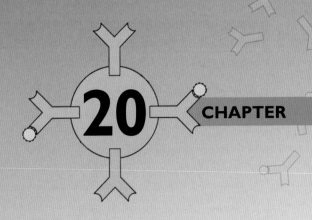

20 CHAPTER

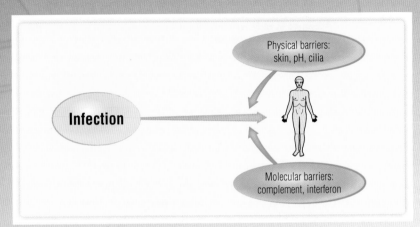

Infections that manage to break through the body's physical barriers activate the molecular barriers of innate immune system. Two of these are the interferons and the complement system.

The innate immune system is a series of nonspecific defenses that are in constant readiness to fight off infection. The innate system differs in a number of ways from the adaptive immune system (Table 20.1). The way the innate immune system operates and interacts with the adaptive system is dealt with in the next four chapters. The innate immune system has two key roles: (1) it uses pattern recognition receptors (PRRs) to recognize pathogen-associated molecular patterns (PAMPs) and responds rapidly to invading pathogens, and (2) it activates other parts of the immune system and tissues throughout the body. To do this, the innate immune system secretes cytokines and several other inflammatory mediators referred to as *danger signals*.

▨ BARRIERS TO INFECTION

The skin and the respiratory and gastrointestinal tracts have evolved as specialized barriers to infection.

Skin

Although many organisms live on the surface of the skin, the dense outer layer of dead keratinocytes prevents penetration of these organisms into deeper tissues. The deeper-layer living keratinocytes are active components in the innate immune system. These keratinocytes secrete cytokines such as interleukin

8 (IL-8) and tumor necrosis factor (TNF) if they are damaged in any way. Such cytokines are responsible for the inflammation that occurs after exposure to ultraviolet light, for example.

Skin also contains Langerhans cells, sentinel cells of the dendritic cell lineage. After exposure to microorganisms, these cells migrate to the local lymph node and present antigen to T cells.

The skin is typical of innate immune system components in its ability to respond rapidly to stimulation and activate and inform the adaptive immune response.

Respiratory Tract

From the point of view of the innate immune system, the respiratory tract is divisible into upper and lower segments. The upper airway begins at the nose and ends in the bronchioles and is protected by the mucociliary escalator. Mucus secreted by goblet cells forms a fine layer that lines the airway and traps microorganisms. Cilia waft the mucus toward the mouth and nose, where trapped organisms are cleared by sneezing or coughing. Mucus secretion is abnormal in cystic fibrosis, and cilia are defective in primary ciliary dyskinesia. Patients with these conditions have recurrent respiratory tract infections.

In the lower respiratory tract, in terminal bronchioles and alveoli, layers of cilia and mucus can obstruct oxygen diffusion. The main defenses here are surfactants secreted by specialized cells that line the alveoli, type II pneumocytes. Surfactants are a mixture of proteins and phospholipids that prevent alveoli from collapsing during expiration. Surfactant also contains

TABLE 20.1   Differences Between the Innate and Adaptive Immune Systems

Innate System	Adaptive System
Distinguishes danger from homeostasis	Distinguishes self from nonself
Preformed (constitutive) or rapidly formed components	Relies on genetic events and cellular growth
Response to infection occurs within minutes.	Response develops over days.
No specificity: The same molecules and cells respond to a range of pathogens.	Very specific: Each cell is genetically programmed to respond to a single antigen.
Uses pattern-recognition molecules	Uses antigen recognition molecules
Uses germlike genes to produce collectins (MBL, surfactant), complement, CRP, and TLR	Uses hypervariable regions in Ig and TCRs and genetic recombination to produce Ig and TCR
Probably fewer than 100 receptors exist.	Up to 10^{18} different receptors are possible.
Pattern-recognition molecules detect molecules unique to pathogens, such as lipopolysaccharide.	Conformational structures (Ig) or short peptides bound to MHC molecules (TCR) are recognized.
No memory: The response does not change after repeated exposure.	Immunologic memory: On repeated exposure, the response is faster, stronger, and qualitatively different.
The older system, seen in all members of the animal kingdom	Evolved in early vertebrate kingdom many millions of years after the innate immune system
Can recognize only molecules that signal infection or injury	Cannot distinguish host from pathogens
Rarely malfunctions	Frequently malfunctions and may cause autoimmunity

CRP, C-reactive protein; Ig, immunoglobulin; MBL, mannan-binding lectin; MHC, major histocompatibility complex; TCR, T-cell receptor; TLR, Toll-like receptor.

pathogen-binding proteins, which are members of the collectin family (Fig. 20.1). The collectins have globular lectin-like heads that can bind to sugars on microorganisms and long collagen-like tails that bind to phagocytes or complement. These molecules have a pattern recognition role.

Both segments of the respiratory tract are also reliant on immunoglobulins, as shown by the frequency of respiratory infections in patients with antibody deficiency.

Respiratory mucosa also responds to signals from the adaptive immune system. As you read in Chapter 16, IL-17 secreted by T-helper 17 (TH17) cells in response to extracellular pathogens stimulates the respiratory epithelium. On the other hand, during TH2 responses, IL-4 also stimulates the hyperplasia and secretion of mucus by goblet cells and hypertrophy of smooth muscle surrounding the airways. These effects of IL-4 evolved to deal with large pathogens such as worms, but in the developed world, they are more often seen in allergy.

Gastrointestinal Tract

The low pH of the stomach is one of the main defenses against infection of the gut. For example, patients who are unable to secret gastric acid have a high risk for *Salmonella* infection. The lower gut is colonized by trillions of bacteria, which are normally harmless and inhibit the growth of pathogenic bacteria. However, the gut epithelium also secretes transformation growth factor beta (TGF-β), as described in Chapter 18. Rather than defend against pathogenic bacteria, TGF-β induces T-regulatory cells (Tregs), which help the host immune system tolerate the presence of harmless commensal bacteria.

■ EXTRACELLULAR MOLECULES OF THE INNATE IMMUNE SYSTEM

The innate immune system relies on families of proteins that can provide a very rapid response to infection. The type I interferons (IFNs) are produced locally in response to infection and directly

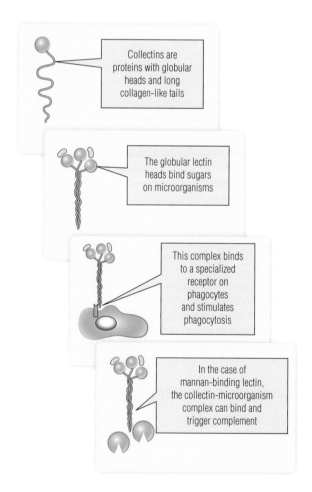

Fig 20.1 The collectin family includes surfactant proteins and mannan-binding lectin; both are important pattern-recognition receptors. C1q is a related protein. These proteins have both lectin-like and collagen-like domains. Lectins are sugar-binding proteins that can bind to microorganisms. The collagen-like domains bind to cellular receptors or activate complement.

 T-cell receptor (TCR)   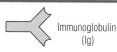 Immunoglobulin (Ig)   Antigen   MCH I inhibit the growth of pathogens. Collectins, complement, and C-reactive protein (CRP) are constitutively produced proteins, although they are found at higher levels during infections, and they bind onto pathogens.

Interferon

Interferons are so named because cells treated with interferon become resistant to viral infection; in other words, interferon *interferes* with viral replication. The antiviral effects are most potent with type I IFN (IFN-α and IFN-β) and less so with IFN-γ, the only type II interferon in humans. IFN-γ is more potent at activating the TH1 arm of the adaptive immune response than at inhibiting viral replication (Chapter 16).

- Type I IFNs are secreted by a wide range of cells at front-line tissues, such as epithelial cells lining the gut. Many cells produce IFNs in response to nonspecific injuries, such as trauma or radiation injury. However, the most efficient producers of type I IFNs are a type of antigen-presenting cell (APC) called *plasmacytoid dendritic cells,* which secrete IFNs in response to infection. These specialized APCs, described in Chapter 12, secrete type I IFNs in response to double-stranded RNA, which they recognize using a PRR called *Toll-like receptor 3* (Chapter 19). Double-stranded RNA is not present in mammalian cells but is produced by viruses during intracellular infection of cells. Double-stranded RNA is a good example of a PAMP; its presence indicates that viral infection is taking place, but it does not indicate the exact type of virus. Type I IFNs have a range of actions (Fig. 20.2).
- Type I IFNs inhibit viral replication by activation of two intracellular enzyme pathways that degrade the viral genome and inhibit transcription of viral messenger RNA (mRNA). This effect of type I IFNs works only on neighboring cells,

but it effectively inhibits viral replication. Such a short-range effect is described as a *paracrine action.*
- Type I IFNs stimulate activity of transporter associated with antigen presentation (TAP), peptide transporters, and proteasomes (Chapter 10) and increased expression of major histocompatibility complex (MHC) class I (Chapter 8); these increase the availability of peptides for binding to MHC class I and promote the effects of CD8⁺ T cells.
- Type I IFNs promote the development of TH1 cells (Chapter 15).
- Type I IFNs activate natural killer (NK) cells (Chapter 21).

Within hours of viral infection, type I IFN secretion is induced and inhibits viral replication, and it arms NK cells to destroy infected cells. Although IFNs improve antigen presentation on MHC class I, primary T-cell and antibody responses may take as long as a week to develop. Consequently, IFNs provide a rapid response that bridges the period required to initiate the innate immune response.

Recombinant IFN-α is used as a biopharmaceutical—also known as a *biologic medical product,* or *biologic*—to treat viral hepatitis, in combination with more conventional antiviral drugs. The benefits of IFN-α are mediated mainly by its antiviral effects and partly through stimulation of the adaptive immune system. Recombinant IFNs can be synthesized in high quantities in mammalian cells. Unlike the conventional antiviral drugs, IFN-α has to be given by injection, it causes side effects, and, because it is a protein molecule, it can eventually be stopped by neutralizing antibodies. Some of the clinical side effects and manufacturing problems of biopharmaceuticals are discussed in Chapter 36.

IFN-α has also been used to treat malignancies, most often chronic myeloid leukemia. The exact mode of action is unclear, although IFN seems to induce either apoptosis or maturation of malignant cells.

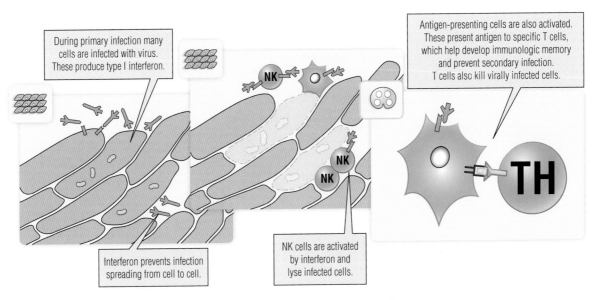

During primary infection many cells are infected with virus. These produce type I interferon.

Antigen-presenting cells are also activated. These present antigen to specific T cells, which help develop immunologic memory and prevent secondary infection. T cells also kill virally infected cells.

Interferon prevents infection spreading from cell to cell.

NK cells are activated by interferon and lyse infected cells.

Fig 20.2 Interferons include alpha, beta, and gamma forms. Interferon gamma has more potent immunostimulatory effects and less potent direct effects on viral replication. *NK,* natural killer; *TH,* T helper.

 MCH II

  Cytokine, chemokine, etc.

 Complement (C′)

 Signaling molecule

During infections, macrophages and other innate immune system cells secrete other cytokines such as IL-1, IL-6, and TNF. These cytokines activate the specific immune system and cause the acute-phase response (see Box 20.1).

Complement

Although a large number of complement components exist, the overall system is simple and easy to understand. There are nine basic complement components, numbered C1 to C9. When they become activated, complement components are split into small and large fragments; the *small fragments* are referred to as *C3a, C4a,* and so on. A simple way of remembering an overview of complement is that three different activators detect pathogens and activate a key component, C3, which is required to switch on three different types of effector molecules (Fig. 20.3).

Complement can be activated by interactions between antibody and antigen. Complement facilitates the effects of antibody and is so named because antibody alone will not kill most bacteria; these molecules are required to *complement* the bactericidal effects of antibody.

Activation of Complement

The complement C3 can be activated in three pathways (Fig. 20.4): (1) the lectin pathway, (2) the classical pathway, and (3) the alternative pathway.

Lectin Pathway

Mannan-binding lectin (MBL) is a collectin that is able to bind, through its lectin portions, onto carbohydrates present on bacteria. Although MBL has no enzyme activity of its own, after

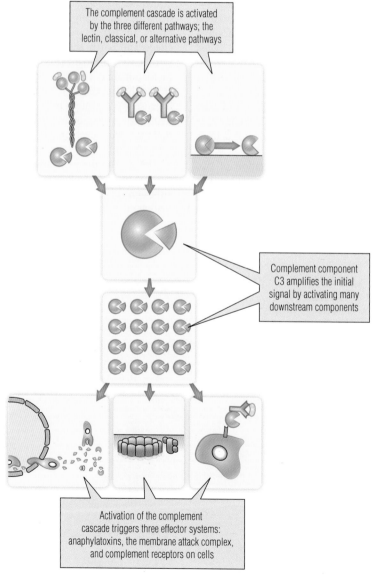

The complement cascade is activated by the three different pathways; the lectin, classical, or alternative pathways

Complement component C3 amplifies the initial signal by activating many downstream components

Activation of the complement cascade triggers three effector systems: anaphylatoxins, the membrane attack complex, and complement receptors on cells

Fig 20.3 An overview of the complement cascade.

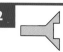 T-cell receptor (TCR)

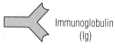 Immunoglobulin (Ig)

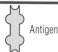 Antigen

 MCH I

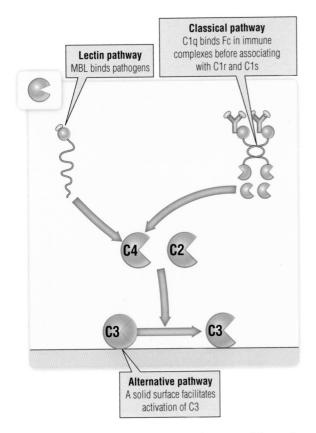

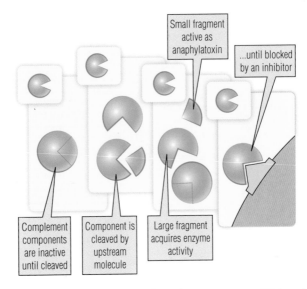

Fig 20.4 Activation of C3 can take place through any one of three pathways. *MBL,* mannan-binding lectin.

Fig 20.5 After cleavage, fragments of complement components C2 through C6 acquire enzyme activity and activate downstream components.

the lectin portions bind to bacteria, the MBL collagen-like domain indirectly activates the next complement components, C2 and C4, which together activate several hundred C3 molecules.

Classical Pathway

The classical pathway is so named because it was discovered first, although it was probably the last to evolve. This pathway is triggered by immune complexes of antibody and antigen. C1 is the initiating protein, and it is able to recognize the Fc portion of immunoglobulin (Ig) molecules when sufficient Fc portions are in sufficiently close proximity. This is most likely to occur when an antigen binds several Ig molecules. Because it has five Fc portions, IgM is particularly good at C1 binding. C1 also has no enzyme activity, but after binding to an Fc, it is able to activate C2 and C4, which in turn activate multiple C3 molecules.

Alternative Pathway

C3 is not a stable molecule, and it is constantly undergoing spontaneous low-level activation, which is most likely to happen on cell surfaces. Normal cells express surface complement inhibitors that prevent spontaneous C3 activation (see Fig. 20.10). The surfaces of pathogens lack complement inhibitors, so the spontaneous activation of C3 can go ahead. People who have mutations in these membrane-bound complement inhibitors develop atypical hemolytic uremic syndrome. They have

uncontrolled activation of C3 on the surface of their endothelial cells and platelets, which causes widespread thrombus formation throughout the body.

The early part of the complement system can also detect cells dying as a result of necrosis, usually secondary to physical or metabolic damage. Cell death from necrosis is an uncontrolled process, and dying cells appear to leak several types of molecules that are able to activate the complement cascade. In this way, some inflammation is a consequence of any type of damage done to tissues. Another type of cell death—programmed cell death, also known as *apoptosis*—is described in Chapter 22. This process is strictly controlled and does not activate complement in the same way as necrosis. Inflammation is thus not a consequence of apoptosis.

Summary of Complement Activation

The alternative pathway activates complement on the surface of any cell that lacks complement inhibitors, whereas the lectin and classical pathways provide focused complement activation to molecules that have been bound by MBL or antibody.

Amplification Steps

Each complement component is constantly present in blood and on activation becomes capable of activating several downstream components. Complement activators are sensitive to small stimuli, such as very few bacteria, and the subsequent amplification steps ensure a dramatic, but usually local, response. This is obtained through the enzyme activity of complement components throughout the complement cascade: C2, C3, C4, C5, and C6. These molecules are activated by cleavage into small and large fragments (Fig. 20.5). The large fragments may become enzymes themselves and may cleave and activate the next molecule in the cascade. These fragments may also interact with inhibitors that switch off the amplification steps.

 MCH II

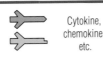 Cytokine, chemokine, etc.

 Complement (C′)

 Signaling molecule

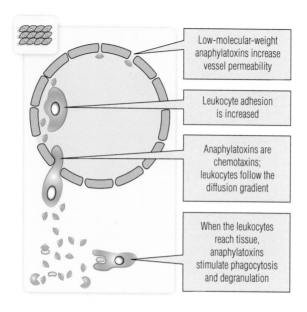

Low-molecular-weight anaphylatoxins increase vessel permeability

Leukocyte adhesion is increased

Anaphylatoxins are chemotaxins; leukocytes follow the diffusion gradient

When the leukocytes reach tissue, anaphylatoxins stimulate phagocytosis and degranulation

Fig 20.6 Anaphylatoxins.

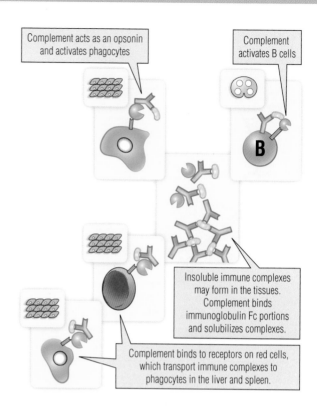

Complement acts as an opsonin and activates phagocytes

Complement activates B cells

Insoluble immune complexes may form in the tissues. Complement binds immunoglobulin Fc portions and solubilizes complexes.

Complement binds to receptors on red cells, which transport immune complexes to phagocytes in the liver and spleen.

Fig 20.7 Complement receptors.

The small fragments of C3 and C5 have biologic activity and are known as *anaphylatoxins*, which are discussed in later sections.

Complement Effectors

Activation of complement produces a number of effector molecules: the anaphylatoxins, complement fragments that bind and activate complement receptors, and the membrane attack complex (MAC).

Anaphylatoxins

The activation of complement components C3 and C5 produces small fragments C3a and C5a. Because they have a low molecular weight, these peptides diffuse away from the site of complement activation and cause the effects shown in Figure 20.6. The C2a low-molecular-weight peptide is cleaved to produce a small kinin, which has marked effects on making endothelial cells contract, which increases vascular permeability.

Complement Receptors

Several complement receptors (CRs) are present on a variety of cells; these bind early complement components (MBL, C1, and activated C4 and C3). CRs serve the following functions (Fig. 20.7):

- *Opsonization.* This is the process by which bacteria and other cells are made available for phagocytosis. Molecules that help to bind pathogens to phagocytes and stimulate phagocytosis are known as *opsonins.* Because so much activated C3 is produced during complement activation, it is the most important opsonin and binds to three different receptors present on a range of phagocytes. IgG can also act as an opsonin when it binds to Fc receptors on phagocytes. Because phagocytes do not have Fc receptors for IgM,

complement-mediated opsonization is particularly important during a primary antibody response, when an IgM response dominates.
- *B-cell stimulation.* Binding of C3 to the CR2 receptor on B cells provides costimulation and decreases the threshold for B-cell activation a thousandfold (see Table 20.1, Chapter 11). Hence, complement binding to antigen promotes the production of antibody. CR2 has been subverted by the Epstein-Barr virus (Chapter 34), which uses it as its receptor.
- *Immune complex clearance.* Immune complexes are insoluble lattices of antigen bound to antibody that can form in tissues or in the blood. These trigger inflammation, and immune-complex disease (Chapter 30) will occur if they are not removed. Complement helps to remove immune complexes in two ways:
  - Large insoluble complexes are particularly difficult to remove from tissues; high numbers of activated C3 interrupt the lattice of the immune complex, making them soluble.
  - C4 and C3 present in solubilized immune complexes can bind to complement receptor CR1 on red cells, which transport the immune complexes to organs rich in fixed phagocytes, such as the liver and spleen. Using their own complement and Fc receptors, these phagocytes remove the immune complexes from the red cells and then phagocytose and destroy the immune complexes. The red cells are not harmed by this process.

Patients with complement deficiency are at high risk for disease caused by immune complexes, such as systemic lupus erythematosus (SLE; see Box 20.2).

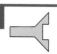 T-cell receptor (TCR)

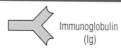 Immunoglobulin (Ig)

 Antigen

 MCH I

Membrane Attack Complex

Activated C3 activates the final part of the cascade of complement components C5 through C9. These components form the MAC. C5 and C6 have enzyme activity, which allows components C7, C8, and C9 to insert themselves into the plasma membrane of the target cell. A group of 10 to 16 molecules of C9 form a ring, which creates a pore in the plasma membrane (Fig. 20.8). This allows free passage of water and solutes across the membrane, killing the cell. The MAC attacks pathogens directly but in humans appears to be crucial only for defenses against *Neisseria* (see Box 20.2). Figure 20.9 summarizes how complement is involved in the response to bacterial infection.

Complement Inhibitors

Complement tends to undergo spontaneous activation, especially by the alternative pathway. Excessive complement activation is undesirable because it causes inflammation and widespread cell death. To prevent inadvertent complement activation, complement inhibitors exist. Their site of action is shown in Figure 20.10.

The importance of these inhibitors is indicated by the fact that deficiency can lead to illness. Atypical hemolytic uremic syndrome has already been described. In hereditary angioedema, a mutation in the C1 inhibitor has dramatic effects (see Box 20.3).

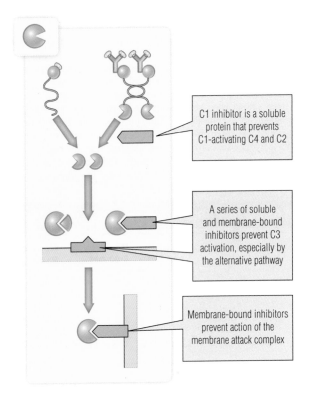

C1 inhibitor is a soluble protein that prevents C1-activating C4 and C2

A series of soluble and membrane-bound inhibitors prevent C3 activation, especially by the alternative pathway

Membrane-bound inhibitors prevent action of the membrane attack complex

Fig 20.10 Complement inhibitors.

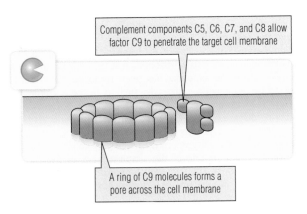

Complement components C5, C6, C7, and C8 allow factor C9 to penetrate the target cell membrane

A ring of C9 molecules forms a pore across the cell membrane

Fig 20.8 The ring of C9 molecules forming a pore in the attacked cell is very similar to perforin, a substance produced by natural killer cells.

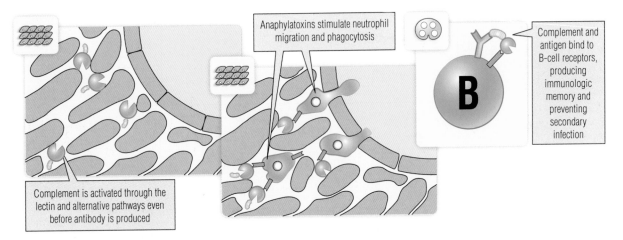

Anaphylatoxins stimulate neutrophil migration and phagocytosis

Complement and antigen bind to B-cell receptors, producing immunologic memory and preventing secondary infection

Complement is activated through the lectin and alternative pathways even before antibody is produced

Fig 20.9 Complement is particularly important in dealing with bacterial infections, and some parallels are found in the ways by which interferons inhibit viral infections. Both complement and interferon can directly attack pathogens, and each recruits different cells in the innate and adaptive immune response.

 MCH II

 Cytokine, chemokine, etc.

 Complement (C')

 Signaling molecule

BOX 20.1 Acute-Phase Response

An 11-year-old girl presents at the emergency department late at night because of a 12-hour history of abdominal pain and vomiting. On examination, her temperature and pulse are normal (Fig. 20.11), and the only sign in the abdomen is some tenderness in the right iliac fossa. The attending surgeon orders some blood tests, the results of which are shown in Table 20.2. He thinks appendicitis is possible but not certain. In any case, the girl has eaten in the past few hours, and a general anesthetic would not be safe. The patient is kept on the observation ward overnight.

The following morning, her temperature and pulse are up slightly, and the nurses ask the surgeon to review the patient. Tenderness is still the only sign in the abdomen, but repeat blood tests show an elevated neutrophil count, raised C-reactive protein (CRP), and a raised erythrocyte sedimentation rate (ESR). These are all characteristics of an acute-phase response, which is often used clinically to distinguish inflammation from other types of clinical problems. In this case, the presence of an acute-phase response convinces the surgeon that he needs to do a laparotomy, during which he finds and removes an inflamed appendix. The girl recovers over the next few days.

The acute-phase response is triggered by the release of interleukin 1 (IL-1), IL-6, and tumor necrosis factor (TNF) from macrophages. These have a direct effect on the hypothalamus (Fig. 20.12) and increase the body temperature, which impairs pathogen reproduction. This effect is mediated by these cytokines, which induce the synthesis of prostaglandin in the hypothalamus. Aspirin can block prostaglandin synthesis and can prevent fever. IL-1, IL-6, and TNF also stimulate the production of a series of proteins by the liver:

- Innate immune system molecules: C3, C4, and CRP
- Damage-limiting proteins: α1-antitrypsin, haptoglobin
- Clotting factors: fibrinogen

Granulocyte-colony stimulating factor (G-CSF) produced during the acute-phase response leads to a rapid increase in the production of neutrophils in the bone marrow. The acute-phase cytokines also contribute to a general activation of the adaptive immune response, which leads to an increase in the production of polyclonal immunoglobulins.

CRP is a protein produced in the liver that binds to phospholipids on the surface of bacteria such as pneumococcus. CRP then acts as an opsonin, stimulating phagocytosis. CRP also activates the complement system through the lectin pathway, and CRP production increases dramatically during inflammation through the actions of TNF and is a particularly good indicator of inflammation. For example, CRP levels are increased up to a thousandfold in acute inflammation, such as appendicitis, and they fall rapidly after the appendix has been removed. CRP is also increased by noninfectious diseases, such as in the autoimmune disease rheumatoid arthritis—and it provides a good way of monitoring disease activity and response to treatment.

The increased synthesis of the proteins mentioned above increases plasma viscosity, which is reflected by an increased ESR. Measuring the ESR is one of the simplest ways of showing an acute-phase response. The ESR takes longer than CRP to become abnormal during an inflammatory response.

TABLE 20.2 Blood Test Results

	Day 1, 12:00 AM	Day 2, 8:00 AM	Normal Range
Erythrocyte sedimentation rate	12	38	<7
C-reactive protein	4	122	<12
Neutrophil count	5.1×10^3/mL	13.4×10^3/mL	$3-6 \times 10^3$/mL

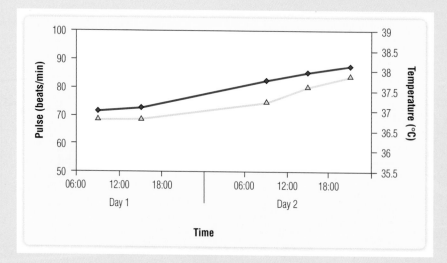

Fig 20.11 This chart shows the vital signs for the patient. Blue diamonds represent the pulse, and the yellow triangles show temperature.

 T-cell receptor (TCR)

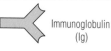 Immunoglobulin (Ig)

 Antigen

 MCH I

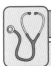

BOX 20.1 Acute-Phase Response—cont'd

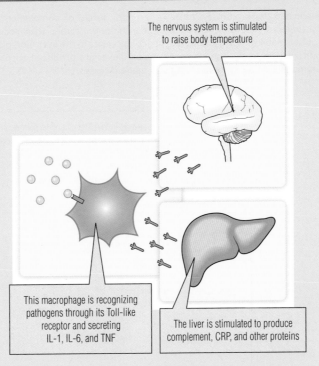

The nervous system is stimulated to raise body temperature

This macrophage is recognizing pathogens through its Toll-like receptor and secreting IL-1, IL-6, and TNF

The liver is stimulated to produce complement, CRP, and other proteins

Fig 20.12 The acute-phase response has widespread effects throughout the body. *CRP,* C-reactive protein; *IL,* interleukin; *TNF,* tumor necrosis factor.

BOX 20.2 Complement Deficiency

A 16-year-old boy presents at the emergency department with severe headache. He is found to be feverish (with a fever of 39.2° C; normal is below 37.0° C) and has marked neck stiffness. The attending doctor thinks he might have meningitis and orders blood cultures and a lumbar puncture. The cerebrospinal fluid (CSF) should be clear, but in this case, it is slightly cloudy. Examination of the CSF shows dramatically increased numbers of neutrophils, some of which contain diplococci (Fig. 20.13). The doctor starts the patient on intravenous broad-spectrum antibiotics, and the boy improves over the next few hours. The following day, culture of the CSF sample confirms infection with *Neisseria meningitidis.*

When the doctor talks to the patient's parents the next day, he finds that two of the boy's siblings have also had *N. meningitidis* infection. This type of family history is typical of hereditary complement deficiency. Further tests confirm deficiency of C8 in the patient and his two affected brothers.

Deficiencies of complement components cause recurrent bacterial infection, partly because the innate immune system clears opsonized bacteria and partly because complement is involved in initiating antibody production (Fig. 20.14). Deficiencies of the membrane attack complex (MAC) lead to a specific higher risk for infection with *Neisseria* species, as in this case. It is currently not known why people with MAC deficiencies are several

thousand times more likely than the general population to get *Neisseria* infection.

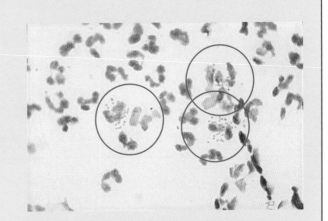

Fig 20.13 Gram stain of the cerebrospinal fluid (CSF) taken from the patient. Normal CSF contains fewer neutrophils. In addition, three neutrophils in this image have phagocytosed *Neisseria meningitidis.* The neutrophils with phagocytosed *Neisseria* are highlighted.

Continued

 MCH II

 Cytokine, chemokine, etc.

 Complement (C')

 Signaling molecule

BOX 20.2 Complement Deficiency—cont'd

Deficiencies in the early lectin and classic pathways cause type III hypersensitivity (immune complex disease) because immune complexes cannot be solubilized or transported to phagocytes (Chapter 30). Deficiency of early complement components can cause the autoimmune disease systemic lupus erythematosus (SLE).

Low levels of complement are more usually the result of consumption, rather than reduced production, of complement components in the liver. Complement is consumed when immune complexes are produced, such as during infections or in autoimmune diseases.

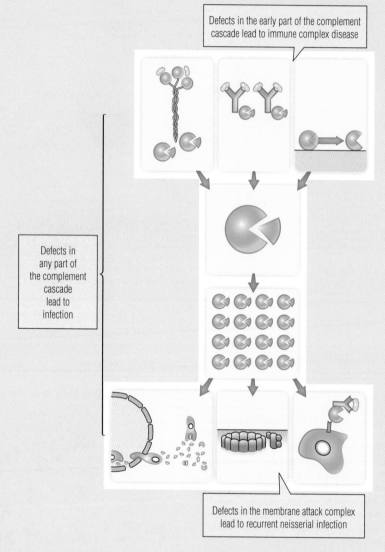

Defects in the early part of the complement cascade lead to immune complex disease

Defects in any part of the complement cascade lead to infection

Defects in the membrane attack complex lead to recurrent neisserial infection

Fig 20.14 The clinical features of complement deficiency depend on exactly which components are defective.

 T-cell receptor (TCR)

Immunoglobulin (Ig)

 Antigen

 MCH I

BOX 20.3 Hereditary Angioedema

A 20-year-old man has had several bouts of facial swelling and unexplained severe abdominal pain throughout his life (Fig. 20.15). During one such bout, his complement C4 level was determined to be low, although C3 is normal. A sample is analyzed for levels of C1 inhibitor, which is found to be very low. A diagnosis of hereditary angioedema is made, and on this occasion he is treated with purified C1 inhibitor. His swelling subsides over a few hours.

Hereditary angioedema is an autosomal-dominant disease caused by deficiency of C1 inhibitor, which is a member of a plasma protein family called *serpins*—serine protease inhibitors. The deficiency of C1 inhibitor means that the early complement cascade is very easily activated. The activation of the complement cascade is halted at the level of C3 because an appropriate surface for complement activation is missing. C4 and C2 are cleaved in the activation, and excessive amounts of the C2a kinin are produced. C1 inhibitor also normally inhibits the production of another kinin, bradykinin, from kininogen. In patients with hereditary angioedema, activation of the complement and kinin cascades by minor triggers—such as trauma, infection, or even psychological stress—cannot be inhibited by C1 inhibitor. The result is excessive amounts of C2a kinin and bradykinin production that leads to increased capillary permeability at any site, causing swelling that is painful and sometimes life threatening.

Purified C1 inhibitor can prevent and treat attacks of hereditary angioedema. An alternative is to give anabolic steroids, which increase C1 inhibitor levels.

Another important serpin is α1-antitrypsin, which normally releases proteases released by phagocytes. Patients who inherit genes for abnormal α1-antitrypsin develop emphysema (lung destruction caused by the unopposed action of proteolytic enzymes) and liver disease (caused by the accumulation of abnormal α1-antitrypsin molecules).

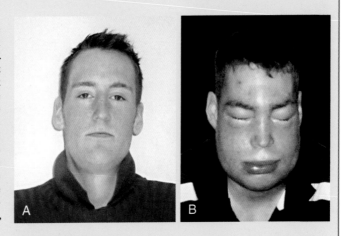

Fig 20.15 The patient as he normally appears and how he appears during an attack of angioedema. (From Helbert M. *Flesh and Bones Immunology.* Edinburgh: Mosby; 2006.)

LEARNING POINTS Can You Now …

1. List the differences between the innate and adaptive immune response?

2. Explain how interferons work and give two examples of how they are used as treatments?

3. Draw a diagram of the complement system?

4. List two consequences of complement deficiencies?

5. Describe how the acute-phase response can best be measured?

 MCH II

 Cytokine, chemokine, etc.

 Complement (C′)

 Signaling molecule

21 Phagocytes

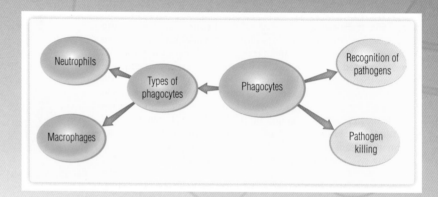

This chapter discusses the next component of the innate immune system, phagocytes, including the differences between the two types of phagocytes, neutrophils and macrophages, and how they recognize and kill pathogens.

Phagocytosis is the internalization of particulate matter by cells into cytoplasmic vesicles and is triggered when phagocytes recognize pathogens. Phagocytes contain lysosomes, granules that contain enzymes that fuse with the vesicles and degrade the particulate matter. In addition, activation of a cascade of phagocyte enzymes leads to the production of toxic molecules, the *oxidative burst,* which is necessary to kill phagocytosed organisms. Phagocytes are therefore mainly concerned with clearing small extracellular pathogens such as bacteria, protozoa, fungi, and cellular debris. A second important role is that phagocytes can also produce cytokines and cell-surface molecules, which alert the adaptive immune system to the presence of infection.

■ PHAGOCYTIC CELL TYPES

Phagocytes are bone marrow–derived (myeloid) cells. A range of phagocytic cells have evolved in humans, and each has specific functions.

Neutrophils

Neutrophils have a distinctive, recognizable morphology (Fig. 21.1). The numbers of neutrophils in the blood vary considerably (see Fig. 21.1A). During homeostasis, neutrophils are produced each day but do not survive more than a few hours. During infection, production of neutrophils is increased, and the numbers in blood go up (see Box 20.1). During infection, neutrophils migrate rapidly to sites of infection, where they kill pathogens. Even when neutrophils successfully kill pathogens, they do not survive. Pus formed at the site of infection is largely composed of dead neutrophils. Neutrophils play a crucial role in early defenses against bacterial infections; consequently, patients with defective neutrophils or low levels of neutrophils (neutropenia) are at particular risk for serious bacterial infection (see Box 21.1).

Monocytes/Macrophages

Monocytes (see Fig. 21.1B) are also myeloid cells but are very different from neutrophils (Table 21.1). Monocytes in the blood are immature cells migrating to their site of activity. Monocytes migrate into tissues where they mature into macrophages (see Fig. 21.1C) and take on a number of specialized forms (Fig. 21.2). All macrophage forms have long life spans and survive in the tissue for months or years.

Tissue Macrophages

Tissue macrophages are large cells with specialized granules and cytoplasmic compartments that are found in a wide range of sites. In some tissues, such as bone marrow and lymph nodes, these active macrophages are referred to as *histiocytes.*

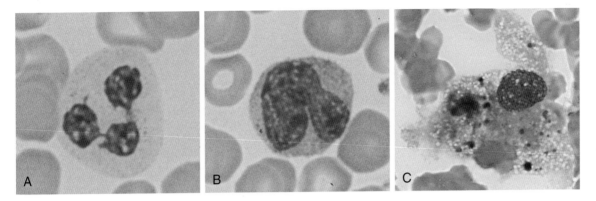

Fig 21.1 Phagocytic cells. **A,** Neutrophils have a distinct appearance because of their multilobed nucleus and their granules, which contain proteolytic enzymes. They can easily be counted by automated instruments when the acute-phase response is being measured. **B,** Monocytes are immature macrophages that have a much more distinctive appearance (**C**).

TABLE 21.1 Comparison of Neutrophils and Macrophages

	Neutrophils	Monocytes/Macrophages
Life cycle	Highly variable production, increase in infection Blood levels vary, increase in infection Migrate only into inflamed tissue Die a few hours after migrating into tissue and encountering pathogen Single mature form	Produced at a steady level Blood levels steady Migrate into tissue when no inflammation is present May survive many years after encountering pathogen Various mature forms depending on tissue
Killing of pathogens	Phagocytosis Kill pathogens using toxic molecules and enzymes Produce NETs	Phagocytosis Kill pathogens using toxic molecules and enzymes Do not produce NETs
Communication with other parts of the immune system	Short-lived secretion of chemokines recruits more neutrophils to the site of inflammation Respond to IL-17 from the adaptive immune system Do not provide many signals to the adaptive immune system	Recruit neutrophils to the site of inflammation by secreting IL-8, TNF, and IL-1 Respond to IFN-γ from the adaptive immune system Stimulate the adaptive immune system by presenting processed antigen, providing costimulation, and secreting cytokines such as IL-12 and TNF

IFN, interferon; IL, interleukin; NETs, neutrophil extracellular traps; TNF, tumor necrosis factor.

Giant and Epithelioid Cells

In sites of chronic inflammation, macrophages undergo further maturation and become multinucleated giant cells or epithelioid cells under the influence of T-cell cytokines. Epithelioid and giant cells are characteristic of granuloma formation (Chapter 23) and participate in prolonging the inflammatory response by presenting antigen to T cells and by secreting cytokines. Unlike neutrophils, macrophages live for many years, and pus is not formed during this type of inflammation.

Fixed Macrophages

These specialized phagocytes line sinusoids in the spleen and liver. In the liver, these macrophages are referred to as *Kupffer cells*. Their role is to phagocytose circulating particulate matter and, in some situations, to phagocytose entire cells (see *hemolytic anemia* in Chapter 29).

Alveolar Macrophages

Alveolar macrophages contribute to the lung's innate defenses. They are involved in disease processes such as chronic obstructive pulmonary disease (COPD).

Glial Cells

Glial cells are long-lived macrophages resident in the nervous system. They are involved in clearing dead neuronal cells.

Osteoclasts

The most specialized macrophages are the osteoclasts in bone, which participate in regulating calcium metabolism by resorbing bone and releasing calcium into the blood.

 MCH II

  Cytokine, chemokine, etc.

 Complement (C')

 Signaling molecule

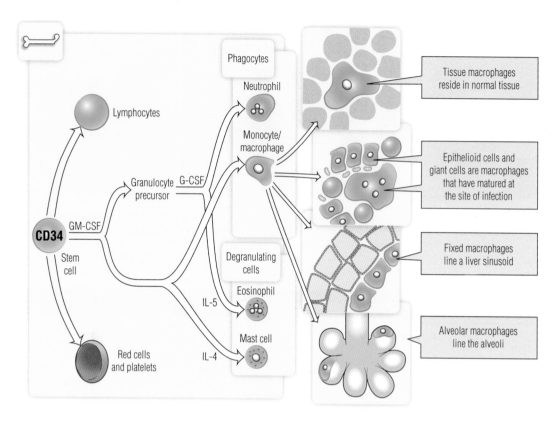

Fig 21.2 Neutrophil production is increased during the acute-phase response by granulocyte colony-stimulating factor (G-CSF). Macrophages are produced constantly at low levels and develop into specialized types in different tissues. *GM-CSF,* granulocyte-macrophage colony-stimulating factor (Chapter 12); *IL,* interleukin.

PHAGOCYTE PRODUCTION

Neutrophils and monocytes are produced from the same stem cells in the bone marrow (see Fig. 21.2 and Chapter 12). Many more neutrophils than monocytes are produced each day. This rapid production is especially vulnerable to the effects of cytotoxic drugs, which can give rise to neutropenia and vulnerability to infection (see Box 21.1). Production of these cells is stimulated by colony-stimulating factors (CSFs), which are produced by tissue macrophages as part of an acute-phase response. CSFs ensure that neutrophils are produced in increasing numbers during infection. Recombinant granulocyte CSF (filgrastim, lenograstim) can be used to boost neutrophil numbers, such as after stem cell transplant.

PHAGOCYTE RECRUITMENT

Monocytes constantly migrate into healthy tissue and differentiate into the specialized macrophages previously mentioned. Macrophages remain in a resting state unless they are stimulated by signals binding to their receptors, described later.

Although neutrophils make up the majority of phagocytes circulating in the blood, they are absent from normal tissues and will migrate only into inflamed tissue (Fig. 21.3). Neutrophils are recruited to sites of inflammation by interleukin 17 (IL-17) secreted by T-helper 17 (TH17) cells and by cytokines and chemokines secreted by resident macrophages. For example,

cytokines produced by local macrophages stimulate endothelial cells in local capillaries to increase expression of P-selectin and integrins such as intercellular adhesion molecules (ICAMs), which then attract neutrophils in a fashion similar to that described for lymphocytes in Chapter 13.

Chemokines are low-molecular-weight chemotactic cytokines that direct cells to specific sites; a dozen or so chemokines and a similar number of chemokine receptors exist. Macrophages at the site of infection secrete chemokines such as IL-8. These modify neutrophil integrins to make the neutrophils more adherent, which allows them to bind to endothelium and undergo *diapedesis* (passage through intact vessel walls into tissues) (Chapter 13). The final chemokine-mediated step is *chemotaxis,* the directional migration of cells along a gradient of chemokines. The net result of chemokine secretion is the attraction of neutrophils into tissues. Interestingly, the same chemokines that attract neutrophils into inflamed tissue stimulate the departure of local dendritic cells for lymph nodes to stimulate the adaptive immune system.

Anaphylatoxins (Chapter 20) produced by activation of the complement cascade are also chemotactic for phagocytes.

To summarize, resident macrophages at the site of infection secrete cytokines and chemokines, which stimulate neutrophil production, neutrophil and endothelium expression of selectins and integrins, neutrophil adherence to endothelium in local vessels, and, finally, chemotaxis to the site of infection. TH17 cells at the site of infection support this role by secreting IL-17.

 T-cell receptor (TCR)

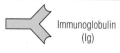 Immunoglobulin (Ig)

 Antigen

 MCH I

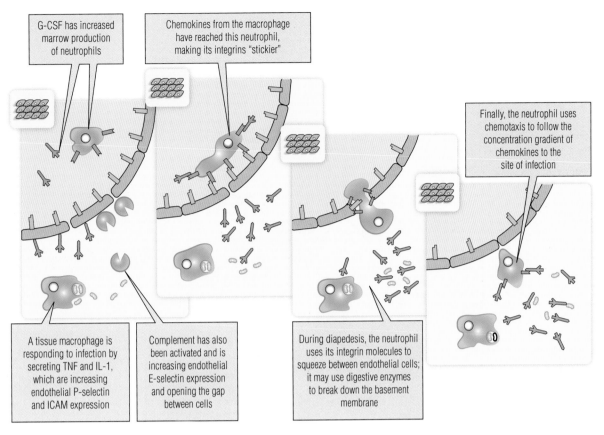

Fig 21.3 Neutrophil migration. *G-CSF,* granulocyte colony-stimulating factor; *ICAM,* intercellular adhesion molecule; *IL-1,* interleukin 1; *TNF,* tumor necrosis factor.

■ RECEPTORS ON PHAGOCYTES

Phagocytes use a variety of receptors on their cell membranes during their journey through the tissues and in their encounters with pathogens or damaged cells (Fig. 21.4).
- Receptors for chemokines and cytokines direct phagocytes to the site of inflammation and, once there, prepare them for action.
- Phagocytes use at least two different types of pattern recognition receptors to recognize pathogen- and damage-associated molecular patterns.

■ MOLECULAR PATTERNS

Toll-Like Receptors

Toll-like receptors (TLRs; Chapter 19) are a family of at least 10 different membrane molecules, each of which recognizes different classes of pathogen molecules, as shown in Table 21.2. The different TLRs have overlapping roles, and it is likely that several different receptors would be triggered by any given infection. TLRs are found on macrophages and other antigen-presenting cells (APCs) such as dendritic cells and B cells—as well as other cells, such as epithelial cells—that have a role in recognizing infection. On binding to the pathogen molecule, TLRs initiate an intracellular signal that leads to cytokine

TABLE 21.2 Toll-Like Receptors and Their Ligands

TLR	Expressed on	Ligand	Associated Pathogen
TLR-2	Widespread	Sugars and lipoproteins	A wide range of bacteria
TLR-3	Dendritic cells, epithelial cells	Double-stranded RNA	Viruses
TLR-4	Macrophages	LPS (TLR-4 forms a complex with CD14)	Gram-negative bacteria
TLR-5	Macrophages	Flagellae	Wide range of motile bacteria
TLR-7	Dendritic cells, macrophages	Single-stranded RNA	Viruses
TLR-9	Dendritic cells, B cells	Unmethylated cytosine and guanine sequences (CpG)	Bacteria

LPS, *lipopolysaccharide;* TLR, *Toll-like receptor.*

 MCH II   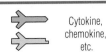 Cytokine, chemokine, etc.   Complement (C′)   Signaling molecule

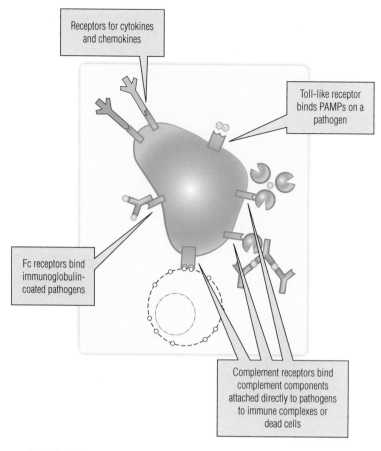

Fig 21.4 Phagocyte receptors. *PAMPs,* pathogen-associated molecular patterns.

production. The TLRs have such potent effects that they may have considerable roles as targets for drugs, as described in Box 21.2 at the end of this chapter.

C-Lectin Receptors

Lectins are sugar-binding proteins. The sugars are recognized by C-lectin receptors as sequences on glycolipids or glycoproteins on pathogen cell surfaces or dying mammalian cells. Binding of C-lectin receptors activates the macrophages that lead to cytokines production. They also firmly bind pathogens. In this way, the C-lectin receptors capture pathogens and deliver them to endocytic pathways. In professional APCs such as macrophages and dendritic cells, C-lectin receptors are required for the degradation of pathogens and subsequent presentation to T cells.

Receptors for Complement Components

By being able to recognize and bind complement (Chapter 20), phagocytes can bind the following:
- Pathogens coated in (opsonized by) complement components
- Complexes of antigen-antibody and complement (immune complexes)
- Dead cells

Receptors for Immunoglobulin

Phagocytes can recognize immunoglobulin G (IgG) through their Fc receptors. IgG stimulates phagocytosis and thus acts as an opsonin.

▌ ACTIONS OF PHAGOCYTES

Macrophages and neutrophils have different actions (see Table 21.1). Both cell types kill pathogens using phagocytosis and the release of toxic molecules and enzymes. However, only neutrophils can produce neutrophil extracellular traps (NETs). Neutrophils do not live long enough after encountering pathogen to do much else apart from killing. During their extended lives, macrophages have a critical role in communicating with both the innate and adaptive immune systems.

Phagocytosis

Phagocytosis is a metabolically active process triggered by binding through one of the receptors mentioned above. Phagocytosis is most effectively triggered by pathogens that have been opsonized by complement or IgG (Fig. 21.5). A phagosome is formed by the ingestion of particulate matter. A number of pathogens have developed defense mechanisms to avoid destruction by phagocytes.

 T-cell receptor (TCR) 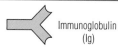 Immunoglobulin (Ig)   Antigen   MCH I

Oxidative Burst

After phagocytosis, three interrelated enzyme pathways are activated that produce toxic molecules, which further damage pathogens (Fig. 21.6). The enzymes produce hydrogen peroxide (phagocyte nicotinamide adenine dinucleotide phosphate [NADPH] oxidase), hypochlorous acid (bleach [myeloperoxidase]), and nitric oxide (inducible nitric oxide synthetase [macrophages but not neutrophils]).

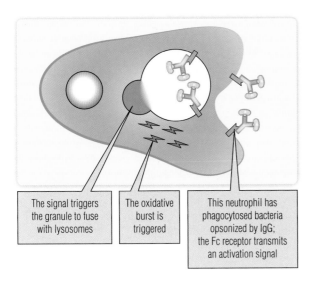

Fig 21.5 Phagocyte killing. *IgG,* immunoglobulin G.

The phagocyte NADPH oxidase enzymes are defective in a type of primary immunodeficiency known as *chronic granulomatous disease* (see Box 21.3).

Nitric oxide is a special molecule because, in addition to being toxic to pathogens, it also acts as an important messenger. Nitric oxide is constitutively produced at low levels by neuronal and endothelial cells and has a role as a neurotransmitter and in maintaining vascular tone. Macrophages can produce high levels of nitric oxide when inducible nitric oxide synthetase is activated. High levels of nitric oxide reduce vascular tone and cardiac output and contribute to the low blood pressure of septic shock (see Box 21.1). Evidence also suggests that nitric oxide acts as a messenger molecule that can promote the effects of T cells and contribute to chronic inflammation.

Proteolytic Enzymes

Macrophages contain enzymes in lysosomes, which can be regenerated during the long life of these cells. In neutrophils, the proteolytic enzymes are contained in granules, which give the cell its characteristic appearance. Neutrophils cannot regenerate granules, and when these have been used up, the cell dies. The main enzymes present are proteolytic and are able to digest bacteria in the acid pH of the lysosomes. In the case of macrophages, the digested peptides can be presented to T cells.

The proteolytic enzymes are usually held retained in lysosomes. Enzymes that leak out of phagocytes are usually prevented from damaging tissues by serpins such as α_1-antitrypsin (see Box 20.3).

Other substances are released into the phagosome, including defensins and lactoferrin. Defensins are low-molecular-weight

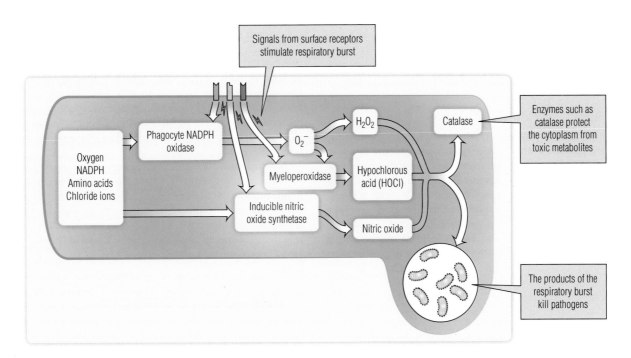

Fig 21.6 Oxidative burst. *NADPH,* nicotinamide adenine dinucleotide phosphate.

 MCH II   Cytokine, chemokine, etc.   Complement (C')   Signaling molecule

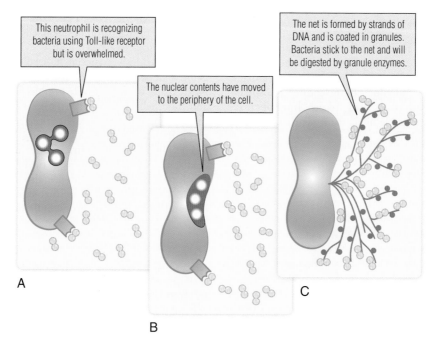

This neutrophil is recognizing bacteria using Toll-like receptor but is overwhelmed.

The nuclear contents have moved to the periphery of the cell.

The net is formed by strands of DNA and is coated in granules. Bacteria stick to the net and will be digested by granule enzymes.

A

B

C

Fig 21.7 This neutrophil is producing an extracellular trap in response to bacteria it is unable to phagocytose.

peptides that punch holes in bacteria. Lactoferrin binds to iron, depriving bacteria of this important nutrient.

A third killing mechanism, used only by neutrophils, is the formation of NETs. This may be helpful when the pathogen is either too large or too numerous to be phagocytosed. Upon activation, the neutrophil breaks down its own cell membrane and extrudes chromatin, a mixture of DNA and histones (Fig. 21.7). The chromatin unravels to produce a trap that physically captures pathogens. The toxic molecules and proteolytic enzymes are also restricted by the NETs, and so the pathogens are destroyed. This is a risky strategy: when present in the extracellular space, DNA becomes a potential antigen, and therefore its presence in NETs may contribute to the development of systemic lupus erythematosus (SLE; Chapter 29).

Inflammatory Signaling

Neutrophils and macrophages produce inflammatory mediators called *prostaglandins* and *leukotrienes*. These are discussed in Chapter 22. Although neutrophils secrete chemokines and nitric oxide, their short life span prevents them from contributing to a stable, long-lasting inflammatory response. Instead, a short-lived response is produced, usually with pus formation. This type of response may be called a *pyogenic* (pus-forming) reaction.

By comparison, macrophages have a key role in stimulating chronic inflammation, largely through secretion of soluble messengers with local and systemic effects. Macrophages are also important APCs because they process antigen, secrete cytokines, and express high levels of costimulatory molecules and major histocompatibility complex (MHC) class II molecules (Chapters 16 and 8, respectively). If antigen is not cleared, the inflammation becomes chronic, and a granuloma is the result. Granulomata are discussed more fully in Chapter 23, but Figure

21.8 shows how mediators produced by macrophages and T cells contribute to chronic inflammation.

Acute-Phase Response

Macrophages secrete IL-1, IL-6, and tumor necrosis factor (TNF) after they have recognized pathogens using pattern recognition molecules. These cytokines increase production of complement and arm the adaptive immune system (Chapter 19). TNF has direct effects on metabolism and increases the breakdown of fat in the body's stores.

IL-1, IL-6, and TNF also affect the central nervous system through receptors in the hypothalamus. The main response is an increase in body temperature, which is seen very rapidly after the beginning of the response to infection. The role of increased body temperature is to inhibit the replication of viruses and bacteria. There is also an increased metabolic rate and anorexia, all of which contribute to the weight loss characteristic of serious infection.

Macrophages also secrete cytokines that activate other parts of the immune system. IL-8 is a chemoattractant that attracts neutrophils to the site of infection. These cytokines all predominantly activate the innate immune system, but dendritic cells stimulated through their TLRs can secrete IL-12, which has a role in activating nearby T cells of the adaptive immune system. IL-12 alerts the adaptive immune system to the presence of infection.

■ PHAGOCYTE DEFECTS

Primary disorders of phagocytes are rare but include important problems such as chronic granulomatous disease (see Box 21.3). Secondary phagocyte defects are much more common. The most

T-cell receptor (TCR)

Immunoglobulin (Ig)

Antigen

MCH I

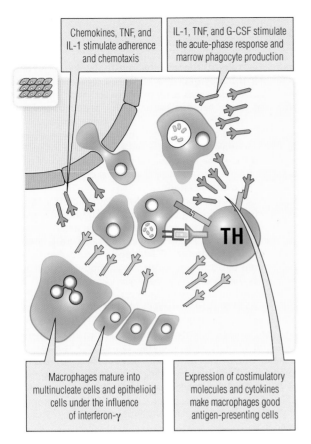

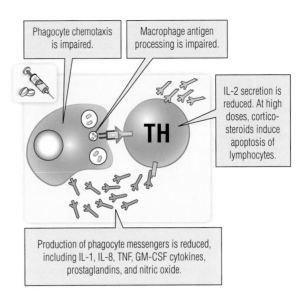

Fig 21.8 The result of mediator release by macrophages can be granuloma formation. A granuloma is a site of chronic inflammation where macrophages may mature into giant or epithelioid cells. Lymphocytes are also present and support macrophages by secreting interferon-γ. *G-CSF*, granulocyte colony-stimulating factor; *IL-1*, interleukin 1; *TH*, T-helper; *TNF*, tumor necrosis factor.

Fig 21.9 Effects of corticosteroids on phagocyte function. *GM-CSF*, granulocyte-macrophage colony-stimulating factor; *IL*, interleukin; *TH*, T helper; *TNF*, tumor necrosis factor.

important is neutropenia, in which numbers of neutrophils are reduced, usually as a result of drug treatment (see Box 21.1). Phagocyte function is impaired secondary to a number of other disorders, such as diabetes and renal failure, and during corticosteroid treatment (Fig. 21.9). At the usual doses, corticosteroids act on phagocytes; at higher doses, they act on lymphocytes. Because they effectively reduce inflammation, corticosteroids are used widely for many diseases. Unfortunately, they also have many side effects; for example, they suppress immunity to infection and cause metabolic problems and hypertension.

■ MOLECULAR RECOGNITION BY THE INNATE AND ADAPTIVE IMMUNE SYSTEMS

It is useful at this point to review the ways in which the two arms of the immune system recognize different molecules. The adaptive immune system can recognize many millions of possible antigens using MHC molecules, T-cell receptors, and Ig molecules, and it can distinguish self from nonself.

However, cells of the adaptive immune system are incapable of distinguishing the normal homeostatic environment from danger. This means that if the adaptive immune system were able to initiate a response autonomously, it could react to self peptides and initiate autoimmunity (Chapter 28). By comparison, the innate immune system recognizes "danger" whether it is due to tissue damage or infection. The pattern recognition receptors (PRRs) used by the innate system can recognize only *pathogen-associated molecular patterns* (PAMPs) or *damage-associated molecular patterns* (DAMPs). Recognition systems, such as the TLRs, activate the cells that express them, such as macrophages, to express increased amounts of MHC molecules and costimulatory molecules, such as CD80, and to secrete cytokines. The expression of costimulatory molecules and cytokines is referred to as a *danger signal*. T cells can respond to antigen only when they have received a danger signal. Thus the innate immune system alerts the adaptive system. This forms part of peripheral tolerance (Chapter 18) and reduces the risk of the adaptive immune system responding to self antigen or harmless environmental antigens.

Macrophages also rely on the adaptive immune system, particularly TH1 cells. For example, TH1 help is required to produce IgG, the Ig most effective at opsonizing bacteria for recognition by the Fc receptor. In addition, interferon gamma (IFN-γ) produced by TH1 is required to support and maintain macrophages during chronic infections, as you will discover in Chapter 23.

Many students make the mistake of believing that the more recently evolved adaptive immune system acts autonomously of the older innate system. We have seen now that this is not the case. APCs must first detect invading pathogens before they can costimulate T cells.

 MCH II

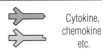 Cytokine, chemokine, etc.

 Complement (C′)

 Signaling molecule

BOX 21.1 Neutropenic Sepsis Leading to Septic Shock

A 12-year-old girl has been receiving cytotoxic chemotherapy for acute lymphoblastic leukemia. Although evidence suggests the leukemia is responding to the drugs, she has become neutropenic (neutrophils <0.5 × 10⁶ mL). Early in the evening, she complained of shivering (rigors) and chills and was found to be feverish. Within half an hour, she collapsed and was found to have the features of shock (tachycardia and hypotension) along with warm peripheries. When she is examined by the physician, no signs of focal organ involvement are found, such as pneumonia, and a diagnosis of neutropenic sepsis complicated by septic shock is made.

Blood is taken for culture, which later grows *Escherichia coli,* and the patient is started on broad-spectrum antibiotics and fluid replacement. She gradually improves over the next 12 hours (Fig. 21.10).

Neutrophils play a crucial role in the early part of bacterial infection. When neutrophils are present and can function normally, they limit infection to the site of entry and produce pus. This creates physical signs, such as pneumonia or abscess formation. In neutropenic patients, neutrophils cannot localize infection, which rapidly spreads to the blood and then to other tissues. Other cells of the immune system, particularly macrophages, are able to function normally; for example, this patient was able to mount an acute-phase response with fever and rigors. Septic shock is an exaggerated part of the normal innate response to infection. Septic shock is an acute state of hypotension often caused by the effects of bacterial lipopolysaccharide. The shock is a result of decreased vascular tone and impaired cardiac output. Septic shock is common in neutropenic patients, in whom gram-negative organisms cause many cases. Septic shock may also be seen in patients with normal immune systems who are overwhelmed by infection because of the massive quantity of organisms present—for example, after a ruptured bowel, when many billions of bacteria are released—or because the individual has no immunity to a high-virulence organism, as with Ebola.

Endotoxin release triggers the innate immune response by activating macrophages through Toll-like receptors (TLRs; Chapter 19). Consequences of macrophage activation include the secretion of tumor necrosis factor (TNF), prostaglandins, and nitric oxide. The TNF triggers more nitric oxide production by smooth muscle and endothelial cells. The very high levels of nitric oxide are responsible for the decreased vascular tone and cardiac output, and it should be remembered that normal levels of nitric oxide help maintain vascular tone. Endothelial cell activation may also trigger the clotting cascade.

Septic shock is often complicated by widespread organ failure, especially when the clotting cascade is also activated. The multiorgan failure is not a direct consequence of the initial infection but is caused by the innate immune system's response to the infection. The syndrome of multiorgan failure consequent to exaggerated innate immune system activation is sometimes referred to as the *systemic inflammatory response syndrome* (SIRS) or *cytokine storm,* and it has a mortality rate of over 70%. Attempts at blocking the effects of gross activation of the innate immune system have largely been unsuccessful (Fig. 21.11). Because treatment of established septic shock is so poor, clinicians pay particular attention to its prevention. This can include measures to reduce the risk of infection taking place, such as by ensuring thorough hand washing and avoiding neutropenia and also monitoring hospitalized patients for early signs of sepsis. Acute blood transfusion reactions are another cause of SIRS (Chapter 29). Toxic shock syndrome is a different entity mediated by cytokines secreted from T cells.

This example illustrates how important it is to respond promptly to very early symptoms of infection in neutropenic patients.

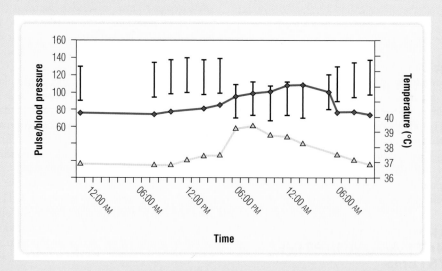

Fig 21.10 Vital signs for the patient. Blue diamonds are the pulse (beats/min), black bars are the blood pressure (mm Hg), and the yellow triangles are temperature.

 T-cell receptor (TCR) 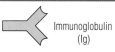 Immunoglobulin (Ig)   Antigen   MCH I

BOX 21.1 Neutropenic Sepsis Leading to Septic Shock—cont'd

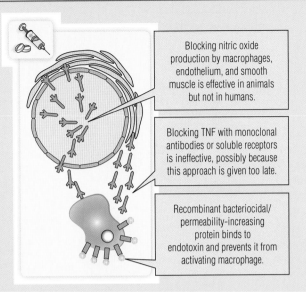

Blocking nitric oxide production by macrophages, endothelium, and smooth muscle is effective in animals but not in humans.

Blocking TNF with monoclonal antibodies or soluble receptors is ineffective, possibly because this approach is given too late.

Recombinant bacteriocidal/permeability-increasing protein binds to endotoxin and prevents it from activating macrophage.

Fig 21.11 Various attempts have been made to reverse the effects of septic shock, but none has been successful, possibly because by the time shock is diagnosed, the mechanisms have often become irreversible. *TNF,* tumor necrosis factor.

BOX 21.2 Drugs Based on Toll-Like Receptor Ligands

Stimulation of Toll-like receptors (TLRs) has potent activating effects on many components of the immune system. In clinical medicine, there are two areas where it is desirable to increase the immune response: in cancer and vaccines, which is discussed further in subsequent chapters. Because cancer and vaccines are not infections, they are not good at producing danger signals, and very often the immune system does not respond as well as we would like it to. Two TLR ligands, unmethylated cytosine and guanosine sequences (CpG motifs) and imiquimod, can safely mimic infections and have been tested in these settings.

CpG motifs are found in bacteria and are absent in human cells. They potently stimulate dendritic cells that express TLR-9 to secrete interleukin 12 (IL-12), which promotes T-helper 1 (TH1) responses and boosts the subsequent production of both immunoglobulin G (IgG) and cytotoxic T lymphocytes (Fig. 21.12).

When combined with existing vaccines, CpG can improve antibody and T-cell responses. When combined with conventional treatments, CpGs have also been found to be effective in clinical trials for some cancers. CpGs appear to have very few side effects.

Imiquimod is a synthetic drug that mimics single-stranded RNA and stimulates TLR-7, also on macrophages and dendritic cells. These then secrete a wide range of cytokines with stimulatory effects on the innate and adaptive immune systems. Imiquimod is widely used to treat wart infections. Like many chronic viral infections, the virus that causes warts is able to replicate slowly inside cells and does not produce a strong danger signal. Imiquimod painted onto warts can be a very effective treatment. Imiquimod can potentiate the effects of vaccines and has been used to treat tumors. It has the advantage that it can be applied directly to some skin tumors with considerable effects.

Continued

  MCH II   Cytokine, chemokine, etc.   Complement (C')   Signaling molecule

BOX 21.2 Drugs Based on Toll-Like Receptor Ligands—cont'd

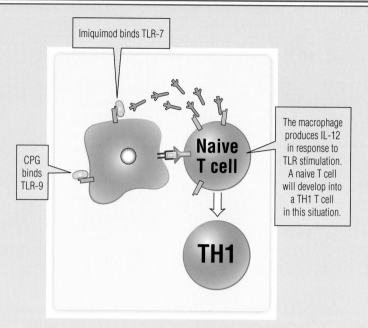

Fig 21.12 Cytosine and guanine sequences (CpGs) and imiquimod mimic danger signals and boost T-helper 1 (TH1) responses to antigens. *IL,* interleukin; *TLR,* Toll-like receptor.

BOX 21.3 Chronic Granulomatous Disease

A 4-year-old boy presents with a high fever and signs of fluid in the left pleural cavity. A sample from the pleural cavity shows pus, from which *Staphylococcus aureus* is grown.

The child has a history of growth retardation and perianal abscesses. He has no siblings and the only family history is of the death of a maternal uncle from infection in his teens.

Blood examination shows a marked neutrophilia of 23×10^6 mL when the normal range is 3 to 6×10^6 mL. A nitro blue tetrazolium test is carried out to determine whether his neutrophils are capable of mounting an oxidative burst (Fig. 21.13). The patient's neutrophils are unable to produce an oxidative burst, consistent with a diagnosis of chronic granulomatous disease (CGD).

CGD is a primary immunodeficiency that affects neutrophil function. This disease is characterized by recurrent bacterial and fungal infections in the presence of neutrophilia. It is caused by mutations in the genes for nicotinamide adenine dinucleotide phosphate (NADPH) oxidase or its regulatory proteins. CGD is usually X-linked. Although neutrophils are produced in abundance and are able to migrate to sites of infection, they cannot produce superoxide radicals, nor can they kill pathogens. Pathogens such as the fungus *Aspergillus* and the bacterium *Staphylococcus*, which would normally lead to short-lived pus-forming infections, are not cleared and lead to the formation of granulomata typical of chronic infection (Chapter 23).

Infection in children with CGD can be prevented by the use of prophylactic antibiotics and antifungal agents, although other approaches such as stem cell transplant have been tried.

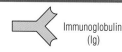 T-cell receptor (TCR)　　 Immunoglobulin (Ig)　　 Antigen　　MCH I

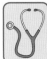

BOX 21.3 Chronic Granulomatous Disease—cont'd

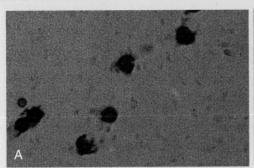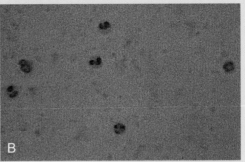

Fig 21.13 The nitro blue tetrazolium (NBT) test. NBT is a pale yellow color but changes to purple in cells that have undergone an oxidative burst. **A,** Neutrophils from a normal donor have been stimulated, and the NBT has produced a black color. **B,** Neutrophils from a patient with chronic granulomatous disease cannot change the color of the dye. No cytoplasmic staining occurs, and it is possible to see the multilobed nucleus.

LEARNING POINTS **Can You Now...**

1. List the differences between the roles of neutrophils and macrophages?
2. List the different types of macrophages and their specialist functions?
3. Describe danger signals and how the innate immune system activates the adaptive immune system?
4. Describe two kinds of problems that arise when quantitative and functional phagocyte defects are present?
5. Describe how phagocytes may contribute to septic shock?

 MCH II   Cytokine, chemokine, etc.   Complement (C′)   Signaling molecule

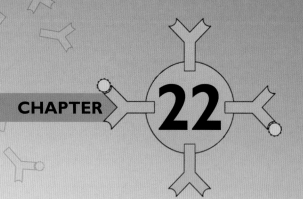

CHAPTER 22

Killing in the Immune System

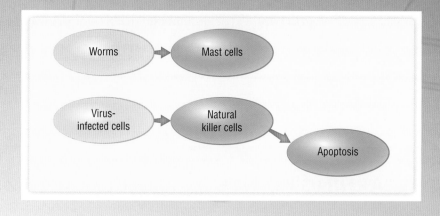

The immune system must be able to destroy a wide range of pathogens. How complement and phagocytes destroy extracellular pathogens has already been described (Table 21.1). The immune system uses the mechanisms shown in the above figure to destroy two special types of pathogen, worms and some viral infections, using mast cells and natural killer (NK) cells. This chapter describes apoptosis, a generic killing mechanism used by many parts of the immune system, in greater detail.

RESPONSE TO PARASITE WORMS

During human evolution, parasitic worms were a major threat to the species. Probably because of improved sanitation, worms are no longer considered a problem to people in the developed world, although one-third of the world's population is still infested with these parasites. Worms come in a variety of shapes and sizes (from 1 mm to 10 m) and tend to have complicated life cycles that involve eggs, larvae, and adult forms. Worm eggs are resistant to low pH and proteolytic digestion in the stomach and do not hatch until they reach the lower gut. Adult worms living inside the lower gut are protected from many of the components of the immune response. To overcome this, mast cells and eosinophils have evolved to respond to worms that live in the gut (Fig. 22.1). On activation these cells discharge toxic substances into the gut lumen, increase mucus secretion, and cause smooth muscle contraction, which results in expulsion of

the worm. These responses are summarized in Figure 22.2. The same mechanisms has evolved in the airways.

MAST CELLS

Mast cells are derived from an unknown precursor cell in the bone marrow under the influence of the T-helper 2 (TH2) cytokines interleukin (IL)-3 and IL-4. Like macrophages, mast cells home into a range of normal tissues, including the submucosa, skin, and connective tissue (Fig. 22.3). Recruitment to these frontline sites is increased during worm infestations.

Like macrophages, mast cells reside in the tissues for several weeks. During this time, they produce granules that contain a range of mediators. The mast cells also acquire immunoglobulin E (IgE) on their specialized Fc receptors (FcεRI), which have a very high affinity for IgE; therefore even IgE produced at a very low level elsewhere in the body will bind with mast cells. Consequently, the mast cells can bind a range of IgE molecules against a number of different antigens (Table 22.1). Mast cells become activated when these surface IgE molecules are cross-linked by antigen (Fig. 22.4). Mast cell FcεRIs are different from other types of Fc receptor; they bind Ig that is not bound to antigen and do not induce activation until they have been cross-linked by antigen. Mast cells are also activated by anaphylatoxins C3a and C5a (Chapter 20) and by a number of drugs.

Innate Immunity • Killing in the Immune System | **22**

Mast cell activation results in degranulation, release of pre-formed substances from the granules, and activation of arachidonic acid metabolism to produce a range of freshly made mediators (Table 22.2).

Granule Contents

Mast Cell Enzymes

Mast cell granules contain a number of proteolytic enzymes, including tryptase and chymotrypsin. These enzymes increase mucus secretion and smooth muscle contraction in, for example, bronchi. In addition, they cleave and activate components of the complement and kinin pathways, which promotes inflammation. Blood levels of mast cell tryptase can be used in the diagnosis of serious allergic reactions (Box 22.1).

Histamine

Histamine causes smooth muscle contraction in the gut and lungs in an attempt to expel worms. Histamine increases

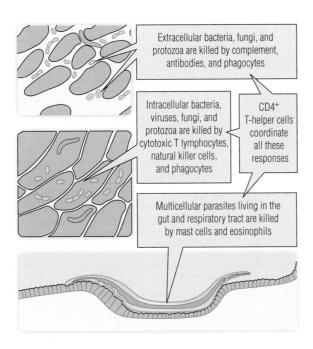

Fig 22.1 Targets for killing by the immune system. In immunodeficiency states, the type of defect is reflected by the infections patients develop. For example, antibody-deficient patients suffer mainly from bacterial infections.

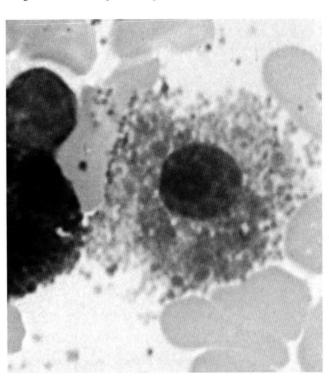

Fig 22.3 Mast cell. The granules in this mast cell contain cytokines, histamine, and proteolytic enzymes. *FcεRI,* Fc receptor; *Ig,* immunoglobulin.

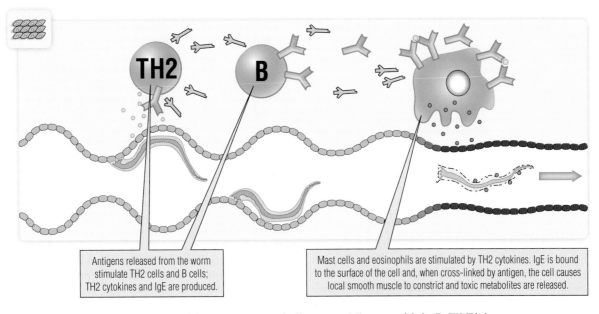

Fig 22.2 Summary of the response to a gut-dwelling worm. *IgE,* immunoglobulin E; *TH,* T-helper.

 MCH II   Cytokine, chemokine, etc.   Complement (C′)   Signaling molecule

163

TABLE 22.1 Different Pathogens Induce Different Immune Receptors

	Extracellular Pathogens	Intracellular Pathogens	Surface Pathogens
Examples of pathogens	Bacteria (eg, *Staphylococcus*) Fungi (eg, *Candida*)	Mycobacteria (eg, TB) Viruses Protozoa	Helminths Arthropods
Innate immune system components	Neutrophils Complement	Interferon Macrophages Natural killer cells	Mast cells Eosinophils
Adaptive immune system components	TH17 T cells IgG, IgM	TH1 T cells Cytotoxic T lymphocytes IgM, IgG, IgA	TH2 T cells IgE

Ig, *immunoglobulin*; TB, *tuberculosis*; TH, *T helper.*

TABLE 22.2 Mast Cell Mediators

Mediator	Actions
PREFORMED MEDIATORS PRESENT IN GRANULES	
Proteolytic enzymes, tryptase and chymotrypsin	Activate components of the complement and kinin pathways (for example, cleaving kininogen to bradykinin), which promotes inflammation
Histamine	Promotes smooth muscle contraction in the gut, lungs, and blood vessels and increases vascular permeability
Cytokines	
TNF	Activates endothelium to enhance diapedesis
IL-4	Activates TH2 cells
IL-3, IL-5	Stimulate eosinophil production and activation
ARACHIDONIC ACID METABOLITES	
Cyclooxygenase Pathway	
Prostaglandins, thromboxane	Vasodilation, increased vascular permeability, and constriction of smooth muscle in the gut and bronchi
Lipoxygenase	
Leukotrienes, platelet-activating factor	Bronchial and gut smooth muscle contraction, chemotactic stimuli for neutrophils and eosinophils

IL, *interleukin*; TH, *T-helper cell*; TNF, *tumor necrosis factor.*

Cytokines

Like activated macrophages, mast cells produce a range of cytokines to promote and extend the inflammatory response. Tumor necrosis factor (TNF) is preformed and present in granules and will activate local endothelium to enhance diapedesis of more inflammatory cells. Mast cells also produce other cytokines after stimulation, and unlike those produced by macrophages, these stimulate TH2 responses. IL-4 activates TH2 cells, and IL-3 and IL-5 stimulate eosinophil production and activation. IL-4 and IL-5 also skew the adaptive immune response away from a TH1 response.

Arachidonic Acid Metabolites

Metabolites of arachidonic acid metabolism are produced by mast cells and phagocytes. Arachidonic acid metabolism is activated by mast cell exposure to antigen and can follow two different pathways (Fig. 22.5):

1. *The cyclooxygenase pathway produces prostaglandins.* These act within seconds to stimulate vasodilation, increase vascular permeability, and constrict smooth muscle in the gut and bronchi. Prostaglandins may have other slower effects, such as inhibition of TH1 cells.
2. *The lipoxygenase pathway produces leukotrienes.* These have rather slower effects than prostaglandins but contribute to bronchial and gut smooth muscle contraction. In addition, leukotrienes act as chemotactic stimuli for neutrophils and eosinophils and thus contribute to increasing the cellularity of the immediate reaction and converting it to a delayed or chronic reaction.

Mast cells reside in a number of tissues that are at the front line of parasitic infection. Although activation of mast cells depends on preformed IgE antibodies, they respond very rapidly to antigen stimulation. The immediate response is caused by histamine, proteolytic enzymes, and prostaglandins and consists of smooth muscle contraction, increased vascular permeability, and mucus secretion. The cytokines and leukotrienes promote a late-phase response to antigen characterized by an influx of eosinophils and TH2 cells. This late-phase inflammation may become chronic but is distinct from the granulomata, which are characterized by the presence of macrophages and TH1 cells.

vascular permeability by causing endothelial cell contraction, which leads to a widening of intercellular gaps and subsequent tissue edema. Histamine provides a chemotactic signal to attract more white cells to the site of worm infestation. Histamine also causes marked itching in the skin, possibly to draw the attention of an infested host to the presence of skin parasites.

 T-cell receptor (TCR)

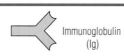 Immunoglobulin (Ig)

 Antigen

 MCH I

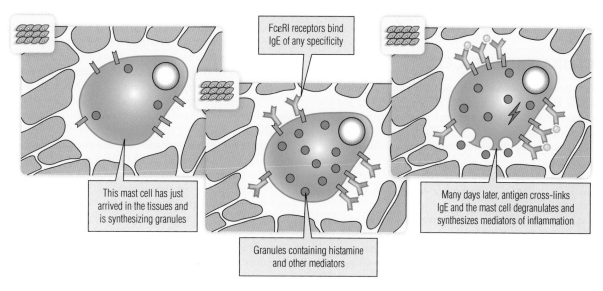

FcεRI receptors bind IgE of any specificity

This mast cell has just arrived in the tissues and is synthesizing granules

Granules containing histamine and other mediators

Many days later, antigen cross-links IgE and the mast cell degranulates and synthesizes mediators of inflammation

Fig 22.4 Mast cell activation.

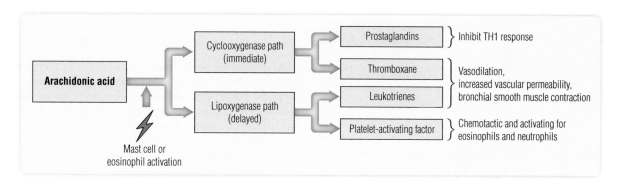

Arachidonic acid

Cyclooxygenase path (immediate)

Lipoxygenase path (delayed)

Mast cell or eosinophil activation

Prostaglandins } Inhibit TH1 response

Thromboxane

Leukotrienes } Vasodilation, increased vascular permeability, bronchial smooth muscle contraction

Platelet-activating factor } Chemotactic and activating for eosinophils and neutrophils

Fig 22.5 Arachidonic acid metabolism. Several of these pathways are affected by drugs. For example, aspirin and other nonsteroidal antiinflammatory drugs inhibit the cyclooxygenase pathways, blocking the immediate effects of mast cell degranulation. However, these drugs do not block the lipoxygenase pathway and can lead to increased production of leukotrienes, which can exacerbate the delayed features of mast cell degranulation.

Eosinophils

Eosinophils are broadly similar to mast cells; however, two factors make them unique: they are specifically recruited to tissues during some types of inflammation, and their granules contain particularly toxic substances.

Eosinophils are derived from precursors that are similar to neutrophils, and their production is stimulated by IL-3 and IL-5. Eosinophils are normally present in blood in small numbers, but their numbers increase dramatically in response to IL-3 and IL-5 secreted by TH2 cells and mast cells. The causes of increased numbers of eosinophils in the blood, known as *eosinophilia,* are discussed in Box 22.2. Eosinophils are recruited to parasite-infested sites by the chemokine eotaxin, which is produced by epithelial cells and leukotrienes produced by mast cells.

Eosinophils are activated by cytokines, chemokines, and perhaps by cross-linked IgE on FcεRI. Activated eosinophils release the same mediators as mast cells (except histamine) and also release three special mediators:

1. A peroxidase that is released onto the surface of parasites and then generates hypochlorous acid
2. Major basic protein, which damages the outer surface of parasites and host tissues
3. Cationic protein, which damages the parasite's outer surface and acts as a neurotoxin, damaging the simple nervous system of the parasite

Immediate (Type I) Hypersensitivity

Because the effects of eosinophil and mast cell degranulation are so rapid, this type of response is sometimes referred to as *immediate,* or *type I, hypersensitivity,* although the cytokines and other mediators released can also set up delayed and chronic inflammatory responses.

People living in the developed world are no longer challenged by worms. In these populations, mast cells and eosinophils cause immediate hypersensitivity in response to innocuous antigens such as pollens—the hallmarks of allergy

 MCH II

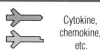 Cytokine, chemokine, etc.

 Complement (C')

 Signaling molecule

(Chapter 27). Eosinophils and mast cells secrete a wide range of mediators, many of which are targets in the treatment of allergy.

■ NATURAL KILLER CELLS

NK cells have two important roles. As their name suggests, they are excellent killers of cells infected by some viruses, but like macrophages, they have an additional role of stimulating the adaptive immune response.

The word *natural* in this context means these cells are capable of recognizing and interacting with a target without any priming or previous sensitization. *Natural* is given the same meaning when used in *natural antibodies* (Chapter 14) or *natural T-regulatory cells* (Chapter 18).

NK cells are part of the innate immune system and fill a potential gap in the specific immune response. Most cells infected with viruses such as influenza are killed when cytotoxic T lymphocytes (CTLs) recognize viral peptides bound to major histocompatibility complex (MHC). Some infectious agents, notably members of the herpesvirus family, downregulate MHC expression on infected cells to evade detection by T cells. Herpesviruses can also block intracellular antigen-presentation pathways (Chapter 10). These evasion mechanisms prevent CTL recognition, but NK cells are still able to recognize and kill cells infected with herpesviruses because they have evolved to recognize and kill cells with low MHC expression (Fig. 22.6). Similarly, some tumor cells have acquired mutations that result in decreased MHC expression, and they are able to evade tumor-specific T cells but not NK cells.

NK cells develop and acquire their receptors in the bone marrow. Although they are not generated in the thymus, they share some characteristics with T cells. For example, they share some T-cell surface molecules, such as CD2, and have an appearance similar to lymphocytes. An alternative name for NK cells is *large granular lymphocytes* (Fig. 22.7). NK cells also use the same generic killing mechanisms as CTLs. However, NK cells do *not* have rearranged T-cell receptor molecules and are thus classified as belonging to the innate immune system. NK cells also share some characteristics of macrophages: they are capable of recognizing antibody-coated target cells, but they do not kill these by phagocytosis.

NK cells arise from the same lymphoid progenitor cells as T and B cells, although it is not clear how their production is regulated. NK cells constitute approximately 5% to 15% of lymphocytes in peripheral blood. They are activated by cytokines (Fig. 22.8), but killing is regulated by signaling through special receptors.

Natural Killer Receptors

Natural killer cells express over 20 different receptors that fall into two different families, *inhibitory* and *activating* receptors.

Natural Killer Inhibitor Receptors

Killer immunoglobulin-like receptors (KIRs) are members of the immunoglobulin superfamily and recognize specific MHC α-chains. NKG2 and CD94 are C-lectin molecules that recognize the nonclassic human leukocyte antigen E (HLA-E) molecule. Both types of receptor are special because they can inhibit killing. This dominant signal overrides all other signals: an NK cell that has detected MHC will not kill.

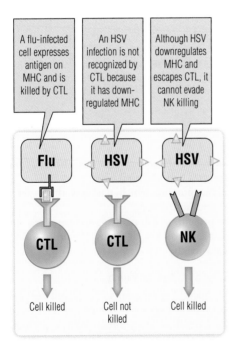

| A flu-infected cell expresses antigen on MHC and is killed by CTL | An HSV infection is not recognized by CTL because it has down-regulated MHC | Although HSV downregulates MHC and escapes CTL, it cannot evade NK killing |

Flu — **CTL** — Cell killed

HSV — **CTL** — Cell not killed

HSV — **NK** — Cell killed

Fig 22.6 Comparison of the killing of cells infected with influenza and herpes simplex virus (HSV). Because HSV downregulates major histocompatibility complex (MHC) expression, cytotoxic T lymphocytes (CTLs) cannot kill infected cells. Natural killer (NK) cells are stimulated by the absence of MHC and kill the infected cell as a result.

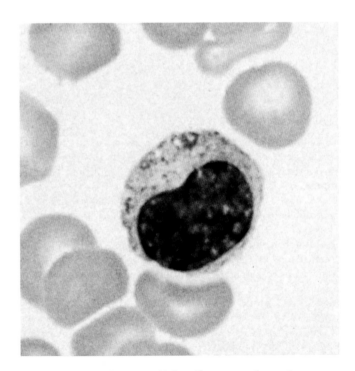

Fig 22.7 The granules in natural killer cells contain perforin and granzyme.

 T-cell receptor (TCR) 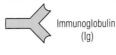 Immunoglobulin (Ig)   Antigen   MCH I

Natural Killer Activating Receptors

NK cells also express a number of activating receptors. In NK cells, a special Fc receptor, FcγRIII, recognizes IgG-bound viral antigen on the surface of infected cells and triggers killing. IgG-mediated NK killing is referred to as *antibody-dependent cellular cytotoxicity* (ADCC) and is illustrated in Figure 22.9. FcγRIII is also expressed by some macrophages, in which case IgG acts as an opsonin that triggers phagocytosis.

When an NK cell encounters a virally infected cell, two outcomes are possible (Fig. 22.10):

1. The NK cell recognizes that the cell is infected using an innate immune system pattern recognition molecule. The NK cell uses its receptors to check that MHC is present on the surface of the cell. If MHC is present at an adequate level,

the receptor delivers a negative signal, which prevents the NK cell killing. Because the virally infected cell expresses MHC, it will in any case be killed by a CTL.

2. If the NK recognizes that a cell is infected by a virus and confirms that levels of MHC are reduced, it will go ahead and kill the target cell.

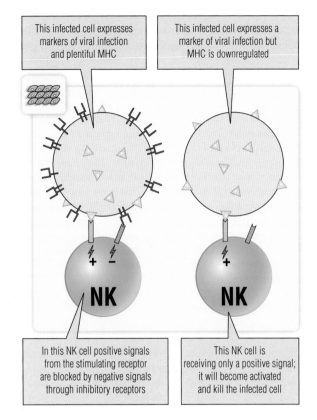

Fig 22.8 Cytokine regulation of natural killer (NK) cells. Like T cells, NK cells proliferate in response to interleukin 2 (IL-2). *TNF,* tumor necrosis factor.

Fig 22.10 Natural killer (NK) cells will not kill the infected cell on the left because it is still expressing major histocompatibility complex (MHC). The infected cell on the right has stopped expressing MHC and will be killed.

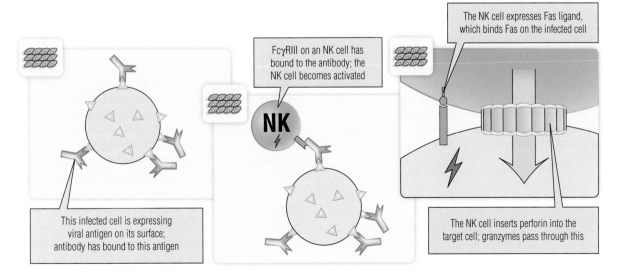

Fig 22.9 Antibody-dependent cellular cytotoxicity (ADCC). Binding of antibody to Fc εRIII stimulates the natural killer (NK) cell. This process is similar to opsonization by immunoglobulin G (IgG).

 MCH II    Cytokine, chemokine, etc.   Complement (C′)   Signaling molecule

The balance between the stimulatory and inhibitory signals determines the outcomes of NK cell activation; NK preferentially kill cells absent MHC expression.

Cells may have absent MHC expression because of viral infection or because of mutation in cancer cells. Either process enables abnormal cells to escape killing by CTLs. NK cells overcome this potential flaw in the immune response by killing cells with absent MHC expression. This type of killing is especially important when interferon gamma (IFN-γ) is present; this cytokine maximizes MHC expression by normal cells and at the same time increases NK cell activity. Reduced expression of MHC acts as a danger signal that alerts NK cells to the presence of infection.

NK cells have one more important role in the placenta, where both paternal and maternal MHC genes may be expressed. NK cells are the major cell of the immune system in the pregnant uterus. Uterine NK cells have a role in preventing viral infection of the uterus and fetus during pregnancy. They have the added advantage of not attacking fetal tissue even though it expresses foreign (paternal) HLA molecules. This is because NK cells are inhibited from killing by MHC, regardless of whether it has a maternal or paternal genetic origin. CTLs would also be able to kill virally infected cells, but only if antigens were presented on maternal MHC. In contrast, CTLs would attack placental cells that express paternal MHC in an allogeneic reaction, similar to a transplant reaction.

CTLs and Natural Killer Cell Effector Mechanisms

The cytotoxic mechanisms used by NK cells are identical to those used by CTLs. Both populations use perforin, granzyme, and Fas ligand (FasL) expression and secretion of TNF, all of which can induce programmed cell death (apoptosis). NK cells and CTLs also secrete immunoregulatory cytokines, such as IFN-γ, and these promote the TH1 inflammatory response.

Perforin

Perforin is contained within the cytotoxic granules of NK cells and CTLs. When CTLs or NK cells are activated, the actin cytoskeleton is reorganized so that perforin molecules are moved to the cell surface. Perforin polymerizes and forms a pore that is inserted into the target cell membrane, rather like the complement membrane-attack complex (MAC; see Fig. 22.9). These pores allow salts and water to flow into the target cell; more importantly, they give granzyme access to the cytoplasm.

Granzyme

Granzyme consists of three separate proteolytic enzymes transported by the activated cytoskeleton and transferred into the target cell. As well as degrading host cell proteins, they specifically activate the **caspase** enzyme system, which results in apoptosis.

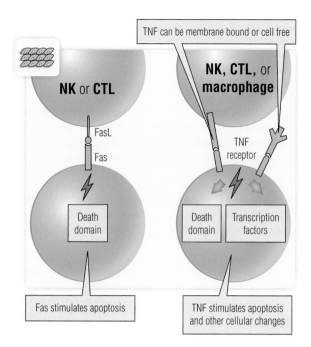

Fig 22.11 Fas and tumor necrosis factor (TNF) receptor can both induce cell death. *CTL*, cytotoxic T lymphocyte; *FasL*, Fas ligand; *NK*, natural killer.

Fas Ligand

Fas ligand (FasL) is a potent inducer of apoptosis and is used by NK cells and CTLs to kill infected cells and tumor cells. Fas is a member of the same family of receptors as the TNF receptor (Fig. 22.11). Fas and FasL are expressed on cells of the immune system during activation. FasL expression is increased on CTLs and NK cells when they become activated; FasL binds Fas on a target cell, which then undergoes apoptosis through the mechanisms described later. T cells may also express Fas and can become targets of Fas-mediated killing. For example, cells in immune-privileged sites, such as the testes, express FasL. Any T cell that accidentally ends up in the testes will be exposed to Fas and undergo apoptosis.

Although NK cells are highly effective at killing in their own right, they also activate the adaptive immune response by secreting cytokines that stimulate TH1 responses. Macrophages behave in a similar way, and this is exactly what we expect from cells of the innate immune system. Both types of cell recognize families of pathogens rather than specific antigens. They attempt to eradicate the pathogen but also activate the adaptive immune system.

NK cells secrete IFN-γ when they encounter target cells. This cytokine stimulates TH1 cells and inhibits TH2 cells. A TH1 response is especially effective at dealing with intracellular infection and can provide immunologic memory to guarantee a strong response should the host be exposed to the same pathogen again.

■ INTRACELLULAR MECHANISMS OF APOPTOSIS

This chapter is most interested in apoptosis that has been induced through the ligation of receptors such as Fas or the TNF receptor (see Fig. 22.11). However, similar intracellular mechanisms lead to apoptosis regardless of the many different triggers.

 T-cell receptor (TCR) 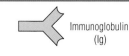 Immunoglobulin (Ig)   Antigen   MCH I

Fas and TNF receptor both have cytoplasmic tails, called *death domains,* which can activate the series of caspase enzymes (Fig. 22.12). Caspases are proteolytic enzymes that cleave proteins after aspartic acid residues. The final result of activation of the caspase is activation of a specific DNAase, which cleaves the DNA of the target cells into 200 base-pair fragments. Caspases are also activated when NK or CTLs inject granzyme into the cell.

Another early effect of apoptosis is the disruption of mitochondria, which causes them to become leaky; the subsequent release of mitochondrial products further activates caspases. Bcl-2 is an antiapoptotic protein that binds to and stabilizes mitochondria and prevents upregulation of apoptosis (Chapter 17). Falling IL-2 levels reduce the intracellular concentration of Bcl-2 and can make apoptosis more likely to occur. This happens at the end of a successful immune response, when antigen levels are falling and IL-2 secretion is diminished.

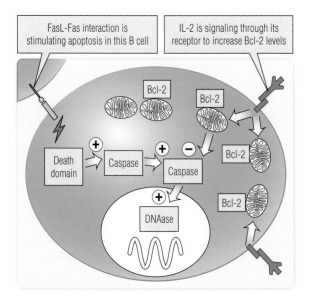

Fig 22.12 Whether this B cell undergoes apoptosis is determined by the balance of signals through Fas, caspases, interleukin 2 (IL-2), and Bcl-2.

Apoptosis in the Immune System

Apoptosis is the process of programmed cell death, in which cells are deliberately killed as a part of physiologic processes. Apoptotic cells are recognized by phagocytes, which usually clear the cell remains without stimulating inflammation. By comparison, *necrosis* is the inadvertent death of cells, usually caused by exposure to metabolic insults, such as hypoxia or toxins. Necrosis does *not* result in DNA fragmentation, and because it activates the complement cascade, it often results in an inflammatory response (Table 22.3).

Apoptosis is an important physiologic process that affects many body systems. During embryonic life, for example, apoptosis is involved in tissue remodeling, such as in the developing vascular system. In this way, apoptosis determines the shape of the developing fetus.

Apoptosis has a number of very important roles in shaping the adaptive immune repertoire. Autoreactive T and B cells undergo apoptosis soon after they are generated in the thymus and bone marrow. In addition, after an immune response to a pathogen, redundant lymphocytes are also cleared by apoptosis. Each of these uses different mechanisms, but the result is that the specificities of the immune response are shaped by apoptosis (Table 22.4).

Apoptosis is also involved in some pathologic processes; for example, evidence shows that one of the ways that CD4⁺ T cells are destroyed by HIV infection is through induction of apoptosis. When apoptotic debris is not cleared adequately by phagocytes, it can become immunogenic. This can lead to the production of autoantibodies—for example, against DNA—and this may generate autoimmune disease such as systemic lupus erythematosus (SLE).

Defective apoptosis can occur in clones of B cells that have increased levels of Bcl-2 through mutations or chromosome translocations that may be protected from apoptosis and can develop into a B-cell malignancy (Chapter 35). Defective apoptosis can also be acquired by infection with some herpesviruses. For example, Epstein-Barr virus (EBV) evades apoptosis by producing a Bcl-2–like protein. This "immortalizes" the B cells that the virus infects and can also contribute to the development of B-cell malignancy.

TABLE 22.3 **Comparison of Apoptosis and Necrosis**		
	Apoptosis	**Necrosis**
Definition	Programmed cell death	Inadvertent cell death
Causes	Destruction during development (eg, thymocytes) or as a result of the actions of T cells, NK cells, eosinophils, mast cells, or complement	Damage by heat, chemicals, anoxia, or infection
Consequences	DNA breaks down but cell membrane remains intact	Cell membrane breaks down and leaks contents
Causes inflammation?	No	Yes, activates complement
Effects	Usually beneficial	Always detrimental

NK, *natural killer.*

 MCH II   Cytokine, chemokine, etc.   Complement (C′)   Signaling molecule

TABLE 22.4 Apoptosis in the Immune System

Area Involving Apoptosis	Target	Mechanism
Negative selection in the thymus Peripheral T-cell tolerance	T cells Autoreactive T cells	Repeated stimulation leads to activation-induced cell death
At the end of an immune response when only a few cells are required to maintain memory	Responding T cells	Cytokine starvation leads to a reduction in Bcl-2
Negative selection of B cells in bone marrow	B cells	
Low-affinity antibody production	B cells	Changes in Bcl-2
Peripheral T-cell tolerance	Autoreactive T cells	Fas
Protection of immune-privileged sites	T cells	Cells (eg, testicular cells) express FasL, which kills incoming T cells
Intracellular infection	Any cells	Fas, TNF, granzyme
Malignancy	Malignant cell	Fas, TNF, granzyme

FasL, *Fas ligand*; TNF, *tumor necrosis factor*.

BOX 22.1 Serious Problems During a Hip Replacement

A 67-year-old woman is scheduled to undergo a hip replacement. She undergoes general anesthesia, and the surgeon begins the procedure. Four minutes after the skin is incised, the antibiotic cefuroxime is given intravenously to reduce the risk of postoperative infection. About 1 minute later, the anesthetist notices that her blood pressure has fallen dramatically from 150/87 to 65/35 mm Hg. At first, the anesthetist suspects that the fall in blood pressure is due to bleeding at the operation site, but the surgeon says this is unlikely. After a few more seconds, the anesthetist notices that it has become very difficult to ventilate the patient, whose oxygen saturation has fallen from 97% to 63%. The anesthetist suspects that this is anaphylaxis (serious allergy) to cefuroxime and administers epinephrine. The response to epinephrine is incomplete, and eventually the anesthetist has to administer three doses of epinephrine before blood pressure and the obstruction to ventilation recover. The surgery is abandoned. A blood sample is taken for mast cell tryptase (MCT) an hour after the reaction and again 24 hours later.

When the patient is seen a few weeks later by an allergist, the results of the mast cell tryptase are available. An hour after the reaction, the MCT level was 245 µg/L and had fallen to 8.5 µg/L when the second sample was taken the next day. The reference range for MCT is 0 to 13 µg/L. The transiently raised MCT after the reaction confirms the suspicion that this was anaphylaxis. Further tests show that the patient is indeed allergic to cefuroxime (Chapter 27). The operation is attempted again a few weeks later. This time a different antibiotic is given, and no further problems are encountered.

Transiently raised MCT is used as a diagnostic test for anaphylactic reactions. This is important when symptoms have several possible causes. In the case described here, the fall in blood pressure could be caused by bleeding, and the difficulty ventilating the patient could be caused by misplacement of the endotracheal tube. The transiently raised MCT suggests strongly that anaphylaxis was the cause.

T-cell receptor (TCR)　　 Immunoglobulin (Ig)　　Antigen　　 MCH I

BOX 22.2 Eosinophilia

A 43-year-old man has returned from working as an overseas aid worker in Southeast Asia, where he has been involved in developing sewage systems (Fig. 22.13). On his return home, he is required to undergo a medical examination, during which he is found to have a raised eosinophil count (2.5×10^6 mL compared with a normal count of $<0.35 \times 10^6$ mL) and abnormal liver function tests (Fig. 22.14).

Although allergy is the most common cause of eosinophilia in the developed world, this patient has no signs or symptoms of allergies such as asthma, rhinitis, or eczema. Neither does he have any features of any cancers sometimes associated with eosinophilia, such as lymphoma. A liver biopsy is performed, which shows parasite eggs surrounded by granulomata. A diagnosis of the parasitic worm infection schistosomiasis is made, and the patient responds well to treatment.

Schistosoma mansoni is a common parasite in some parts of the world. Humans are infected when larvae penetrate the skin from contaminated water supplies. Adult worms live in the portal veins and discharge eggs, which may lodge in the liver. Mast cells and eosinophils are able to kill schistosomiasis worms and their eggs using the mechanisms described above. The marked eosinophilia is a reflection of the activation of these cells. As the eggs disintegrate, they release peptides that are processed and recognized as conventional antigens by T-helper 1 (TH1) cells. Untreated schistosomiasis leads to chronic inflammation in the liver and is one cause of liver cirrhosis. It is not yet clear whether this damage is caused by the eosinophil response to adult worms, the TH1 cell response to worm eggs, or a combination of both.

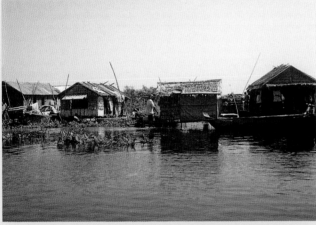

Fig 22.13 In this village in Cambodia, human feces are dropped straight into the water supply. The plant growing in the lake is water hyacinth, which provides the home for the snail that is the host to schistosomes. In this kind of environment, mast cells and eosinophils provide important defenses for the human population.

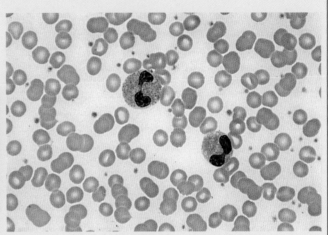

Fig 22.14 Eosinophils. The multilobed nuclei of these cells indicate how closely related they are to neutrophils (see Fig 21.1A). Note the coarse red granules.

LEARNING POINTS   Can You Now...

1. Identify the type of infection that mast cells and eosinophils respond to?
2. List the contents of mast cell and eosinophil granules?
3. Describe the consequences of arachidonic acid metabolism?
4. Describe two ways by which herpesvirus family members avoid being killed?
5. Describe natural killer cell receptors?
6. List NK cell killing mechanisms?
7. Draw the mechanism of apoptosis?

 MCH II

  Cytokine, chemokine, etc.

 Complement (C')

 Signaling molecule

23 # Inflammation

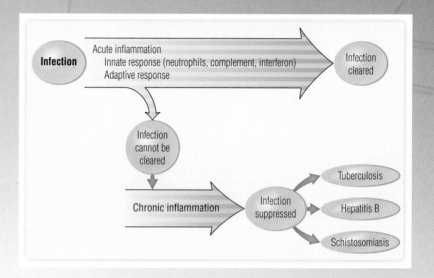

During infection, the innate and adaptive components of the immune system generate inflammation that clears most infections. Some infections cannot be cleared, and chronic inflammation results. Tuberculosis and hepatitis B are common examples of infections that cause chronic inflammation. Although acute and chronic inflammation evolved as mechanisms for responding to infections, they can also contribute to autoimmune disease.

■ TYPES OF INFLAMMATION

Inflammation is clinically defined as the presence of redness, swelling, and pain. Histologically, it is defined as the presence of edema fluid and the infiltration of tissues by white cells. The type of white cells involved—neutrophils, macrophages, eosinophils, or types of lymphocytes—vary with each type of inflammation.

The causes of inflammation are numerous; for example, a burn will cause an acute inflammatory response, and although this is triggered by a physical stimulus, it is at least partially mediated by immunologic mechanisms, such as the release of tumor necrosis factor (TNF) from damaged tissues.

However, most inflammation is a response to infection. Acute infections are those that last a few days and in most cases are cleared by the immune system; they rarely result in death. Examples of acute infections include influenza and staphylococcal abscesses (boils). Clearance of these infections is largely reliant on the innate immune system, although this system is helped in these examples by T-helper 1 (TH1) and TH17 cells, respectively. If the offending stimulus cannot be rapidly removed, the inflammation tends to become chronic. Figure 23.1 and Table 23.1 show some infections that result in either chronic or acute inflammation.

Acute reactions to extracellular bacteria result in *pus* formation; they are *pyogenic*. For example, pustules or larger abscesses in the skin are usually caused by *Staphylococcus.* Yellow sputum also reflects pyogenic infection, this time in the chest, usually caused by pneumococcus or *Haemophilus.* Meningitis due to *Neisseria meningitidis* is another type of pyogenic infection; recall the neutrophils in the cerebrospinal fluid (CSF) sample in Figure 20.13. In pus and infected sputum, the yellow color is contributed by neutrophil granules. Although damage may be severe in the short term, these infections often resolve with minimal scarring.

On the other hand, failure to clear acute infection leads to various types of chronic inflammation (see Fig. 23.1). Chronic intracellular bacterial infections may lead to the formation of granuloma, collections of specialized macrophages surrounded

T-cell response to develop. Granulomatous reactions are sometimes referred to as *delayed hypersensitivity. M. tuberculosis* elicits a typical delayed hypersensitivity reaction, as illustrated by skin testing for TB (see Box 23.1). Granuloma development requires T-cell involvement and therefore has characteristics of adaptive immunity, such as antigen specificity and recall responsiveness.

Chronic viral infection leads to more diffuse inflammation, although macrophages and T cells are still present. This typically occurs in infections with hepatitis B virus (HBV), in which acute inflammation occurs initially as a result of antiviral activity. Chronic inflammation can follow as the inflammatory response continues in a failed attempt to eliminate the pathogen. This chronic stage results in damage to the host organs (see Box 23.2) and is also coordinated by TH1 cells.

Acute inflammation mediated by mast cells is characterized by edema; when it becomes more long lasting, eosinophils enter the inflamed tissue. A good example of chronic inflammation mediated by mast cells and eosinophils is schistosomiasis, discussed in Chapter 22. This is an example of an organism living on a body surface; this type of chronic inflammation is coordinated by TH2 cells.

Although TH17 cells have an important role in the clearance of acute infections caused by extracellular pathogens, there is currently no evidence for their involvement in chronic infections in humans.

■ CYTOKINE NETWORK IN INFLAMMATION

Cytokines are required to initiate acute inflammation and maintain chronic inflammatory responses. These responses require help from $CD4^+$ T cells. The interaction between these and either macrophages or eosinophils is sometimes referred to as the *cytokine network.*

Macrophages secrete interleukin 1 (IL-1), TNF, and granulocyte-macrophage colony-stimulating factor (GM-CSF), which activate the acute-phase response and promote marrow production of neutrophils and monocytes. Macrophage-produced TNF and IL-1 increase adherence of leukocytes to local endothelium. These leukocytes then follow the chemotactic signal of chemokines also produced by macrophages. In addition, macrophages produce cytokines that act on T cells, including IL-1 and IL-12. IL-1 is a general activator of T cells and, along with costimulatory molecules such as CD40, activates all classes of T cells. IL-12 preferentially activates TH1 and natural killer (NK) cells.

In response to these macrophage-derived cytokines, TH1 and NK cells secrete interferon gamma (IFN-γ) and more TNF. The major effects of IFN-γ are to:
- Increase expression of major histocompatibility complex (MHC) on macrophages and other local cells
- Increase antigen processing through proteasomes in macrophages
- Induce macrophage maturation
- Increase NK cell activity
- Inhibit TH2 cells
- Cause mild antiviral effects (Chapter 20).

The effects of IFN-γ on macrophages are to stimulate TH1 cell activity further through antigen presentation and cytokine production. The exchange of cytokines between macrophages

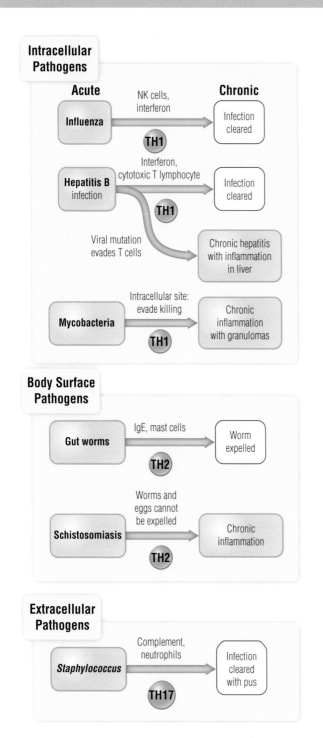

Fig 23.1 Whether chronic inflammation develops depends on pathogen and host factors. For example, in hepatitis B virus infection, both viral mutations and host human leukocyte antigen type may determine whether chronic inflammation occurs. *IgE,* immunoglobulin E; *NK,* natural killer.

by T cells. This occurs in tuberculosis (TB; the infection caused by *Mycobacterium tuberculosis,* described in detail later). Granuloma formation is coordinated by TH1 cells.

Pus formation can develop over a few hours. Granulomata take 2 to 3 days to develop because of the time it takes for the

 MCH II   Cytokine, chemokine, etc.   Complement (C')   Signaling molecule

TABLE 23.1 Key Features of Inflammation Triggered by Intracellular Pathogens, Body Surface Pathogens, and Extracellular Pathogens

	Intracellular Pathogen	Body Surface Pathogen	Extracellular Pathogen
Example	*Acute:* Influenza *Chronic:* Tuberculosis, hepatitis B infection	*Acute:* Worms *Chronic:* Schistosomiasis	Staphylococcal infection
Innate immune system effectors	Dendritic cell, NK cell, macrophage, IFN	Mast cells, eosinophils	Neutrophils, complement
Adaptive immune system effectors	TH1 cells, CD8⁺ T cells	TH2 cells, IgE	TH17 cells
Cytokines	TH1 cytokines: IL-12, IFN-γ	TH2 cytokines: IL-4, IL-5	IL-17

IFN, *interferon;* Ig, *immunoglobulin;* IL, *interleukin;* NK, *natural killer;* TH, *T-helper.*

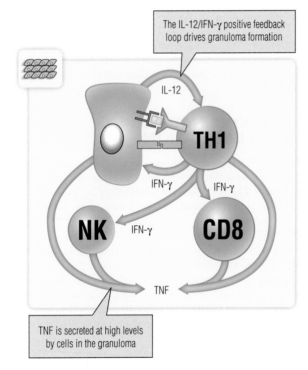

The IL-12/IFN-γ positive feedback loop drives granuloma formation

TNF is secreted at high levels by cells in the granuloma

Fig 23.2 The cytokines interleukin 12 (IL-12) and interferon gamma (IFN-γ) form a positive feedback loop. Tumor necrosis factor (TNF) also contributes to granuloma formation. *NK,* natural killer.

and T cells generates a strong positive feedback loop between these two populations and skews the immune response toward a TH1 pattern (Fig. 23.2).

TNF, produced by macrophages and T cells, has a number of important roles in the development of an inflammatory response. However, high local levels of TNF can cause negative effects such as tissue destruction. TNF also has potent systemic effects, such as fat catabolism, fever, and loss of appetite, that lead to weight loss.

The feedback loop ultimately comes to a halt when phagocytes have cleared all residual antigen. Thus stimulation of T cells ceases, and the level of IFN-γ falls. Costimulation by macrophages is reduced, and the result is that T cells die through apoptosis.

The cytokine network is used to control several intracellular infections, most importantly bacteria of the *Mycobacterium* family. These range from organisms that have adapted to host immunity, such as *M. tuberculosis,* to usually harmless organisms referred to as *opportunist,* or *atypical,* mycobacteria. The opportunist mycobacteria cause disease when the cytokine network has failed in a variety of separate situations:

- Rarely, some individuals inherit mutations in the genes for IL-12, IL-12 receptor, or IFN-γ receptor. These individuals are highly prone to infection with all types of mycobacteria.
- More frequently, the cytokine network is disrupted by drugs. For example, monoclonal antibodies against TNF are used to treat rheumatoid arthritis (Chapter 31). Mycobacterial infection is a recognized complication of anti-TNF treatment.
- Most importantly, HIV infection is a frequent cause of mycobacterial infection, particularly in Africa. This is because HIV infects and damages both T cells and macrophages, as discussed in Chapter 33. Early in HIV infection, when the immune deficiency is not severe, infection with *M. tuberculosis* is characteristic. In later HIV infection, with more severe immune deficiency, infection with opportunist mycobacteria is common.

■ TUBERCULOSIS

In the late 20th century, TB was thought to be under control. However, it has reemerged as a major threat to global health and now kills 2 to 3 million individuals per year.

M. tuberculosis stimulates macrophages by binding Toll-like receptors (TLRs) 2 and 4, which recognize mycobacterial lipoproteins and polysaccharides. This stimulates phagocytosis and secretion of inflammatory mediators, such as IL-12 and nitric oxide. Mycobacterial peptides presented by macrophages elicit strong TH1 responses. The most important of these are secretion of TNF and IFN-γ, which stimulate the formation of granuloma during primary infection.

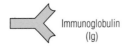 T-cell receptor (TCR)   Immunoglobulin (Ig)   Antigen   MCH I

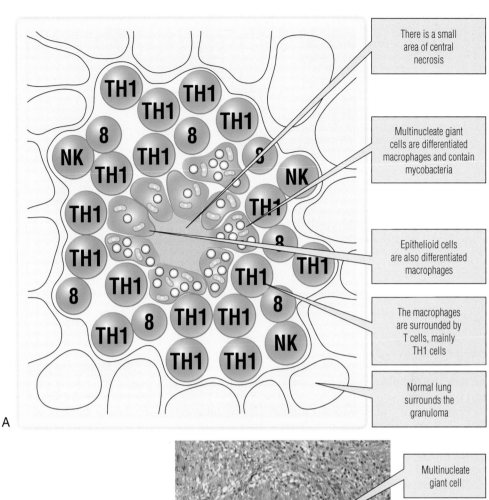

There is a small area of central necrosis

Multinucleate giant cells are differentiated macrophages and contain mycobacteria

Epithelioid cells are also differentiated macrophages

The macrophages are surrounded by T cells, mainly TH1 cells

Normal lung surrounds the granuloma

A

Multinucleate giant cell

Cuff of lymphocytes surrounding granuloma

Central area of caseous necrosis

B

Fig 23.3 A, The major features of a tuberculous granuloma. In this particular case, necrosis is minimal. If necrosis becomes more severe, the granuloma will break down and *Mycobacterium tuberculosis* could be coughed up. **B,** Micrograph of a tuberculous granuloma. Note the central necrosis, two giant cells on either side of this, and the cuff of lymphocytes in the periphery. *NK,* natural killer; *TH1,* T-helper 1.

Mycobacteria, such as *M. tuberculosis,* have waxy coats that block the effects of phagocyte enzymes. They also secrete catalase, which prevents the effects of the oxidative burst. Because it is hard to kill them, macrophages seal off mycobacteria inside phagosomes. This sealing-off process requires help from T cells in the form of TH1 cytokines such as IFN-γ.

Initial exposure to TB results in primary infection. In most patients with primary TB, mycobacterial growth is contained within the granuloma (Fig. 23.3).

Here, macrophages mature under the influence of IFN-γ into giant and epithelioid cells. Granulomata seal off infected macrophages so well that the center of a granuloma occasionally

 MCH II

 Cytokine, chemokine, etc.

Complement (C')

 Signaling molecule

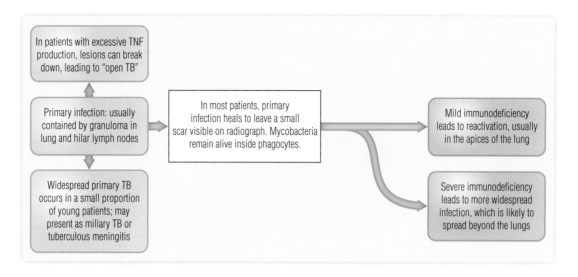

Fig 23.4 Infection with *Mycobacterium tuberculosis* can have a number of short- and long-term outcomes. *TB,* tuberculosis; *TNF,* tumor necrosis factor.

becomes hypoxic, and the cells may become necrotic. The necrotic area resembles cheese; this caseous necrosis is a hallmark of TB infection.

Fewer than 10% of patients with primary TB have any symptoms, and even fewer develop widespread infection. In very young or immunodeficient patients, primary TB is not contained within the granuloma. In these patients, infection may be widespread (miliary TB; Fig. 23.4).

Even when infection is contained and controlled in the lungs, many mycobacteria may survive inside macrophages or other cells for several years. This is referred to as *latent infection*. Tests for latent TB infection are described in Box 23-1.

Paradoxically, patients who respond to primary TB infection with excessive production of TNF may develop extensive local tissue damage and become infectious to other people.

Postprimary (reactivation) TB occurs in about 10% of patients, especially if macrophage function is moderately impaired. This commonly happens when patients are treated with high doses of corticosteroids or if malnutrition is present, such as in alcoholics. Reactivation of TB is also a common problem in HIV infection.

Antibodies have a negligible role in the protection from or response to *M. tuberculosis*. Unlike hepatitis B infection (see below), preexisting antibodies do not prevent TB infection. In established *M. tuberculosis* infection, the mycobacteria reside inside cells and are not susceptible to antibody-mediated destruction.

■ HEPATITIS B INFECTION

Hepatitis B infection is a major global health problem, with 350 million individuals across the world infected. The virus causes hepatitis that often leads to cirrhosis and liver cancer (hepatoma). HBV replicates only in hepatocytes but does not damage these cells directly; the virus is not cytopathic.

The immune response to HBV is important at two different stages. If antibodies to the HBV surface protein (HBsAg) are present when the virus first enters the blood, the antibodies can bind on to the virus, preventing it from attaching itself to hepatocytes. Thus anti-HBsAg can protect from infection; such antibodies are usually the result of vaccination. HBV vaccination was discussed in Box 17.1 and will be explained further in Chapter 25. Antibodies against HBsAg can also be given as passive immunity after known exposure to HBV, as described in Box 4.2.

Once HBV is actively replicating in the liver, antibodies become less important than the cellular immunity mediated by TH1 cells. In established infections, antibodies still provide a degree of control over HBV because drugs or disease that prevent antibody production can lead to a flareup of HBV replication. In established disease, antibodies play an important role in diagnosis (Box 23.2; see also Box 6.1).

Cellular immunity is important in people who do not have protective antibodies and in whom virus is already replicating in hepatocytes. HBV is susceptible to the antiviral effects of interferons, as described in Chapter 20. During hepatitis B infection, the specific immune system responds to infection with a TH1-type response, as would be expected for a viral infection, and hepatitis B–specific CD4$^+$ and CD8$^+$ T cells migrate to the liver. These cells secrete IFN-γ and TNF, cytokines that promote the inflammatory response, and evidence shows that the antiviral effects of IFN-γ inhibit viral replication. Nearly all infected patients develop transient hepatitis, which is life threatening in fewer than 1% (see Box 6.1). However, most infected patients (80% to 90%) manage to suppress viral replication through the antiviral effects of IFN-γ. Unlike the type I interferons, IFN-γ has potent stimulating effects on inflammation, and a mild inflammatory response develops, during which some hepatocytes are damaged by the immune response rather than by the virus itself. The result is acute hepatitis. In the majority of patients, viral replication is subsequently controlled. Although

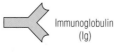
T-cell receptor (TCR)

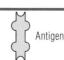
Immunoglobulin (Ig)

Antigen

MCH I

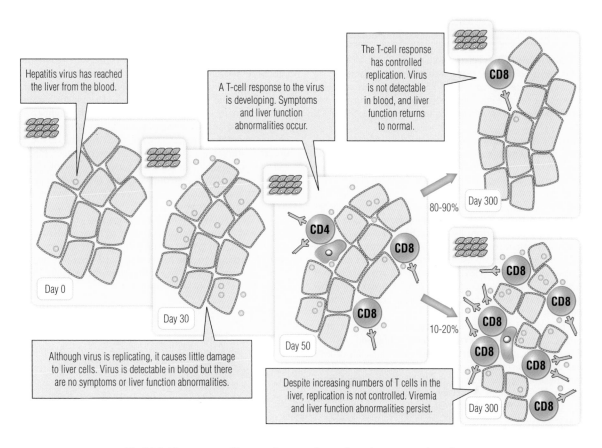

Fig 23.5 The outcome of hepatitis B virus infection depends on immunologic factors.

virus is not eradicated, ongoing T-cell responses are enough to minimize virus replication so that, for example, the patient stops being infectious to other individuals (Fig. 23.5).

In approximately 10% to 20% of infected people, the virus is not cleared through these means. This can happen when the initial inoculum of virus was particularly large. Failure to clear the virus is also more likely when an individual is exposed to it at a very early age; this is a type of tolerance. Host factors, such as the human leukocyte antigen (HLA) type, may affect the risk of not clearing virus. In these individuals the inflammatory response persists, although it is unable to inhibit viral replication completely. Unlike TB, chronic hepatitis B infection does not produce granulomata. In hepatitis B patients, production of IFN-γ is a double-edged sword; it is the best hope for inhibiting viral replication but will promote a chronic inflammatory response that results in chronic active hepatitis. The recruitment of NK cells, macrophages, and T cells that are not even specific for HBV eventually leads to chronic inflammation inside the portal areas. The resulting tissue destruction causes scars that can lead to liver cirrhosis and, through unknown mechanisms, can set the scene for liver cancer. In these individuals, the inflammation is overzealous in the sense that it is causing more damage than benefit.

Individuals who have been infected with HBV but have successfully suppressed viral replication can be compromised in a number of ways. For example, you will read in later chapters how monoclonal antibodies against B cells or against TNF are used to treat some diseases. Both of these antibodies can reactivate hepatitis B infection. For this reason, it is important to check whether patients have latent infection with HBV before treatment with these antibodies.

■ "OVERZEALOUS" INFLAMMATION

During inflammation, granuloma formation and cytokines may have negative effects. Some of the negative effects of TNF have already been mentioned, such as weight loss. A specific example of an overzealous response is excessive granuloma formation in the lung in response to *M. tuberculosis*. The blood supply to the centers of large granulomata is poor. The central part of granulomata may die and become necrotic, and this is then coughed up by the patient. Lung cavities are produced when necrotic material is coughed up. Coughing up necrotic material allows the mycobacteria contained in it to be spread from person to person. These infectious patients are described as having *open TB*. Another type of overzealous response occurs when the immune system causes fibrosis and cirrhosis in patients with hepatitis B infection. This is referred to as *hypersensitivity*.

 MCH II

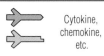 Cytokine, chemokine, etc.

 Complement (C′)

 Signaling molecule

BOX 23.1 Tuberculosis Outbreak in a Prison

Tuberculosis (TB) is relatively common in prison inmates.

An infection control team is called into a prison after a prisoner has developed symptoms of TB. She has been coughing and has experienced weight loss and sweats. Her chest radiograph shows destruction of normal tissue and is suggestive of TB (Fig. 23.6).

Culture of her sputum is positive for *Mycobacterium tuberculosis,* confirming the diagnosis and the significant risk to other inmates. The index patient is transferred to the prison hospital for treatment and to prevent her from infecting other patients.

During her stay in prison, she has shared cells with 36 other prisoners. These prisoners require screening for exposure to TB and development of infection. Because chest radiographs and sputum cultures are insensitive to early TB infection, tests of immunity to *M. tuberculosis* are used to screen individuals exposed to patients with "open TB." Tests for latent TB are carried out in the prison and, in this case, four of the 36 prisoners show evidence of latent TB and are treated with combinations of antibiotics.

Unlike hepatitis B infections and many other infections, antibody testing is not used to diagnose latent infection with *M. tuberculosis*. This is in large part because all humans produce antibodies against harmless mycobacteria living in the environment, and these antibodies cannot easily be distinguished from those against *M. tuberculosis*. Antibody testing for latent TB is so unreliable that the World Health Organization has taken the unusual step of banning such tests.

Two types of test are used safely to test for latent TB, and both evaluate cellular immunity to tuberculosis. Immunity to TB implies either exposure to TB itself or that the patient has been vaccinated. These tests are most often used to screen individuals who have been exposed to patients with open TB. The older test is a skin test that relies on the delayed hypersensitivity reaction. Skin testing is gradually being replaced by a blood test that measures interferon gamma (IFN-γ) secreted in response to mycobacterial antigens (Fig. 23.7).

The IFN-γ release assay (IGRA) is reliant on the presence of effector T cells circulating in the blood, which are able to secrete IFN-γ within 24 hours of the addition of antigen in patients with latent TB. Delayed hypersensitivity skin testing is carried out with intradermal injection of tuberculin, a sterile mixture of proteins and lipoproteins derived from *M. tuberculosis*. This type of skin test is also known as the *Mantoux* or *Heaf* test, depending on the type of injection technique used. The reaction starts when Toll-like receptors (TLRs) on dermal macrophages recognize the mycobacteria and in response secrete tumor necrosis factor (TNF) and chemokines, which increase the expression of local endothelial adhesion molecules (Fig. 23.8).

At the same time, dendritic cells migrate from the site of injection to draining lymph nodes. The migrating dendritic cells are loaded with mycobacterial antigens, which can be presented to T cells in the draining lymph node if adequate numbers exist from a primary response. Remember that the number of T cells for a specific antigen increases during the acquisition of immunologic memory. The activated T cells migrate to the injection site and interact with local activated macrophages. Macrophages will also accumulate and mature as a result of cytokines secreted by the T cells. When a strong response (Fig. 23.9) is produced at 48 hours, more than 80% of the cells present in the skin lesion are activated macrophages.

The delayed hypersensitivity skin test is cheap to do because it does not require a laboratory test to measure IFN-γ. However, the skin test will give a positive result after exposure to TB or after TB vaccination. The IGRA blood test does not give a positive result after vaccination and is therefore more useful in countries where TB vaccine is given routinely.

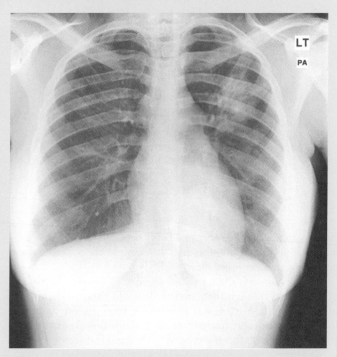

Fig 23.6 This chest radiograph shows changes typical of tuberculosis that tend to affect the apices of the lungs. An opacity in the upper zone of the left lung is clearly seen. (Courtesy Dr. Mark Woodhead, Manchester Royal Infirmary, United Kingdom.)

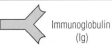 T-cell receptor (TCR)   Immunoglobulin (Ig)   Antigen ⊔ MCH I

BOX 23.1 Tuberculosis Outbreak in a Prison—cont'd

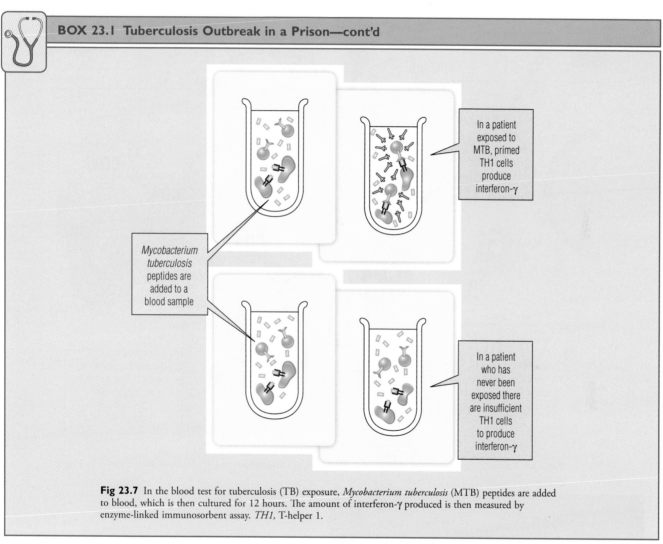

Mycobacterium tuberculosis peptides are added to a blood sample

In a patient exposed to MTB, primed TH1 cells produce interferon-γ

In a patient who has never been exposed there are insufficient TH1 cells to produce interferon-γ

Fig 23.7 In the blood test for tuberculosis (TB) exposure, *Mycobacterium tuberculosis* (MTB) peptides are added to blood, which is then cultured for 12 hours. The amount of interferon-γ produced is then measured by enzyme-linked immunosorbent assay. *TH1*, T-helper 1.

Continued

 MCH II

 Cytokine, chemokine, etc.

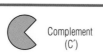 Complement (C′)

 Signaling molecule

BOX 23.1 Tuberculosis Outbreak in a Prison—cont'd

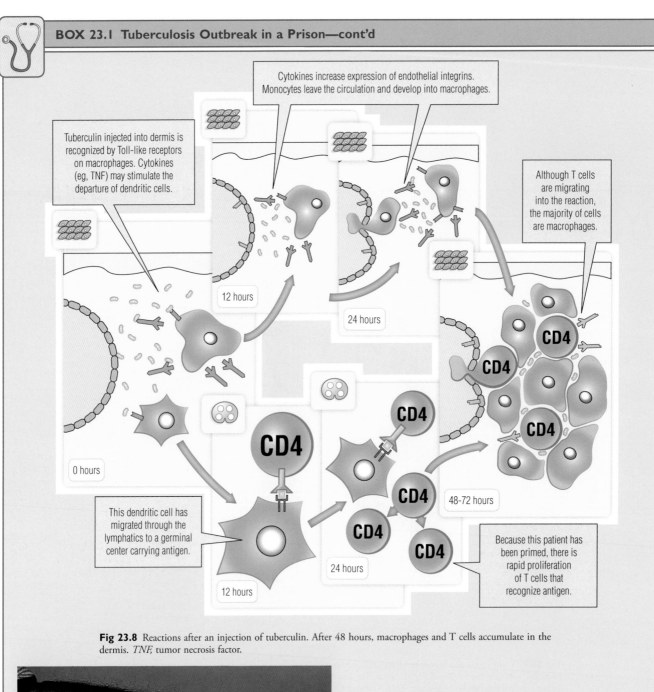

Cytokines increase expression of endothelial integrins. Monocytes leave the circulation and develop into macrophages.

Tuberculin injected into dermis is recognized by Toll-like receptors on macrophages. Cytokines (eg, TNF) may stimulate the departure of dendritic cells.

Although T cells are migrating into the reaction, the majority of cells are macrophages.

This dendritic cell has migrated through the lymphatics to a germinal center carrying antigen.

Because this patient has been primed, there is rapid proliferation of T cells that recognize antigen.

0 hours

12 hours

24 hours

48-72 hours

12 hours

24 hours

Fig 23.8 Reactions after an injection of tuberculin. After 48 hours, macrophages and T cells accumulate in the dermis. *TNF,* tumor necrosis factor.

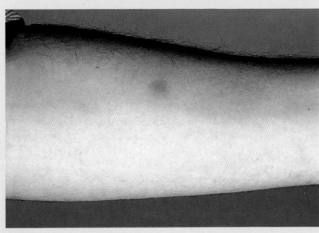

Fig 23.9 This is a positive tuberculin skin test in one of the prisoners described in Box 23-1, shown 48 hours after injection. This prisoner had never had the tuberculosis (TB) vaccine; therefore the positive test confirms exposure to TB and possible latent infection.

 T-cell receptor (TCR)

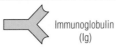 Immunoglobulin (Ig)

 Antigen

 MCH I

BOX 23.2 Chronic Active Hepatitis B Infection

In Box 6.1, you read about a woman who was diagnosed as having been recently infected with hepatitis B virus (HBV). Although she initially had evidence of viral replication and felt unwell, she began to feel better spontaneously, and levels of viral DNA and hepatitis B surface antigen (HBsAg) fell (see Fig. 6.8C). This indicated that she had entered a phase of immunologic control of her hepatitis B infection, which was *not* damaging her liver.

However, 9 years later, she begins to feel unwell again. Liver function tests are abnormal, and once again her HBV viral DNA is present, along with HBsAg, in blood. A liver ultrasound scan is carried out and reveals no evidence of hepatoma, the worst complication of HBV infection. A liver biopsy is carried out and this shows a diffuse inflammatory infiltrate of mainly T cells. There is also evidence of early liver scarring, referred to as *fibrosis* or *cirrhosis*.

Taken together, these tests show that viral replication is active and is not being controlled by her immune response. Furthermore, her immune response appears to be causing damage to the liver. This can happen if the virus mutates and a change in the amino acid sequence of viral peptides enables it to evade the immune system.

Figure 23.10 shows the treatments available to prevent or treat HBV infection. The patient decides to start treatment with interferon (IFN)-α. In hepatitis B infection, the aim is to suppress viral replication but not to increase immune activation or inflammation. IFN-α is a type I interferon that has more potent antiviral effects than immune-stimulatory effects (Chapter 20). Interferon gamma (IFN-γ) has more proinflammatory effects than antiviral effects and in this setting is a "bad guy." Box 24.1 describes what happens next.

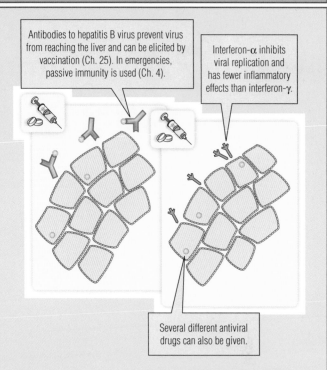

Antibodies to hepatitis B virus prevent virus from reaching the liver and can be elicited by vaccination (Ch. 25). In emergencies, passive immunity is used (Ch. 4).

Interferon-α inhibits viral replication and has fewer inflammatory effects than interferon-γ.

Several different antiviral drugs can also be given.

Fig 23.10 Hepatitis B virus infection can be prevented or treated in a number of ways.

LEARNING POINTS   Can You Now...

1. Define inflammation?
2. Describe the outcomes of tuberculosis infection?
3. Describe the consequences of hepatitis B infection and how they are affected by the immune response?
4. Draw the cytokine network?
5. Describe two immunologic tests for latent tuberculosis?

 MCH II

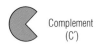 Cytokine, chemokine, etc.

Complement (C')

 Signaling molecule

Cytokines in the Immune System

CHAPTER **24**

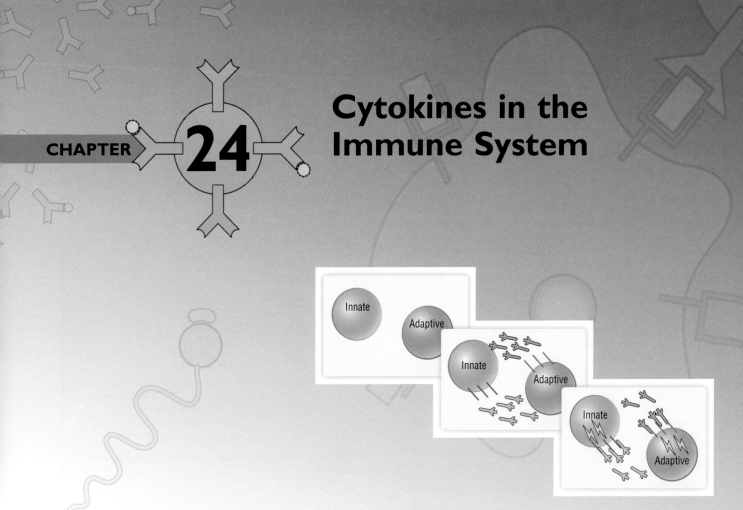

The cells of the adaptive and innate immune systems cannot function in isolation. Immune cells use cytokines to communicate with each other and with different tissues in the body. This chapter discusses cytokines further: how they are recognized by specific receptors and how they activate special signaling molecules in their target cells. No new cytokines are discussed in this chapter, and the interactions described have already been covered. Use this chapter to review what you have learned about immune responses. At the end of this chapter, some important clinical applications for cytokines are described.

▓ OVERVIEW

This section reviews what has been discussed so far about the adaptive and innate immune systems and focuses on the types, structure, and role of cytokines and their receptors. Some of the material in this chapter will be familiar, but you will need to develop a good working knowledge of cytokines because of their increasing significance in clinical medicine.

Cytokines are soluble messenger molecules usually secreted by cells of the immune system. Some cytokines such as type I interferons (IFNs) and tumor necrosis factor (TNF) are secreted by nonimmune cells (eg, epithelial cells). Although some cytokines are constantly secreted at a low level (*constitutively secreted*), most are secreted only when cells become activated as part of the response to infection.

Cytokines are secreted at extremely variable levels. Adaptive immune system cytokines are secreted at very low levels and affect only neighboring cells (*paracrine effects*) or even the secreting cell itself (*autocrine effects*). This low-level secretion is to maintain the specificity of the adaptive immune system. For example, interleukin 2 (IL-2), secreted by activated T cells, has potent effects that induce T-cell proliferation. Most of these effects are mediated on the cell that is secreting IL-2. If IL-2 were secreted at high levels, it might activate cells that were not recognizing specific antigen. Because of the low level of secretion, however, adaptive immune system cytokines are almost impossible to detect in fresh blood samples.

Cytokines of the innate immune system are often secreted at low levels over a short range, such as chemokines directed at attracting neutrophils to the site of infection, but they can also be secreted at high enough levels to be measurable in blood samples. When they are secreted at high levels, they act like hormones of the endocrine system. For example, IL-1, IL-6, and TNF secreted during an acute-phase response can have distant effects such as induction of fever (Chapter 20).

Because most cytokines are secreted in response to infection, they are secreted only transiently. For example, IL-2 is secreted only by activated T cells for about 8 hours. Any longer secretion would cause inappropriate and potentially dangerous prolonged immune system activation. Once infection is resolved, cytokine secretion tends to fall. In addition, toward the end of an immune response, inhibitory cytokines such as IL-10 and transforming growth factor beta (TGF-β) may be produced to ensure the immune response does not continue.

Cytokine receptors are also often only expressed transiently. The complete IL-2 receptor is only transiently expressed by activated T cells. Again, this mechanism has evolved to prevent inappropriate activation of the immune system.

Cytokines have two more important features, redundancy and pleiotropism. *Redundancy* refers to the fact that, in general, several cytokines secreted during an immune response have very similar properties. For example, TNF and IL-1 have similar effects. These cytokines synergize with one another; in other words, the impact of both cytokines being secreted together is greater than the sum of the effects of the individual cytokines. This is important clinically because attempts to block the effects of cytokines may not always guarantee clinical outcomes. Anti-TNF monoclonal antibodies are successful at preventing joint damage in rheumatoid arthritis, for example, but do not completely prevent disease because IL-1 is also mediating damage.

Pleiotropism refers to the fact that many cytokines affect several different types of cells. This is also clinically important: the antiviral effects of interferon-α are used to treat hepatitis B virus (HBV) infection, but interferon-α makes patients feel unwell because it induces an acute-phase response. How pleiotropism causes side effects of cytokine treatment is described in Box 24.1.

Cytokines act as part of a complex network. Apart from synergizing with one another, cytokines can also inhibit each other. For example, IFN-γ promotes T-helper 1 (TH1) cell responses and also inhibits the development of TH2 responses, mediated by IL-4. This can contribute to the unexpected effects seen when cytokines are administered or blocked during treatment.

Finally, the nomenclature of cytokines can be hard to follow. The largest group, interleukins, were so named because they were initially thought to act between leukocytes. In fact, they often have much wider effects on many different types of cells. The interleukins (IL-1, IL-2, etc) were named in the order they were discovered, so their numbering has no relation to function.

Some of the originally discovered cytokines were named after their presumed function. The interferons, for example, were so named because they interfere with viral replication, but they also have potent effects activating the immune system. TNF was so named because it can induce necrosis in cancers when injected into animals at high concentrations. Its effects in vivo are usually far more subtle.

Table 24.1 lists the important cytokines by their general effects. Note how many cytokines link the adaptive and innate immune systems.

CYTOKINE RECEPTORS AND SIGNALING MOLECULES

Most cytokines use receptors that belong to one of three families. Each of these families of receptors is linked to different signal-transduction molecules that convey signals from the receptor to the inside of the cell. These share some properties with the signal-transduction machinery connected to T- and B-cell receptors (Chapter 11). The three main types of receptor are (1) the

common cytokine receptor family, (2) the chemokine receptor, and (3) the TNF receptor.

Most cytokines use the common receptor molecules, sometimes called the *hemopoietin receptors*. This includes cytokines that act as growth factors and the interferons. Common cytokine receptors consist of one or more transmembrane molecules with extracellular domains that confer specificity for particular cytokines (Fig. 24.1). The receptors for IL-2, IL-4, and IL-7 consist of three separate polypeptide chains but share a common γ-chain. The gene for the γ-chain is defective in X-linked severe combined immunodeficiency disease (SCID). The clinical consequences of this are described in Box 12.2.

Most of the common cytokine receptors are not expressed in high numbers in completely resting cells; they tend to be upregulated after a cell has been activated, such as after a T cell has been activated through its T-cell receptor. After upregulation, the cytokine receptors are normally spread across the surface of the cell. When cytokine binds to its receptor, it causes aggregation of the receptors at the cell surface. One of several tyrosine kinases, called *Janus kinases (JAKs),* are normally loosely associated with the cytoplasmic portion of the cytokine receptors. JAKs remain inactive when they are spread under the cell's surface. The JAK enzymes become activated when the receptors are brought together by cytokine binding, and then they phosphorylate one of several transcription factors called *signal transducers* and *activators of transcription* (STATs). Once STAT molecules have become phosphorylated, they form a dimer, migrate to the nucleus, and activate transcription of specific genes.

There are several JAK and STAT molecules. For example, when IL-2 binds to receptors on the surface of activated T cells, it activates JAK5, STAT1, and STAT3. When these migrate to the nucleus, they activate genes that initiate T-cell proliferation.

When extracellular levels of cytokines fall toward the end of the immune response, they cease binding to receptors, and the events leading to gene transcription will come to an end.

Chemokines are a large family of cytokines that have already been mentioned in relation to attracting cells into inflamed tissues (Chapters 13 and 21). They also have a role in leukocyte homing. For example, chemokines secreted by cells in lymph nodes attract B cells to germinal centers and dendritic cells and attract T cells to the T-cell areas (Chapter 13). To achieve these complex signals are approximately 50 different chemokines and approximately 20 different receptors. Most of the receptors can bind several different chemokines, and many chemokines can bind different receptors. The chemokine receptors are α-helices that span the cytoplasmic membrane seven times (Fig. 24.2). On binding chemokines, the receptors catalyze the replacement of guanosine diphosphate (GDP) by guanosine triphosphate (GTP). One specific chemokine receptor is used as a coreceptor for HIV (Chapter 33).

TNF uses a special family of receptors. TNF is secreted and can be active as a membrane-bound form. It can also be cleaved from the secreting cell membrane and is then free to cause local or remote effects. Both cell-bound and cell-free TNF are present as a trimer and bind to one of two types of receptor, which are also trimers.

Two other important members of the TNF–TNF receptor family, CD40 and CD40-ligand (CD154), have already

 MCH II

 Cytokine, chemokine, etc.

 Complement (C′)

 Signaling molecule

TABLE 24.1 Cytokines and Their General Effects

General Effects	Cytokine	Secreted by	Targets	Receptor Family	Chapter Reference
Proinflammatory	TNF	Macrophages, T cells, other cells	Many cell types	TNF receptor	21, 22, 23
	IL-1	Macrophages	Endothelial cells, liver cells, hypothalamus	Ig superfamily molecule	21
	Chemokines (including IL-8)	Macrophages, endothelial cells, T cells	All leukocytes	Chemokine receptor	13, 21, 33
	Type I interferons	Macrophages, dendritic cells, many other cells	Many cell types	Common cytokine receptor family	20, 23
	IL-6	Macrophages, T cells	Liver, B cells		20, 21
Growth factors	IL-7	Bone marrow stromal cells	Lymphoid progenitors		12
	G-CSF	Macrophages	Neutrophils		12, 21
	IL-2	T cells	T cells and NK cells		11, 12, 15, 16, 22
TH1	IFN-γ	TH1	Macrophages, B cells, T cells, and NK cells		16, 17, 23
	IL-12	Macrophages	TH1 cells and NK cells		16, 17, 23
TH2	IL-4	TH2 cells and mast cells	T cells, B cells, and mast cells		16, 17, 23
	IL-5	TH2 cells	Eosinophils and B cells		16, 17, 23
TH17	IL-23	Dendritic cells and epithelial cells	TH17 cells		16, 17, 23
	IL-17	TH17 cells	Neutrophils and epithelial cells	Specialized receptor	16, 17, 23
Inhibitory/regulatory	IL-10	Macrophages and Tregs	T cells and macrophages	Common cytokine receptor family	18
	TGF-β	Macrophages and Tregs	B cells, T cells, and macrophages	Specialized receptor	13, 18

Blue *indicates cells of the innate immune system, pink indicates cells of the adaptive immune system, and orange indicates cells of both systems.*
G-CSF, *granulocyte colony-stimulating factor;* IFN, *interferon;* IL, *interleukin;* NK, *natural killer;* TGF, *transforming growth factor;* TH, *T helper;* Tregs, *T regulatory (cells).*

been discussed. This pair of costimulatory molecules is involved in interactions between T cells and either B cells or antigen-presenting cells (APCs). The other pair is Fas and Fas ligand (FasL; Table 24.2).

The effects of TNF depend on the target cell it binds to. When TNF binds to infected cells, it induces apoptosis by inducing caspases through death domain engagement, as described in Chapter 22. On the other hand, when TNF binds macrophages or endothelial cells, it induces transcription of genes by engaging a special set of adaptor molecules that activate nuclear factor kappa B (NF-κB). Fas-FasL ligation induces apoptosis only in target cells, but it does so in a wide range of situations. CD40/CD154 (CD40 ligand) binding induces gene transcription and has an important role in communication between T cells and either APCs or B cells (Fig. 24.3). Chapter 16 discussed that mutations in the *CD154* gene can lead to antibody deficiency.

■ REVIEW OF SOME OF THE ROLES OF CYTOKINES IN IMMUNE RESPONSES

Most of the components of the immune system should now be familiar. It is useful at this stage to review how these components fit together, particularly to understand the role of cytokines in

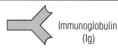

T-cell receptor (TCR)

Immunoglobulin (Ig)

Antigen

MCH I

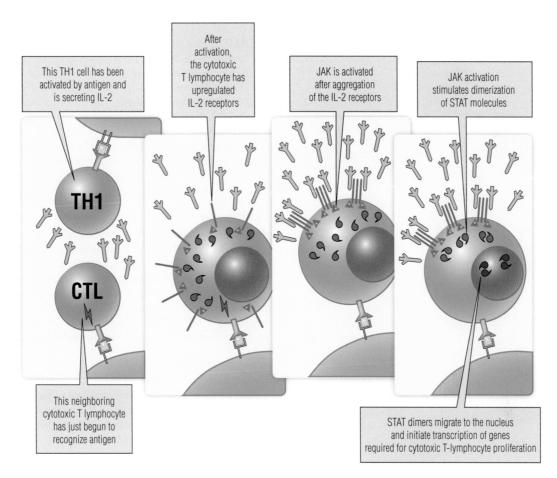

Fig 24.1 The key features of the hemopoietin family of cytokine receptors and associated signaling molecules. *IL,* interleukin; *TH1,* T-helper 1.

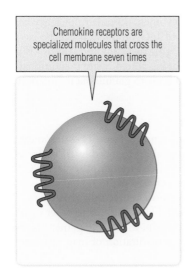

Fig 24.2 A typical chemokine receptor.

TABLE 24.2 Tumor Necrosis Factor Family Members and Their Receptors

TNF-Like Molecule	TNF Receptor–Like Molecule	Induces Apoptosis	Induces Gene Transcription
TNF	TNF receptor	Yes	Yes
CD40 ligand	CD40	No	Yes
Fas ligand	Fas	Yes	No

TNF, *tumor necrosis factor.*

Acute Inflammation: Initial Response to Infection

Invading pathogens present pathogen-associated molecular patterns (PAMPs) to cells of the innate immune system, which respond by producing danger signals, mainly secreted cytokines. In the case of extracellular bacteria or fungi, phagocyte recognition using Toll-like receptor (TLR) leads to secretion of cytokines, including IL-1, TNF, granulocyte-colony stimulating factor (G-CSF), and IL-6. These stimulate local inflammation and may contribute to the development of an acute-phase response. Often, systemic features of an acute-phase response are present that include fever, high white blood cell count, loss of appetite,

communication between the innate and adaptive immune systems (Fig. 24.4). Be sure you understand the role of cytokines in initiation of inflammation, T-cell priming, development of T-cell specialization, and finally the winding down of the immune response.

 MCH II   Cytokine, chemokine, etc.   Complement (C′)   Signaling molecule

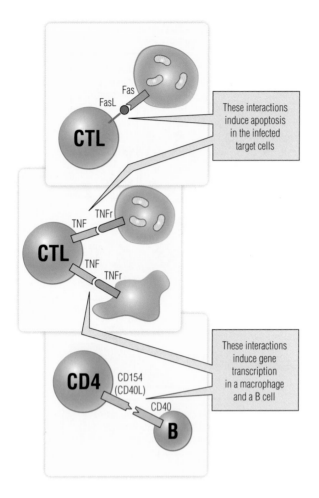

Fig 24.3 The different possible effects of tumor necrosis factor (TNF) family members binding to their receptors. *CD40L,* CD154 (CD40 ligand); *CTL,* cytotoxic T lymphocyte; *FasL,* Fas ligand; *TNFr,* TNF receptor.

and malaise. At its most extreme, an acute-phase response may lead to septic shock (Chapter 21).

Macrophages and other local cells secrete IL-8 and other chemokines, which attract neutrophils to the site of infection. These cells also secrete IL-23, which can stimulate the priming of TH17 cells. If the host is exposed to the same pathogen again, TH17 will secrete IL-17, which is also highly effective at attracting neutrophils and stimulating epithelial cells to secrete antimicrobial peptides.

The situation is different in the case of viral infections; type I IFN secretion predominates. Type I cytokines have direct antiviral effects and enhance antigen presentation and the development of TH1 responses. Type I cytokines also trigger an acute-phase response (see Box 24.1).

T-Cell Priming

The next events take place in the lymph node that drains the site of infection. Antigen is presented by dendritic cells and is recognized by T cells that express the appropriate receptor. As discussed in Chapter 16, TH cells will become activated only if APCs also provide costimulation in the form of surface

molecules (CD40, CD80, intercellular adhesion molecule [ICAM]). APCs also secrete costimulatory cytokines that include IL-1 and type I IFNs, both of which help initiate T-cell responses.

T-helper cells becoming activated upregulate the IL-2 receptor and begin to secrete IL-2. TH cells will not proliferate until IL-2 has bound to its receptor. The IL-2 may have been secreted by the cell itself (*autocrine effect*) or by a neighboring T cell (*paracrine effect*); either can lead to expansion of T-cell clones. The subsequent events depend on the type of pathogen triggering the response and the site of the response.

Development of Specialized T-Cell Responses

Gut Immunity

Gut-derived T cells secrete a cytokine called *transforming growth factor beta* (TGF-β). TGF-β induces an immunoglobulin (Ig) class switch from IgM to IgA, which has a major role in mucosal immunity. TGF-β also has potent antiinflammatory effects and inhibits the effects of most T-cell populations, macrophages, and proinflammatory cytokines. TGF-β can induce T cells to become regulatory T cells (Tregs). The net result is that in the gut, most of the immune response is skewed toward the production of IgA.

TH17 Responses

Extracellular pathogens such as bacteria and fungi stimulate the innate immune system to produce IL-23. This in turn stimulates the generation of TH17 T cells. These secrete IL-17, which has potent effects in attracting neutrophils to the site of infection.

TH1 Responses

Intracellular pathogens stimulate APCs to secrete IL-12 and type I IFNs. As detailed in Chapter 16, these induce the T-cell transcription factor T-bet, which leads to IFN-γ secretion and a TH1 phenotype. TH1 cells favor the production of IgG by B cells, which can then stimulate phagocytosis by activated phagocytes. B-cell IgG production can be supported by IL-6, which acts as a growth factor for B cells. When intracellular pathogens cannot be cleared, there is additional high-level TNF secretion, which leads to granuloma production, as discussed in Chapter 23.

TH2 Responses

Worm infections tend to favor TH2 responses. It is not clear what inducing signal is produced by APCs in response to worm infection, but the T-cell transcription factor GATA3 is induced and leads to the secretion of IL-4. IL-4 favors B-cell production of IgE, which activates mast cells that in turn produce more IL-4. In addition, TH2 cells secrete other cytokines, IL-5, and the chemokine eotaxin, which help perpetuate the TH2 response by stimulating the maturation of mast cells and eosinophils.

Regulatory T Cells

Tregs are part of peripheral tolerance and prevent responses to self antigen. They secrete IL-10 and TGF-β. Tregs use these cytokines to inhibit responses to self antigen.

End of the Immune Response

Once a pathogen is cleared, the amount of danger signal received by the innate immune system falls, and levels of cytokines such

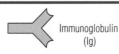 T-cell receptor (TCR)

Immunoglobulin (Ig)

 Antigen

 MCH I

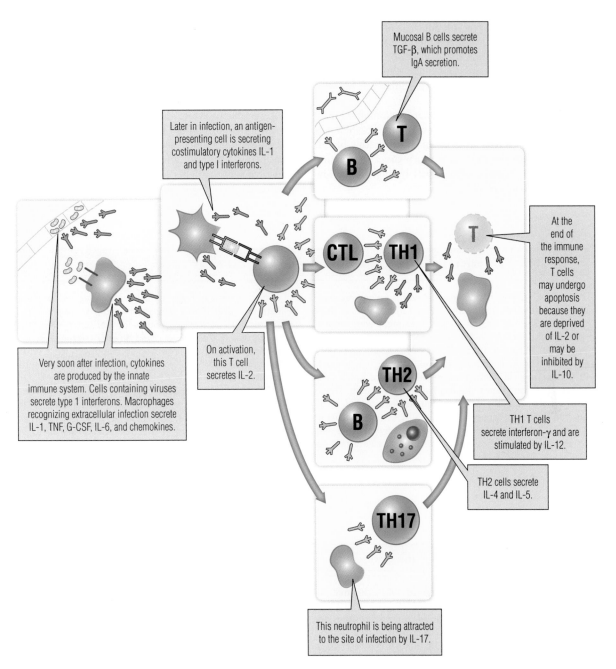

Fig 24.4 The roles of cytokines in the immune response. Note again how cytokines communicate between the adaptive and innate immune systems. *CTL,* cytotoxic T lymphocyte; *G-CSF,* granulocyte colony-stimulating factor; *Ig,* immunoglobulin; *IL,* interleukin; *TGF,* transforming growth factor; *TH,* T helper; *TNF,* tumor necrosis factor.

as IL-1, type I IFNs, and TNF tend to fall. In addition, less antigen is available for presentation, and T-cell stimulation will decline, which leads to lower levels of cytokine production and lower levels of cytokine-receptor expression. As levels of IL-2 in particular fall, T cells produce less Bcl-2 and are prone to undergo apoptosis. These factors tend to wind down the immune response.

Although the numbers of memory T cells are probably maintained by low-level constitutive IL-7 secretion, and neutrophil

numbers are maintained by constitutive G-CSF production, the production of proinflammatory cytokines is switched off in between infections.

■ CLINICAL USES FOR CYTOKINES AND CYTOKINE BLOCKADE

Blood levels of hormones are routinely measured in clinical practice. For example, hypothyroidism is diagnosed by showing

 MCH II    Cytokine, chemokine, etc.   Complement (C')   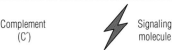 Signaling molecule

low levels of thyroxine. However, blood levels of cytokines are not measured in routine clinical practice. The reason for this is that cytokines usually act over a very small anatomic range—for example, a germinal center in a lymph node—and do not spill over into the blood. This is a fundamental difference between hormones and cytokines.

The one situation in which cytokines are measurable in the blood is in very severe infection, such as toxic shock, when it is possible to find high levels of TNF or IL-6 in the blood. However, even in these situations it is much easier to measure the clinical impact of high cytokine levels by high fever, low blood pressure, or abnormal white cell count.

Note that in the IFN-γ release assay (IGRA) discussed in Box 23.1, IFN-γ is *not* measured in blood; rather it is measured after it has been secreted by patient cells stimulated in vitro.

Cytokines are occasionally used as treatments. For example, hepatitis B virus (HBV) infection can be treated with recombinant interferon-α. But as described Box 24.1, this frequently causes problems. More often, cytokines are blocked, usually with monoclonal antibodies. The next few chapters discuss some of the diseases for which monoclonal antibodies are used. For the time being, it is important to understand how blocking cytokines can predispose patients to specific infections. This is described in Box 24.2.

BOX 24.1 Side Effects of Interferon-α Treatment

Box 23.2 described a 38-year-old woman who was diagnosed with chronic hepatitis caused by hepatitis B virus (HBV) infection. She has chosen to start treatment with recombinant interferon (IFN)-α; however, the product she receives has been "pegylated" (Chapter 36) so that she only needs one injection per week. After the injection she developed a high fever (well over 40°C), had muscle pains, and lost her appetite for 2 days. This happened all four times she has had the treatment. These symptoms would normally be regarded as features of virus infection, but they also happen in about 50% of patients being treated with IFN-α. The patient is switched to antiviral drugs and the side effects go away. Five years later, she has returned to normal health.

IFN-α is used in hepatitis B infection because of its antiviral effects. However, IFN-α also activates the acute-phase response (Chapter 20). There are receptors for IFN-α in the hypothalamus, so it is possible that IFN-α could directly trigger an acute-phase response. Alternatively, IFN-α could stimulate T cells, which then release interleukin 6 (IL-6), which in turn triggers the acute-phase response.

Most cytokines are pleiotropic, and they affect many different cells. This means that cytokines given therapeutically tend to cause side effects. At the current time, although many cytokines have been manufactured in the quantities required to be used therapeutically, the number of licensed indications is very small. This is largely because of the severity of side effects.

BOX 24.2 An Unexpected Infection

A 51-year-old man was diagnosed with rheumatoid arthritis 1 year ago. The details of his diagnosis are given in Box 31.1. His arthritis does not respond to first-line drugs, so the decision is made for him to start treatment with a monoclonal antibody against tumor necrosis factor (TNF). TNF plays an important role in causing joint damage in rheumatoid arthritis (Chapter 31), and anti-TNF antibodies are highly effective in this condition.

Anti-TNF monoclonal antibodies are known to reactivate latent tuberculosis. This is because TNF is important in the cytokine network that maintains the integrity of granulomata (see Fig. 23.2). For this reason, latent tuberculosis must be ruled out before starting anti-TNF treatment. This patient has an interferon gamma release assay (IGRA; Box 23.1). This assay is negative, which indicates that latent tuberculosis is unlikely. The patient starts his anti-TNF treatment.

The patient's anti-TNF antibodies are given intravenously every 4 weeks. After the third infusion, he says his symptoms are about 75% better, and he decides to continue treatment.

Two weeks later, the patient develops an acute illness with high fever, dizziness, low blood pressure, and a rapid heart rate. In the emergency department, a physician diagnoses septic shock, and the patient is started on antibiotics after a blood culture sample is taken. The patient makes a gradual recovery. The bacterium *Listeria monocytogenes* is grown from the blood culture sample.

As well as increasing the risk of reactivating tuberculosis, anti-TNF monoclonal antibodies increase the risk of other intracellular organisms. *Listeria* is one such intracellular bacteria. It is a rare infection contracted by eating contaminated foods. *Listeria* causes death in about 20% of patients. This story illustrates how important it is to consider unusual infections in patients being treated with cytokine blockade.

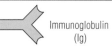 T-cell receptor (TCR)

 Immunoglobulin (Ig)

 Antigen

MCH I

LEARNING POINTS   Can You Now...

1. Define cytokines and explain three of their general principles of action?
2. Predict two different types of clinical problems with using cytokines as treatment?

3. Diagram three different types of cytokine receptors and their associated intracellular signaling pathways?
4. List the roles played by cytokines at different times in the immune response?

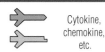 MCH II

 Cytokine, chemokine, etc.

 Complement (C´)

Signaling molecule

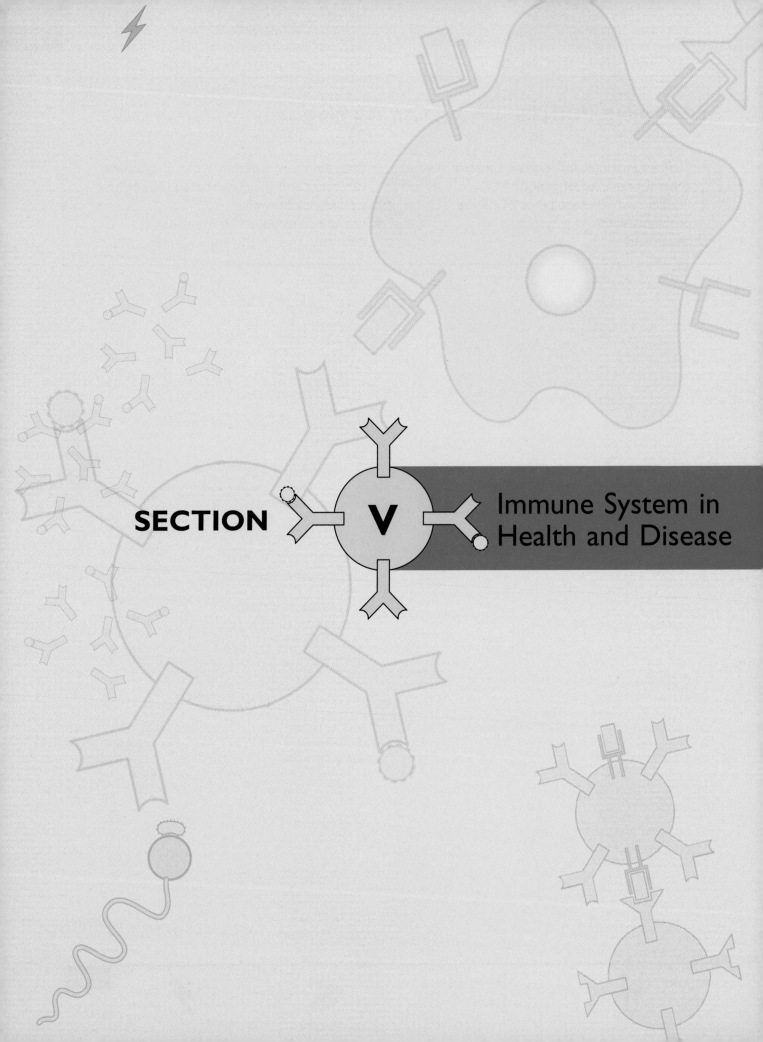

SECTION **V** Immune System in Health and Disease

Infections and Vaccines

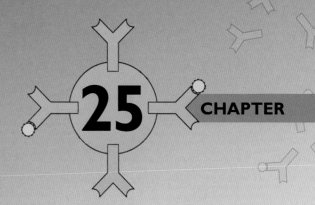

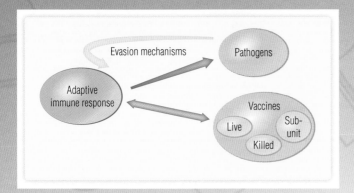

This chapter discusses some of the mechanisms pathogens use to evade the immune response as well as how the three main types of vaccines stimulate the immune response. The boxes in this chapter give more details about four important vaccines.

■ HOW ORGANISMS EVADE THE IMMUNE RESPONSE

To be successful, each type of pathogen has evolved different ways of evading the immune response. Some of these are summarized in Figure 25.1.

Small RNA viruses, such as influenza (Box 25.2) and HIV (Chapter 33), do not have enough capacity in their small genomes to encode proteins that could help evade the immune response. However, a characteristic of the RNA genome is that it tends to mutate, and antigenic proteins that belong to RNA viruses change continually, thus evading immunologic memory. In the case of HIV, this can happen within an individual. After infection with HIV, many different strains will arise within the infected host over just a few months. Influenza mutates more slowly, across a population rather than in an individual.

DNA viruses are larger and have capacity in their genomes for evasion tools. Some DNA viruses, such as members of the herpesvirus family, evade the adaptive immune response by downregulating major histocompatibility complex (MHC) expression, and the innate response is required for their control (natural killer [NK] cells). Because there is no immunologic memory for the innate system, it is hard to prime responses to

viruses such as herpesviruses and to protect individuals from infection.

Bacterial pathogens use a variety of strategies to evade the immune system. Pneumococcus (*Streptococcus pneumoniae*) and *Haemophilus* species evade the innate response (opsonization by complement and phagocytosis) by producing a polysaccharide capsule. These encapsulated organisms are successful pathogens of the respiratory tract.

Mycobacteria, such as *Mycobacterium tuberculosis,* have waxy coats that block the effects of phagocyte enzymes. They also secrete catalase, which inhibits the effects of the respiratory burst. How macrophages control mycobacteria without killing them is discussed in Chapter 23.

Listeria causes meningitis, particularly in pregnant women. *Listeria* secretes listeriolysin, which punches holes in the phagolysosome walls. The bacteria can then escape into the cytoplasm, where they are not exposed to the toxic products of the metabolic burst or to proteolytic enzymes.

■ MECHANISMS OF IMMUNITY

Aside from some of the infections mentioned in the preceding section (tuberculosis [TB], HIV, and herpesvirus infections), most primary infections are completely cleared by the immune system to achieve a state of sterilizing immunity. In addition, immunologic memory develops; subsequent exposure to the same pathogen elicits a memory response by the adaptive immune system so that infection is prevented or symptoms are reduced.

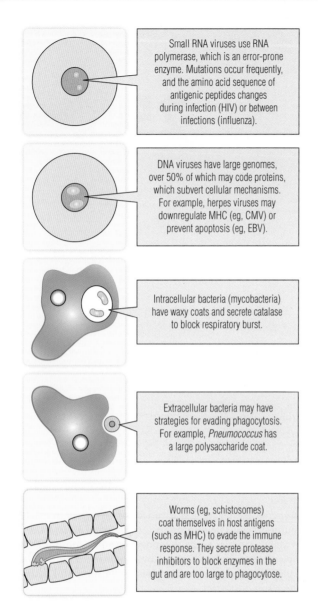

Small RNA viruses use RNA polymerase, which is an error-prone enzyme. Mutations occur frequently, and the amino acid sequence of antigenic peptides changes during infection (HIV) or between infections (influenza).

DNA viruses have large genomes, over 50% of which may code proteins, which subvert cellular mechanisms. For example, herpes viruses may downregulate MHC (eg, CMV) or prevent apoptosis (eg, EBV).

Intracellular bacteria (mycobacteria) have waxy coats and secrete catalase to block respiratory burst.

Extracellular bacteria may have strategies for evading phagocytosis. For example, *Pneumococcus* has a large polysaccharide coat.

Worms (eg, schistosomes) coat themselves in host antigens (such as MHC) to evade the immune response. They secrete protease inhibitors to block enzymes in the gut and are too large to phagocytose.

Fig 25.1 Strategies to avoid the immune system. *CMV,* cytomegalovirus; *EBV,* Epstein-Barr virus; *MHC,* major histocompatibility complex.

TABLE 25.1   Classification Scheme for Vaccines

Types of Vaccine	Component of Vaccine	Examples
Live	Attenuated human pathogen	Oral polio, measles, mumps, rubella, influenza*
	Nonhuman pathogen	Smallpox vaccine, BCG
	Recombinant organism	Experimental; canarypox used as a vector for HIV
Killed		Pertussis*
		Influenza*
Subunit	Purified peptide components	Acellular pertussis*
	Toxoids	Diphtheria, tetanus
	Polysaccharides	*Pneumococcus, Haemophilus, Meningococcus*
	Recombinant peptides	Hepatitis B, human papillomavirus
	DNA vaccines	Experimental (eg, HIV)

*Available in more than one type.
BCG, bacille Calmette-Guérin.

situations, it is possible to give both passive immunotherapy to reduce the immediate risk of infection and the vaccine to induce immunologic memory and reduce the risk for future infection. Antidigoxin Fab fragments (see Box 4.2) are also a type of passive immunity.

Active immunity develops after the immune system has been exposed to antigen in the form of infection or vaccine. Immunologic memory then develops and protects the individual from reinfection. Of the various types and compositions of vaccine (Table 25.1), each has its own advantages and problems. Most vaccines elicit antibodies, and some elicit T-cell responses. Antibodies elicited by vaccines can prevent pathogens from binding onto target cells, or they can prevent the actions of toxins released from pathogens; these are both examples of neutralizing antibodies. Antibodies can also activate complement and stimulate phagocytosis and NK cell–mediated killing. CD8⁺ T cells induced by vaccines can inhibit viral replication by secreting interferons or, more often, by killing infected cells.

This chapter describes the details of each type of vaccine. Boxes 25.1 through 25.4 give more specific information about vaccines for smallpox, whooping cough, influenza, and hepatitis B.

■ TYPES OF VACCINES

Live Vaccines

Live vaccines were the first to be discovered, and they are still the most effective; for example, the successful vaccines against smallpox and polio are live vaccines. Live vaccines use organisms that are not virulent; although they replicate in healthy vaccine recipients, they do not cause disease. One way of obtaining nonvirulent organisms is to use organisms that have evolved to grow in animals. For example, the virus that causes cowpox has

After maternal antibody has been lost, early childhood is characterized by a series of primary infections while effective immunologic memory is developed. Vaccination can act as a substitute for primary infection, allowing immunologic memory to develop without a symptomatic primary infection. Vaccines are a success story; smallpox is one lethal infection that has been completely eradicated by vaccination. Many other infections—such as polio, diphtheria, and pertussis—have become relatively rare.

Before we discuss vaccines in detail, we need to mention *passive immunotherapy,* the transfer of adaptive immunity— usually antibodies—from one individual to another. Passive immunotherapy is often used to give protective antibodies to an individual who has been exposed to a pathogen. Examples include an individual exposed to tetanus (see Box 30.2). In these

 T-cell receptor (TCR)   Immunoglobulin (Ig)   Antigen   MCH I

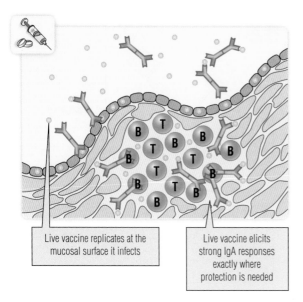

Live vaccine replicates at the mucosal surface it infects

Live vaccine elicits strong IgA responses exactly where protection is needed

Fig 25.2 Live vaccines, such as polio or influenza, replicate at the site of infection. *IgA,* immunoglobulin A.

been used very successfully as a vaccine for smallpox (see Box 25.1). Antibodies against live vaccines, such as measles and mumps, persist for many decades after vaccination. Other live vaccines use human pathogens that have been attenuated (ie, weakened) so that they are incapable of causing disease. Attenuation has been conventionally carried out by growing the organism in special conditions in vitro. In the future, more live vaccines are likely to be attenuated by direct manipulation of their genomes.

Live vaccines are highly effective for three reasons (Fig. 25.2):

- They replicate and thus deliver sustained doses of antigen.
- They replicate intracellularly so they deliver antigenic peptides to MHC class I molecules and thus stimulate cytotoxic T lymphocytes (CTLs).
- They replicate at the anatomic site of infection, which further focuses the immune response. For example, live vaccines given by nose or by mouth elicit immunoglobulin A (IgA) antibodies.

Live vaccines also may be excreted and passed on to other, unvaccinated individuals.

Attenuated live vaccines can cause serious infections in two types of situations. In patients with immunodeficiency, they can cause infection despite attenuation. Occasionally, the viruses in live vaccines spontaneously revert to the virulent wild-type organism. Attenuated polio vaccine differs from the wild-type virus in only 10 base pairs. Such small differences make it easy for the virus to mutate back to the virulent form. Poliovirus that has reverted from the attenuated to the virulent form has been identified in water supplies. As a result of concerns raised by this finding, the United States has started to use killed polio vaccine once more.

Organisms can also be deliberately altered genetically. For example, viral vectors are viruses that have been made safe for use in humans and can be used as vectors to take the required genes from another organism for expression in cells. These vaccines are largely experimental but have been used in clinical trials. For example, canarypox virus has been used as a vector for HIV genes.

Killed Organisms

Killed organisms are generally not as effective as live vaccines at eliciting a protective immune response, although they are theoretically much safer. These differences are attributable to the fact that killed vaccines do not replicate in hosts and cannot enter intracellular antigen-presenting pathways. Influenza vaccine is available as a live virus but is more frequently given as a killed virus. This is discussed in Box 25.2.

Subunit Vaccines

Subunits are components of pathogens and induce predominantly antibody responses. Subunits can be prepared by destroying virulent organisms, purifying the subunit, and then inactivating it so that it cannot cause disease. Other subunits are prepared using recombinant technology.

Subunits purified from organisms and then inactivated are referred to as *toxoids.* They are usually bacterial toxins that have been chemically altered to make them safe, although they retain their antigenicity. The neutralizing antibodies produced block the effects of the toxins. Diphtheria and tetanus toxoid are good examples of this approach. Subunit and toxoid vaccines are generally of low immunogenicity compared with intact organisms, and they may need adjuvants to work effectively. The antibody response induced by subunit vaccines is also of relatively short duration compared with that of live vaccines. For example, antibody to tetanus only persists for about 10 years after vaccination. This is why a booster may be required for this type of vaccine.

Hepatitis B vaccine is a subunit antigen that has been produced using recombinant techniques (Box 25.3). Hepatitis B vaccine is made up of recombinant virus surface peptide. Antibodies raised against surface peptide will prevent the virus attaching to and then entering liver cells. Up to now, hepatitis B vaccine has been highly effective. Reasons that peptide vaccines may not remain successful are described in Box 25.4.

Polysaccharides are very poor immunogens, largely because they rely on the response of T-independent B cells (Chapters 14 and 16) and do not make good vaccines. To overcome this, effective vaccines contain polysaccharide that has been chemically conjugated to a peptide antigen, and tetanus toxoid is often used. T cells that respond to the peptide then provide help for B cells that respond to the polysaccharide (see also Box 16.3).

A final type of subunit vaccine is the DNA vaccine. In this experimental approach, the gene for the immunogenic protein is coated onto gold microspheres and injected directly into cells (eg, of the skin). In mice, this has resulted in antibody production, indicating that the genes were transcribed (see also Box 10.3). So far in humans, it has not been possible to deliver sufficient DNA for this approach to be used routinely.

Adjuvants

Adjuvants are defined as substances given to increase the immune response (antibodies or T cells) to an antigen.

 MCH II

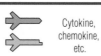 Cytokine, chemokine, etc.

 Complement (C')

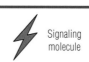 Signaling molecule

Adjuvants provide the pathogen- or damage-associated molecular patterns (PAMPs or DAMPs) required to drive the innate immune system to release danger signals to drive antibody and T-cell responses. Live vaccines generally do not require adjuvants because they are capable of providing danger signals and stimulating Toll-like receptors (TLRs) themselves. For example, bacille Calmette-Guérin (BCG), the live vaccine for tuberculosis, produces large quantities of bacterial sugars that activate TLRs 2 and 4. Killed whole vaccines also contain substances that activate TLRs and can act as adjuvants. Vaccines that use recombinant or purified proteins do not contain sufficient natural adjuvant; therefore synthetic adjuvant must be added.

Up until the 21st century, aluminum hydroxide (alum) was the only synthetic adjuvant used routinely in humans. It is still used to boost the effects of a wide variety of subunit vaccines. Alum was introduced empirically as an adjuvant to vaccines, and it was not known how it worked at the time of introduction. Alum activates macrophages, which then secrete inflammatory cytokines and present antigen to T and B cells. Alum probably does this by causing local tissue damage, which then activates DAMPs on the macrophages. Alum is not a powerful adjuvant, and research continues to find ways of improving vaccines.

More recently, monophosphoryl lipid (MPL) derived from *Salmonella* polysaccharide was found to be a potent agonist for TLR-4. Macrophages exposed to MPL were found to increase interleukin 12 (IL-12) secretion and to upregulate MHC class II expression. These actions theoretically increase antigen presentation and skew the immune response toward T-helper 1 (TH1). MPL is now used in important licensed vaccines, such as against human papillomavirus (HPV) and malaria (see Box 25.4).

Accessing Intracellular Pathways

A second problem with subunit vaccines is that they do not enter the intracellular antigen-processing pathways and so do not elicit CTL responses, which are particularly important in dealing with intracellular infections such as HIV. Live vaccines derived from intracellular pathogens—such as poliovirus and BCG—are able to access intracellular pathways. New technologies help gain access to intracellular pathways:

- Immunostimulatory complexes (ISCOMs) are micelles of lipid and subunit antigen that are lipophilic and can penetrate cell membranes (Fig. 25.3). These vaccines may incorporate viruslike particles (VLPs), which add further structure. Lipid and VLPs have been used in the malaria vaccine (see Box 25.4).
- Vectors are living viruses that have been made safe by genetic modification, such as canarypox. Genes for the pathogen, such as HIV, can be added. These genes are expressed intracellularly, but there is no live pathogen (HIV) replication.
- DNA vaccines as described above could be used as a way of expressing proteins intracellularly, if sufficient DNA could be administered.

Table 25.2 summarizes some of the experimental vaccine approaches that have been mentioned in this chapter.

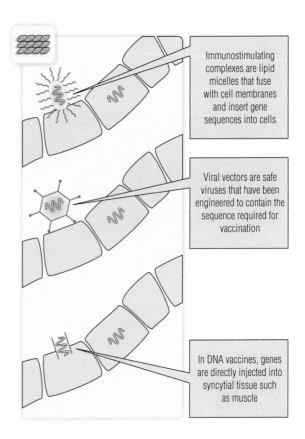

Immunostimulating complexes are lipid micelles that fuse with cell membranes and insert gene sequences into cells

Viral vectors are safe viruses that have been engineered to contain the sequence required for vaccination

In DNA vaccines, genes are directly injected into syncytial tissue such as muscle

Fig 25.3 Technologies that may offer safe vaccines for eliciting cytotoxic T-lymphocyte responses.

TABLE 25.2 How Technologies Are Improving Vaccine Effectiveness

Problem	Tools
Delivery of antigen via intracellular pathways	Live viral vectors DNA vaccines Immunostimulatory complexes
Inadequate stimulation of the innate immune system	Modern adjuvants that agonize Toll-like receptors
Poor responses to polysaccharide antigen	Conjugate vaccines (see Box 16.3)

■ VACCINE SCHEDULES

Vaccine schedules take into account the clinical implications of each type of infection. For example, the main purpose of rubella vaccine is to prevent intrauterine infection, which can cause deformities, so there is little point in giving it before puberty. On the other hand, it would be desirable to protect very young infants against *Haemophilus* because this organism causes the most damage at this age (see Box 16.3). However, even as conjugate vaccines, polysaccharides do not elicit antibodies in

 T-cell receptor (TCR)

 Immunoglobulin (Ig)

Antigen

 MCH I

newborn babies. The aim of human papillomavirus (HPV) vaccines is to prevent the sexual transmission of the strains of HPV that cause cervical cancer. For this reason, these vaccines are given at the time of puberty.

Vaccine schedules also vary in different parts of the world (Table 25.3). For example, measles is a major cause of death in infants in the developing world; therefore the vaccine is given as early as possible. In the developed world, measles has become rare and tends to affect school-age children, so the vaccine can be given slightly later. However, the main factor affecting the use of vaccines in the developing world is cost.

TABLE 25.3   Vaccination Schedules in the Developed and Developing World

Time of Vaccination	Developed World	Developing World
0–6 months	Rotavirus	BCG (tuberculosis)
	Hepatitis B	Malaria
	Diphtheria	Hepatitis B
	Tetanus	Diphtheria
	Pneumococcal conjugate	Tetanus
	Haemophilus conjugate	Pneumococcal conjugate
	Acellular pertussis	*Haemophilus* conjugate
	Inactivated polio	Live polio
6–12 months	Influenza	Measles
1–10 years	Measles	
	Mumps	
	Rubella	
	Varicella	
Early teenage	Human papillomavirus	
	Meningococcus	

This figure compares vaccine schedules in the developed and developing world. Does not include boosters. Live vaccines are shown in yellow, killed vaccines are shown in blue, and subunit vaccines are shown in pink. Influenza can be given as a live or killed vaccine.
BCG, bacille Calmette-Guérin.

BOX 25.1 Smallpox Vaccine

A 32-year-old soldier is required to have smallpox vaccination. What do you know about this vaccine, and why it has to be given to this individual?

Smallpox (variola virus) is a highly contagious viral infection that causes a blistering skin reaction and carries a mortality rate of 10% to 30%. The related cowpox causes a mild, local blistering reaction. It was known for many centuries that cowpox infection could protect against subsequent smallpox infection, but it was not until the end of the 18th century that Edward Jenner formally showed that deliberate inoculation with vaccinia virus would protect against smallpox. This is where the term *vaccination* originates.

Global smallpox vaccination was carried out by the World Health Organization, and the last case of smallpox in the general population occurred in 1977. Since then, the only cases of smallpox reported have occurred in laboratory workers. Some supplies of variola virus were retained in various laboratories across the world, and concern has been raised that these supplies of wild smallpox virus may have been accessed by bioterrorists. Because global vaccination was abandoned at the beginning of the 1980s, most young people are not immune to smallpox; hence, this virus could be used as a biologic weapon. Some governments have therefore recommended smallpox vaccination at least for military personnel.

Vaccinia is a live vaccine that is scraped into the surface of the skin. It replicates in the skin and causes considerable local inflammation. In the first week following vaccination, a blister forms that gradually heals over during the second week. The blister contains viable vaccinia virus, and blister fluid can infect other individuals. In patients with defective immune systems, smallpox vaccination leads to widespread dissemination of the vaccinia virus, a generalized rash, and the risk of serious illness.

Continued

 MCH II

  Cytokine, chemokine, etc.

 Complement (C′)

 Signaling molecule

BOX 25.1 Smallpox Vaccine—cont'd

Because vaccinia replicates inside cells in the skin, it delivers a high level of antigen to the intracellular antigen-presentation pathway and stimulates the development of cytotoxic T lymphocytes (CTLs). Viruses that have budded off into the extracellular space will be phagocytosed, enter the extracellular antigen pathway, and stimulate helper T cells and antibody production. In the days of the global vaccination scheme, considerable data were established on the longevity of the antibody and CTL responses. Because each individual was vaccinated just once, and because natural vaccinia infection is not endemic, the exposure can be pinpointed to vaccinia vaccination. The absence of environmental vaccinia ensures that any responses measured are not maintained by reexposure to this or any cross-reacting organism.

Figure 25.4 shows the longevity of the immune response to vaccinia virus and also the level of protection from infection. The data show that antibody levels are sustained for at least 60 years. Vaccinia-specific B- and T-cell numbers decline in the years immediately after vaccination but are then sustained. Even 50 years after vaccination, vaccinia-specific B cells account for 1:1000 of all circulating B cells. These T and B cells are functional; if the individual is revaccinated, he or she will mount a secondary immune response, indicating the presence of functional memory T and B cells. Although T-cell responses decline, with a half-life of 8 to 10 years, antibody levels and protection from infection last for at least 60 years after vaccination.

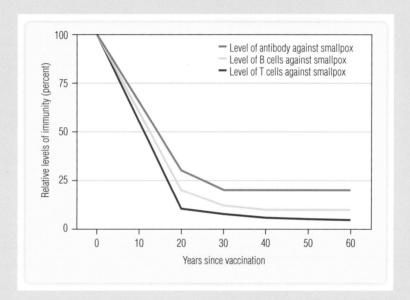

Fig 25.4 The relationship between longevity of antibody and B-cell and T-cell responses to smallpox. The red lines are antibody levels, green lines are B-cell numbers, and blue lines represent levels of T-cell responsiveness.

BOX 25.2 Influenza Vaccine

A 26-year-old doctor working in a busy emergency department has been asked to get vaccinated against the flu. She is not keen on the idea because she had the vaccine last year. Can you explain why she needs to have it again this year?

Influenza is a respiratory virus that causes severe infection in the very young and in the elderly. Each year, influenza causes about 36,000 deaths in the United States during the influenza season, which lasts from October to February. In 1918, just after the first World War, a new influenza virus emerged and caused an influenza pandemic. "Spanish flu" spread around the world in 9 months and caused 40 million deaths.

Influenza is an RNA virus that uses a protein called *hemagglutinin* to bind sugars on respiratory epithelial cells. Influenza is cytopathic; it causes damage to the cells it infects. The presence of double-stranded RNA stimulates respiratory tract cells to secrete interferon-α within a few hours of viral infection, which inhibits viral replication (Chapter 20) and slows the spread of influenza in the lungs.

Dendritic cells migrate to the local lymph node and present antigen to T cells. Under the influence of T-helper type 1 (TH1) cells, cytotoxic T lymphocytes (CTLs) begin to appear after 2 to 3 days. These cells clear the residual infected cells, and sterilizing immunity is thus achieved.

Influenza also elicits an antibody response, and immunoglobulin M (IgM) antibodies begin to appear after about 5 days. These neutralizing antibodies bind to hemagglutinin and prevent virus

T-cell receptor (TCR)

Immunoglobulin (Ig)

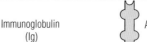
Antigen

MCH I

BOX 25.2 Influenza Vaccine—cont'd

from infecting cells. The antibody response against influenza develops too late to have a major role in helping to clear established infection, and it is most important in preventing reinfection with an identical viral strain.

Influenza is a relatively unstable RNA virus that can undergo spontaneous mutation. Gradual mutations slowly change the viral genome and result in antigenic drift. Because the mutated virus has some antigenic similarity with existing strains, existing immunity is partially protective; this means that no widespread epidemic will occur, and infection is usually mild (Fig. 25.5). More rapid, extensive genetic changes can also occur. These events occur when a host animal is infected with two different strains of flu virus. The two strains exchange segments of genes, and a third, new strain results. This is referred to as *genetic shift* and is believed to cause the flu pandemics that occur every few years. Most of these genetic events occur between human and bird flus. There have been some human infections with new strains of bird flu, but at the time of writing, there is no evidence that a new, shifted, mutant flu virus has emerged from Asia. If a new, shifted virus does emerge that is capable of human-to-human spread, global infection is very likely to arise within a few weeks because of mass air travel.

Influenza vaccine is effective at preventing infection in individuals at risk for severe complications (eg, patients with chronic chest problems). The conventional flu vaccine used killed influenza virus. The flu virus is grown in hen eggs and is then killed and purified. A live vaccine also exists that is sprayed into the nose and can elicit protective IgA antibodies in addition to IgG.

To be effective, the flu vaccine must contain the most up-to-date strains. The World Health Organization provides guidance for vaccine manufacturers with early warnings of changes in the virus. The vaccine manufacturers select viruses to include in the vaccine in January. During the next 6 months, the selected viruses are grown on eggs until there is enough virus to start manufacturing the vaccine. This process requires virus manufacturers to obtain tens of millions of eggs during spring each year. By summer, if production has gone to plan, the vaccine (killed or live) is ready for testing. If the vaccine passes its safety tests, it can then be distributed to users.

In most years, there is enough warning of slightly drifted flu virus to enable the production of updated vaccine. However, if a new virus emerges through antigenic shift after recombination with bird flu, it can take the manufacturers up to 10 months to prepare the new vaccine. In the age of mass air travel, the shifted virus may have spread around the world in this time.

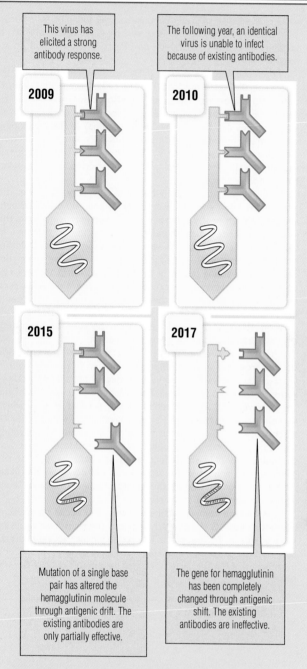

2009 — This virus has elicited a strong antibody response.

2010 — The following year, an identical virus is unable to infect because of existing antibodies.

2015 — Mutation of a single base pair has altered the hemagglutinin molecule through antigenic drift. The existing antibodies are only partially effective.

2017 — The gene for hemagglutinin has been completely changed through antigenic shift. The existing antibodies are ineffective.

Fig 25.5 Single base-pair mutations that cause drift are relatively frequent. Shift occurs much less often, probably when human influenza virus exchanges gene sequences with animal viruses (reassortment). Such events overcome immunity on an enormous scale and trigger global pandemics.

 MCH II   Cytokine, chemokine, etc.   Complement (C')   Signaling molecule

BOX 25.3 Hepatitis B Vaccine

A relative of yours is considering training to be a nurse. She has been told she will have to have hepatitis B vaccine but is worried about side effects. What can you do to reassure her?

When the hepatitis B virus (HBV) invades liver tissue, it triggers a specific T-cell response. These T cells prevent viral replication in the majority of cases but can also cause irreversible liver damage, as described in Chapter 23. A long-term complication of viral hepatitis can be liver cancer (hepatoma). In the developing world, many individuals become infected very early in childhood and maintain a carrier status throughout life. The hepatitis B vaccine was the first recombinant subunit vaccine, and it has been tremendously successful.

In developing countries where HBV is very common, the vaccine has been given to everybody to build up so-called *herd immunity*. When nearly everyone in a community is immune, the number of carriers falls, thereby protecting the nonimmune. In these countries, hepatitis B vaccination programs have almost eradicated hepatoma—the first example of a vaccine being successful at preventing cancer. In the developed world, the strategy up to now has been to vaccinate only high-risk individuals, such as those at risk because their work (eg, medical residents). Increasingly, governments are switching from the selective vaccination strategy to global vaccination because of the safety, effectiveness, and value of global vaccination.

Hepatitis B vaccine consists of a relatively short peptide derived from the hepatitis B surface antigen (HBsAg) grown in yeast cells. The vaccine can be produced on a large scale—somewhat like producing beer. The yeast and other contaminants are removed and alum is added to the purified HBsAg, which forms viruslike particles (VLPs) that have an additional immunostimulatory effect even though they are incapable of replicating (Fig. 25.6). Recombinant subunit vaccines produced in this way are quite safe. Mild side effects such as headache, pain at the injection site, and fever are short lived and common and likely reflect the alum activating the innate immune response. More significant side effects are rare.

This vaccine stimulates T-helper cells and elicits neutralizing immunoglobulin G (IgG), which prevents the virus from entering hepatocytes in the first place. The recombinant vaccine protects 80% to 90% of those vaccinated. Failure to develop protection from hepatitis B after vaccination can be a result of host or viral factors.

Host Factors

The short peptide contains only a few potential T-cell epitopes. Vaccine responses are diminished in individuals who are homozygous at all their major histocompatibility complex (MHC) class II alleles because these individuals have relatively fewer MHC molecules on which they can display a limited number of antigenic peptides. This is referred to as the *heterozygote advantage* and is explained in detail in Chapter 8.

Viral Factors

HBV is prone to undergo gradual mutation. In the face of widespread immunity to HBsAg, viral strains with mutations in this protein are at an advantage and can escape vaccine-induced immunity. These strains were very rare when the vaccine was first introduced, but mutations are becoming increasingly common in viral isolates from the very countries where widespread vaccination has been successful.

Possible solutions are to use either a larger peptide or a mixture of peptides. These approaches decrease the chances of particular human leukocyte antigen alleles being unable to bind epitopes, and they may reduce the risk of successful viral mutations.

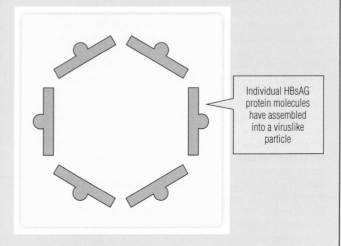

Individual HBsAG protein molecules have assembled into a viruslike particle

Fig 25.6 Compare this hepatitis B surface antigen (HBsAg) viruslike particle with the image of a virus (see Fig. 6.7A). The viruslike particle cannot replicate because it does not contain DNA.

 T-cell receptor (TCR)

 Immunoglobulin (Ig)

 Antigen

MCH I

BOX 25.4 Malaria Vaccine

A 7-year-old girl living in Vietnam has a high fever and is losing consciousness. Malaria parasites are found on a blood film. Fortunately, she responds to antimalarial drugs. Last year her 6-year-old sister died from malaria. What can be done to prevent this happening again?

Malaria kills about 1 million people each year. It is caused by the protozoan *Plasmodium,* which is injected into the human bloodstream by a mosquito bite. *Plasmodium* initially reproduces in the liver and then changes its morphology and undergoes several reproductive cycles in the red cells. Symptoms do not arise until red cells are infected. A mosquito bite at this point may infect the mosquito, where the protozoan changes its morphology and reproduces again, before reinfecting another human.

Individuals who have inherited the polymorphism in the hemoglobin gene that causes sickle cell trait have a degree of protection from malaria (see Box 3.1). Other than this, most individuals have few defenses against *Plasmodium.* This is largely because considerable antigenic variation exists with each of the different stages in the life cycle of *Plasmodium.* Unlike most other pathogens, natural infection does *not* lead to sterilizing immunity. This means that people who have recovered from malaria may experience further acute infections, albeit somewhat milder. Over time, if the individual is not exposed to malaria again, they will lose any immunity they had and will risk a severe infection on reexposure.

It has proven very challenging to develop a malaria vaccine. Circumsporozoite protein (CSP) has been identified as a useful antigen for vaccines. CSP is used by *Plasmodium* to dock onto hepatocytes, and antibodies against CSP can disrupt this part of the life cycle. CSP has the advantage of not varying across different strains of *Plasmodium.* The CSP protein is expressed in combination with hepatitis B surface antigen (HBsAg), and the CSP HBsAg fusion protein forms a viruslike particle (VLP) to boost the immune response. The adjuvant monophosphoryl lipid (MPL) is also added (Fig. 25.7). Even with these modifications, current malaria vaccines have only about 50% efficacy in preventing acute malaria in vaccinated children.

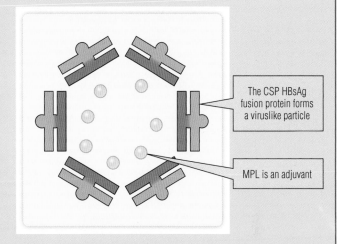

The CSP HBsAg fusion protein forms a viruslike particle

MPL is an adjuvant

Fig 25.7 This diagram shows the best malaria vaccine currently available. *CSP,* circumsporozoite protein; *HBsAg,* hepatitis B surface antigen; *MPL,* monophosphoryl lipid.

LEARNING POINTS Can You Now...

1. Describe three different types of vaccine currently in use and how these vary in their safety and efficacy?

2. Explain how we can measure the longevity of immunologic memory from vaccine responses?

3. Describe two different types of whooping cough vaccine and why they are used in different countries?

4. Explain why influenza vaccine may need to be given every year?

5. Describe two newer approaches to vaccination?

 MCH II   Cytokine, chemokine, etc.   Complement (C')    Signaling molecule

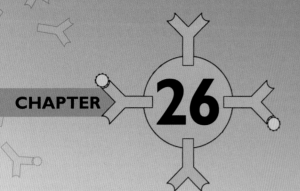

CHAPTER 26

Hypersensitivity Reactions

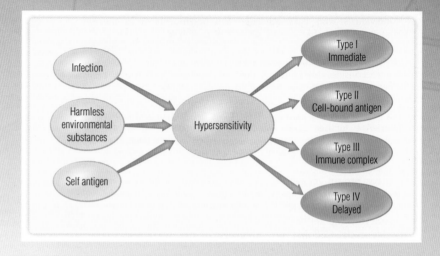

This chapter discusses how hypersensitivity reactions can be triggered by infections, harmless environmental substances, and autoantigens and can lead to four different types of reactions. Examples of each of the four different types of hypersensitivity reactions are given in clinical boxes in this chapter and are explored in much more detail in the next few chapters.

Excessive immune responses that cause damage are called *hypersensitivity reactions*, and they can occur in response to three different types of antigen:

- *Infectious agents*. The immune system sometimes overreacts to infections and causes disease; when an overzealous immune response contributes to the symptoms of infection, the resultant disease is a type of hypersensitivity.
- *Environmental substances*. Hypersensitivity can occur in response to innocuous environmental antigens, one example of which is allergy. For example, in hay fever, grass pollens themselves are incapable of causing damage; the immune *response* to the pollen is what causes the harm.
- *Self antigens*. Normal host molecules can trigger immune responses, referred to as *autoimmunity;* when these cause hypersensitivity, *autoimmune disease* is the result.

Hypersensitivity reactions use four different mechanisms for causing disease; these are the topics of Chapters 26 through 31.

■ TYPES OF TRIGGERS FOR HYPERSENSITIVITY

Hypersensitivity to Infectious Agents

Not all infections are capable of causing hypersensitivity reactions. For example, although the common cold elicits a strong immune response, it never appears to cause harm. Other respiratory viruses such as influenza can cause hypersensitivity. Influenza virus damages epithelial cells in the respiratory tract but can sometimes elicit an exaggerated immune response, which is far more damaging than the virus itself. Influenza can trigger high levels of cytokine secretion, sometimes referred to as a *cytokine storm*. The cytokines attract leukocytes to the lungs and trigger vascular changes that lead to hypotension and coagulation. In severe influenza, inflammatory cytokines also spill out into the systemic circulation, causing ill effects in remote parts of the body, such as the brain. This is analogous to the cytokine response seen in septic shock, described in Chapter 21, which also leads to a type of cytokine storm.

Infections that are capable of eliciting hypersensitivity do not do so in every case. Chapter 23 discusses how hepatitis B virus (HBV) infection can result in chronic hepatitis in some individuals who make an overzealous response. The response depends on the infecting dose of virus and the immune response genes of the individual. Another very different example of an infection causing hypersensitivity is immune complex disease caused by streptococci (Box 26.3).

Hypersensitivity to Environmental Substances

For environmental substances to trigger hypersensitivity reactions, they must gain access to the immune system. Dust triggers a range of responses because it is able to enter the lower extremities of the respiratory tract, an area rich in adaptive immune response cells. Dust can mimic parasites and may stimulate an antibody response. If the dominant antibody is immunoglobulin E (IgE), it may subsequently trigger immediate hypersensitivity, which manifests as allergy symptoms such as asthma or rhinitis. If the dust stimulates IgG antibodies, it may trigger a different kind of hypersensitivity, such as farmer's lung (Chapter 30).

Smaller molecules sometimes diffuse into the skin and may act as haptens, triggering a delayed hypersensitivity reaction. This is the basis of contact dermatitis caused by nickel, discussed in Box 26.4.

Drugs administered orally, by injection, or onto the surface of the body can elicit hypersensitivity reactions mediated by IgE or IgG antibodies or by T cells. Immunologically mediated hypersensitivity reactions to drugs are quite common, and even very tiny doses of drug can trigger life-threatening reactions. These are all classified as *idiosyncratic adverse drug reactions*. We return to this topic in Chapter 31.

A word of caution is needed here. Laypeople, and many clinicians, refer to any hypersensitivity reaction to exogenous substances as "allergy," a term that originally meant any altered reaction to external substances. Most texts define *allergy* as an immediate hypersensitivity mediated by IgE antibodies. This more restrictive definition is used because it helps to explain the specific diagnosis and treatment of hypersensitivities mediated by IgE.

Hypersensitivity to Self Antigens

A degree of immune response to self antigens is normal and present in most people. When these become exaggerated or when tolerance to other antigens breaks down, hypersensitivity reactions can occur. This is autoimmune disease, discussed in Chapter 28.

■ TYPES OF HYPERSENSITIVITY REACTION

The hypersensitivity classification system used here was first described by Gell and Coombs (Table 26.1). The system classifies the different types of hypersensitivity reactions by the types of immune responses involved. Each type of hypersensitivity reaction produces characteristic clinical disease whether the trigger is an environmental, infectious, or self antigen. For example, in type III hypersensitivity, the clinical result is similar whether the antigen is *Streptococcus*, a drug, or an autoantigen such as DNA.

Hypersensitivity reactions are reliant on the adaptive immune system. Previous exposure to antigen is required to prime the adaptive immune response to produce IgE (type I), IgG (types II and III), or T cells (type IV). Because previous exposure is required, hypersensitivity reactions do *not* take place when an individual is first exposed to antigen. In each type of hypersensitivity reaction, the damage is caused by different aspects of the adaptive and innate systems, both of which should now be familiar through discussion of their role in clearing infections.

Type I

Type I hypersensitivity is mediated through the degranulation of mast cells and eosinophils. The effects are felt within minutes of exposure (see Box 26.1). This type of hypersensitivity is sometimes referred to as *immediate hypersensitivity* and is also commonly known as *allergy* (Chapter 27).

TABLE 26.1 Gell and Coombs Classification of Hypersensitivity

	Type I: Immediate Hypersensitivity	Type II: Bound Antigen	Type III: Immune Complex	Type IV: Delayed Hypersensitivity
Onset	Seconds, if IgE is preformed	Seconds, if IgG is preformed	Hours, if IgG is preformed	2–3 days
Infectious trigger	Schistosomiasis	Immune hemolytic anemias	Poststreptococcal glomerulonephritis	Hepatitis B virus
Environmental trigger	House dust mite, peanut	Immune hemolytic anemias	Farmer's lung	Contact dermatitis
Autoimmunity	Not applicable	Immune hemolytic anemias	Systematic lupus erythematosus	IDDM, celiac disease, MS, RA
Adaptive immune system mediators	IgE	IgG	IgG	T cells
Innate immune system mediators	Mast cells, eosinophils	Complement, phagocytes	Complement neutrophils	Macrophages

IDDM, *insulin-dependent diabetes mellitus;* Ig, *immunoglobulin;* MS, *multiple sclerosis;* RA, *rheumatoid arthritis.*

 MCH II   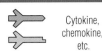 Cytokine, chemokine, etc.   Complement (C')   Signaling molecule

Type II

Type II hypersensitivity is caused by IgG reacting with antigen present on the surface of cells. The bound Ig then interacts with complement or with Fc receptor on macrophages. These innate mechanisms then damage the target cells using processes that may take several hours, as in the case of drug-induced hemolysis (see Box 26.2).

Type III

IgG is also responsible for type III hypersensitivity. In this case, immune complexes of antigen and antibody form and either cause damage at the site of production or circulate and cause damage elsewhere. Immune complexes take some time to form and to initiate tissue damage. Poststreptococcal glomerulonephritis is a good example of immune complex disease (see Box 26.3; see also Chapter 30).

Type IV

The slowest form of hypersensitivity is that mediated by T cells, so-called type IV hypersensitivity. This can take 2 to 3 days to develop and is referred to as *delayed hypersensitivity* (Box 26.4; see also Chapter 31).

■ DIAGNOSIS AND TREATMENT OF HYPERSENSITIVITY

There are major differences in how the types of hypersensitivity reaction are diagnosed and treated. For example, although skin tests are used to diagnose both type I and type IV hypersensitivity, the exact type of testing depends on the type of disease suspected. Treatment for each type of hypersensitivity is also different, as explained in the following chapters.

Because many diseases are caused by an overlap of different types of hypersensitivity, one criticism of the Gell and Coombs classification system is that it is simplistic. However, some knowledge of this system makes it easier to understand how the different disorders come about and how they can be effectively diagnosed and treated.

In this book, we do not provide an exhaustive list of hypersensitivity disorders, nor do we work through the different anatomic systems. This is because an understanding of the mechanisms of hypersensitivity enables students to apply this knowledge to other disease settings. Many more hypersensitivity reactions exist than we have had an opportunity to discuss in detail.

BOX 26.1 Type I Hypersensitivity: Hay Fever

A brother and sister growing up in New England have problems with a runny nose and sore eyes at different times of the year. Both of them notice that their symptoms improve indoors, but they return within minutes of going outside. The girl's symptoms are worse in the spring. The boy has symptoms in the summer, which has made him struggle with exams. Skin-prick testing is carried out (Chapter 27), and it confirms that the girl is allergic to birch pollen and the boy is allergic to grass pollen. The chart (Fig. 26.1) shows why their symptoms happen at different times of the year. It is also important to know where they live. In New England and Northern Europe, grass and birch pollen are notable. In other parts of the United States, ragweed is more notable, whereas in Spain and Italy, olive pollen frequently causes problems.

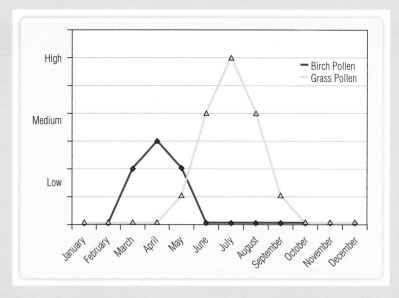

Fig 26.1 The pollen count by month for New England.

 T-cell receptor (TCR) 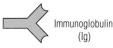 Immunoglobulin (Ig)  Antigen   MCH I

BOX 26.2 Type II Hypersensitivity: Drug-Induced Hemolysis

A woman in her 30s presents with acute fatigue and breathlessness. Two days earlier, she was given penicillin for a urinary tract infection; she has had the same antibiotic once before without problems. She is found to be pale and mildly jaundiced. The laboratory work shows that her red blood cells are being destroyed in the circulation. Further testing shows that her serum contains antibodies that react with her red cells but only when the red cells are coated with penicillin, which confirms the diagnosis of penicillin-induced immune hemolytic anemia.

Penicillin is a low-molecular-weight compound that cannot act as an antigen in its own right, but it can act as a hapten (Fig. 26.2; see also Box 5.1). In penicillin-induced hemolysis, previous exposure to penicillin induces immunoglobulin G (IgG) antibodies. On reexposure, penicillin binds to red cells and becomes a target for IgG. The IgG-coated red cells are taken up and are destroyed by the spleen (Fig. 26.3).

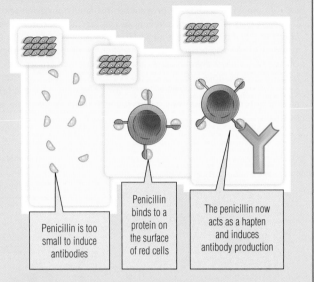

Penicillin is too small to induce antibodies

Penicillin binds to a protein on the surface of red cells

The penicillin now acts as a hapten and induces antibody production

Fig 26.2 Haptens interact with normal proteins from a variety of host tissues.

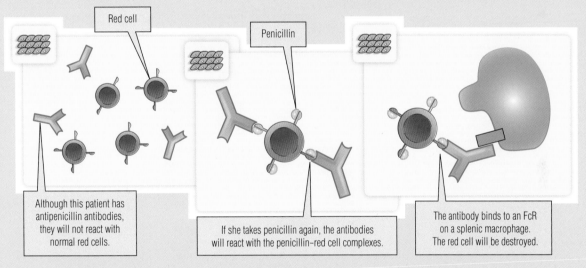

Red cell

Penicillin

Although this patient has antipenicillin antibodies, they will not react with normal red cells.

If she takes penicillin again, the antibodies will react with the penicillin–red cell complexes.

The antibody binds to an FcR on a splenic macrophage. The red cell will be destroyed.

Fig 26.3 Penicillin-induced immune hemolysis. Destruction of red cells takes place within 24 hours of reexposure to the antigen. *FcR,* Fc receptor.

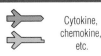 MCH II   Cytokine, chemokine, etc.   Complement (C′)   Signaling molecule

BOX 26.3 Type III Hypersensitivity: Poststreptococcal Glomerulonephritis

An 11-year-old boy presents to his family physician with a 3-day history of swelling of the legs and scrotum. He complained of a sore throat about 2 weeks earlier, and his urine contains blood and protein; taken together, these are the findings of acute glomerulonephritis. A throat swab is taken, and the bacterium β-hemolytic *Streptococcus* is grown. The boy is started on antibiotics for the infection, and during the next 3 weeks his edema improves. When he is reviewed at this stage, his urine is normal.

Circulating immune complexes occur during other infections. Some individuals with hepatitis B virus (HBV) infection are unable to control infection with adequate T-cell responses (Chapter 23), and viral replication is ongoing. Although these individuals produce high levels of antibody, antigen may still be excessive, and circulating immune complexes may form (Figs. 26.4 and 26.5.)

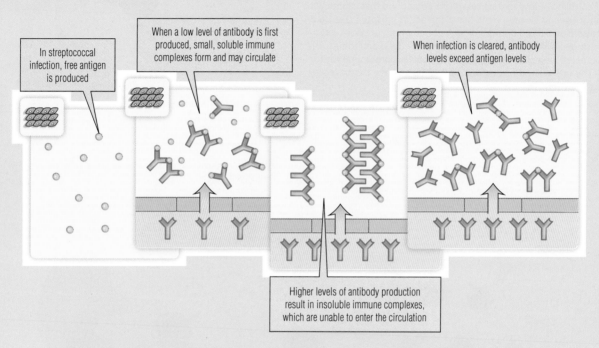

In streptococcal infection, free antigen is produced

When a low level of antibody is first produced, small, soluble immune complexes form and may circulate

When infection is cleared, antibody levels exceed antigen levels

Higher levels of antibody production result in insoluble immune complexes, which are unable to enter the circulation

Fig 26.4 Poststreptococcal glomerulonephritis. Acute infections, such as with *Streptococcus,* can trigger circulating immune complexes until the antigen is cleared.

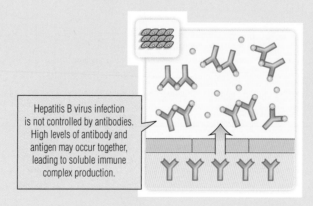

Hepatitis B virus infection is not controlled by antibodies. High levels of antibody and antigen may occur together, leading to soluble immune complex production.

Fig 26.5 Chronic infections, such as with hepatitis B virus, cause more long-lasting immune complex disease.

 T-cell receptor (TCR)

Immunoglobulin (Ig)

 Antigen

MCH I

BOX 26.4 Type IV Hypersensitivity: Contact Dermatitis

A 53-year-old man develops an itchy rash on his ankle. He notices that it is worse in the summertime, and it is particularly bad if he has been gardening (Fig. 26.6). A dermatologist thinks this is contact dermatitis and organizes a patch test to various plant extracts (Fig. 26.7). The patch test is read 3 days after the extracts have been applied and confirms sensitivity to dandelion and related weeds.

Contact dermatitis is an example of type IV delayed hypersensitivity. The skin lesions consist of T cells and macrophages and develop 24 to 72 hours after exposure to the antigen. In this way, the lesions of contact dermatitis are very similar to those induced by a tuberculin skin test.

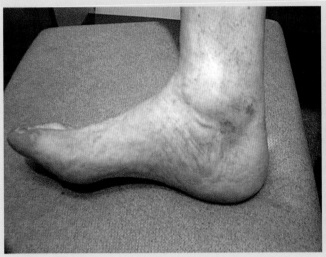

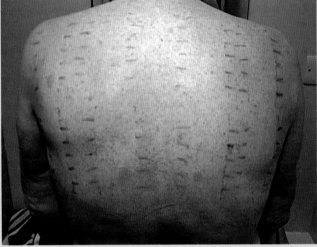

Fig 26.6 The patient has patches of contact dermatitis over his ankle, where fragments of plants have fallen into his gardening boots. (From Helbert M. *Flesh and Bones of Immunology.* Edinburgh: Mosby; 2006.)

Fig 26.7 In the patch test, possible sensitizing antigens are placed on the skin under a dressing. This figure shows a typical positive reaction, in this case to extracts of three plants. At the cellular level, the evolution of this test is very similar to that of a tuberculin skin test. (From Helbert M. *Flesh and Bones of Immunology.* Edinburgh: Mosby; 2006.)

LEARNING POINTS Can You Now...

1. Explain the Gell and Coombs classification of hypersensitivity reactions?
2. Give two examples of infection that causes different types of hypersensitivity?
3. Give three examples of how normally innocuous substances may cause hypersensitivity?
4. Contrast the two different skin tests described in this chapter?

 MCH II   Cytokine, chemokine, etc.   Complement (C′)   Signaling molecule

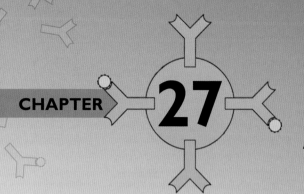

27

Immediate Hypersensitivity (Type I): Allergy

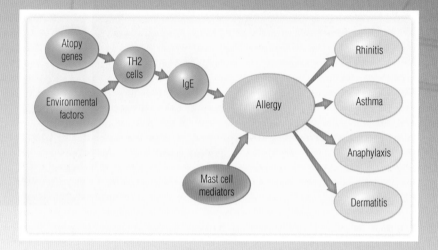

This chapter explains how genes and environmental factors can contribute to the development of an immune system skewed toward T-helper 2 (TH2) responses. Changes in the environment have led to a dramatic increase in the prevalence of allergy. This leads to excessive immunoglobulin E (IgE) production, which, along with mast cell mediators, leads to the symptoms of allergy.

DEFINITIONS

The immunologic definition of *atopy* is an immediate hypersensitivity reaction to environmental antigens mediated by IgE. Such reactions tend to run in families; these families are said to have inherited the *atopy trait*. Although the term *allergy* was originally defined as any altered reactivity to exogenous antigens, it is now often used synonymously with atopy. In this and most texts, *allergy* is defined as immediate hypersensitivity mediated by IgE. Allergic diseases include anaphylaxis, angioedema, urticaria, rhinitis, asthma, and some types of dermatitis or eczema. The distinction between true allergy and other reactions is important because some of the treatments for allergy would be inappropriate for other types of reaction.

Allergies can occur in isolation in an individual. For example, an individual may have allergy to penicillin and no other allergies at all. More often, individuals develop different types of allergy at different times in their lives. Typically, atopic eczema

develops in an infant, then food allergies develop as a toddler, and finally allergic rhinitis and asthma develop in elementary school. About half of toddlers with atopic eczema develop asthma, and two-thirds develop rhinitis. This phenomenon is referred to as the *allergic march*. It is common for allergies to improve spontaneously over time. The best example of this is allergic eczema due to eggs, which disappears in the majority of young children.

Allergies are usually very rapid reactions mediated by IgE; the symptoms develop within minutes of exposure to antigen. However, some allergic reactions continue for a long time, such as when the environmental antigen cannot be easily avoided, and they develop into a late-phase reaction characterized by T-cell infiltrates, discussed later in this chapter.

The beginning of this chapter explains how allergies develop. Some of this material will be familiar from Chapter 16 (TH1 and TH2 cells) and Chapter 22 (mast cells). The second half of the chapter describes the clinical features of allergies in more detail.

ALLERGEN

Antigens that trigger allergic reactions are referred to as *allergens*, which must be able to gain entry to the body. Some allergens are present in the environment as small particles or low-molecular-weight substances that penetrate the body after being inhaled, eaten, or administered as drugs. Inhaled antigens include pollens, fungal spores, and the feces of the house dust mite. Many allergens, including house dust mite feces, are enzymes. This characteristic may allow them to partially digest innate immune system barriers. Some insect venoms, which are injected directly into the skin, are allergens.

An important part of the treatment of allergy is identification and avoidance of allergens, which is facilitated by careful history taking. For example, a patient with a runny nose (rhinitis) is likely to be sensitive to aeroallergens. If symptoms occur predominantly in the summer, grass pollen is the likely culprit. If symptoms occur year-round and mainly indoors, sensitivity to house dust mite feces is likely. House dust mite allergy occurs in areas where a cold climate dictates the need for central heating, heavy bedding, and thick carpets—the habitat of this mite.

Additional clues to the identity of allergens can be provided by knowledge of cross-reacting allergens. Allergists use detailed knowledge about allergens to provide patients with avoidance strategies. Here are some examples:

- Peanut allergy is the most common allergic cause of severe reactions and death. Many people with peanut allergy are allergic to the peanut protein Ara h2. This protein is very stable and is not destroyed by cooking or by gastric acid. In people who are allergic to Ara h2, minute quantities of peanut in food can cause severe systemic reactions (Box 27.2) even in cooked foods.
- Other individuals are allergic to a different peanut protein, Ara h8, which cross-reacts with proteins found in other foods (hazelnut, carrot, apple) and with birch pollen. People with Ara h8 allergy can have nasal symptoms when birch trees are in blossom (see Box 27.1) Importantly, Ara h8 is an unstable protein that *is* destroyed by heating and by gastric acid. This means that cooked foods containing peanut are somewhat less risky for people with allergy to Ara h8. Additionally, because the Ara h8 protein is destroyed by gastric acid, it does not have systemic effects and tends to cause symptoms mainly in the mouth and lips. The coexistence of springtime nasal

symptoms and allergy to this food group is referred to as the *oral allergy syndrome*.
- Another example of cross-reactivity is between latex and some foods (see Box 27.1).
- In penicillin allergy, the allergen is the β-lactam core of the penicillin molecule. Patients experience symptoms with different members of the penicillin family, such as amoxicillin and flucloxacillin. Patients with penicillin allergy can react to other families of antibiotics, such as cephalosporins, which also contain β-lactam ring structures (see Box 5.1).

As shown by these examples, people with allergies often need to be referred to specialists to have their allergies investigated in detail. This can be done by skin-prick (see Box 27.1) or blood testing (see Box 27.2).

■ DEGRANULATING CELLS

The major cells involved in allergy, mast cells, and eosinophils are described in Chapter 22, which explained how these cells evolved to kill parasites. Mast cells are resident in a wide number of tissues, rather like macrophages, whereas eosinophils migrate into tissues where type I hypersensitivity is taking place, rather like neutrophils attracted to sites of inflammation. These cells release the mediators that cause the symptoms of allergy. A third type of degranulating cell is the basophil. These have a similar appearance to mast cells, but they stay in circulation. It is unknown whether they have a special function.

Mast cells are responsible for initiating the symptoms of allergic reactions after allergen and IgE have interacted. Mast cells express receptors for IgE and FcεRI (high-affinity IgE receptor). When allergen cross-links IgE bound to cells by FcεRI, cells release the mediators of the early-phase reaction (Fig. 27.1). However, mast cells, eosinophils, and basophils can also be activated by other stimuli. For example, activated complement generated by infections can activate mast cells, as can signals transmitted by the nervous system—for example, in response to changes in temperature. It is important to remember

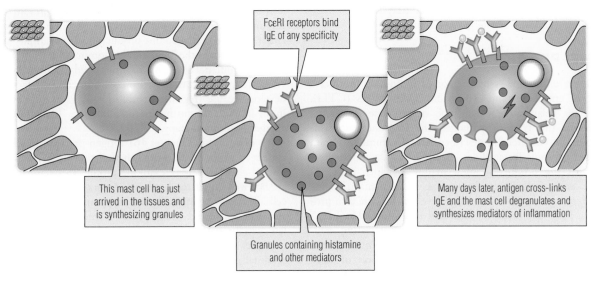

FcεRI receptors bind IgE of any specificity

This mast cell has just arrived in the tissues and is synthesizing granules

Granules containing histamine and other mediators

Many days later, antigen cross-links IgE and the mast cell degranulates and synthesizes mediators of inflammation

Fig 27.1 Immunoglobulin E (IgE) binds to the FcεR on mast cells. Mast cells become activated when allergen cross-links the IgE molecules.

 MCH II

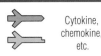 Cytokine, chemokine, etc.

 Complement (C′)

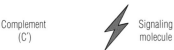 Signaling molecule

TABLE 27.1 Allergic Diseases

System Affected	Clinical Syndrome	Symptoms
Systemic	Anaphylaxis	Low blood pressure, angioedema, and airway obstruction can be fatal (eg, allergies to nuts, antibiotics).
Airways	Asthma	Reversible airway obstruction occurs in the bronchi.
	Rhinitis	Discharge, sneezing, and nasal obstruction often coexist with allergic conjunctivitis.
Skin	Urticaria	Itchy edema of the cutaneous tissues is short lived. Lesion is identical to that induced by skin-prick testing.
	Angioedema	Short-lived, non-itchy edema of the subcutaneous tissues occurs. Some forms, such as lip swelling, may be manifestations of food allergy.
	Atopic eczema	Chronic, itchy inflammation of the skin occurs. Some cases are caused by food allergy.

All the above syndromes can be caused by nonallergic mechanisms. For example, infection can also trigger asthma, rhinitis, and urticaria.

that the symptoms described in detail later in this chapter (Table 27.1) can be caused by other conditions in addition to allergy.

ANTIBODY

IgE is required for type I hypersensitivity reactions. B cells class switch to IgE production when they are costimulated by interleukin 4 (IL-4) secreted by T-helper 2 (TH2) cells. Once IgE is produced, it binds to the high-affinity receptor FcεRI, expressed on resting mast cells resident in tissues and eosinophils that have been activated and that have migrated into tissues (see Fig. 27.1). IgE binds to the FcεRI with such high affinity that although IgE is found at a thousandfold lower concentration than IgG in serum, mast cells are constantly coated with IgE against different antigens.

Very high levels of IgE are seen in patients infected with parasites, such as in schistosomiasis. Total levels of IgE are also high in people who have inherited the atopy trait. Levels of IgE specific for given allergens can be measured using skin-prick testing or enzyme-linked immunosorbent assay (ELISA) when investigating the cause of allergic symptoms.

T-HELPER 2 CELLS

Most adaptive immune system responses in humans produce a mixture of antibodies and cytotoxic T lymphocytes (CTLs). The precise balance of which type of response dominates depends on the type of pathogen the immune system is responding to. Chapter 23, described how the immune system responds to chronic intracellular infection, such as tuberculosis (TB), with the production of a mainly T-helper 1 (TH1) response, with resulting activation of CTLs and macrophages by interferon gamma (IFN-γ). High levels of IgG are also produced in TH1 responses. As described in Chapter 16, TH17 cells respond to extracellular infections by activating neutrophils and stimulating epithelial cells to secrete antimicrobial peptides. However, allergy requires the production of large amounts of IgE, which in turn requires help from TH2 cells that produce IL-4. In TH2 responses, production of IgG and CTLs is inhibited. TB and allergy represent opposite poles of the adaptive immune response. Most responses are much less extreme and involve a mix of TH1, TH17, and TH2 cells.

TH1-polarized cells are characterized by expressing the transcription factor TBX21, which promotes the secretion of IFN-γ. TH17 cells are regulated by the transcription factor RORγt. TH2 cells express the transcription factor GATA3, which promotes the secretion of IL-4 and associated cytokines IL-5 and IL-13. All CD4+ T cells arise from developing T cells, which have the capacity to differentiate into either a TH1, TH17, or a TH2 direction. Which direction this differentiation takes is dictated by whether TBX21, RORγt, or GATA3 becomes the dominant transcription factor (see Box 16.1).

A fourth population of CD4+ T cells is the regulatory T cells (Tregs; Chapter 18). Tregs play an important role in peripheral tolerance and inhibit both TH1 and TH2 cells in an antigen-dependent fashion. Tregs inhibit other T cells by secreting cytokines, such as transforming growth factor beta (TGF-β) and IL-10. Tregs may also have a role during infection; for example, they may prevent overzealous responses that would otherwise lead to hypersensitivity. In most people, Tregs prevent T-helper responses from becoming overpolarized toward extremes of either TH1 or TH2 cytokine production. For example, in nonallergic individuals, the Tregs are the dominant T-cell type specific for environmental allergens. In other words, in nonallergic individuals, a polarized response to environmental allergens cannot develop because Tregs would inhibit it. Tregs can also be induced in an individual who has become allergic. This is the basis of allergen immunotherapy.

As discussed in Chapter 16, antigen-presenting cells (APCs) appear to make the decision whether precursor T cells develop toward a TH1 or TH2 cytokine profile. In circumstances that are not well understood, an APC favors the production of TH2 cells. This may be more likely to happen if the antigen is present at a mucosal surface or is associated with molecules that stimulate certain pattern recognition molecules on the APC. For example, stimulation of Toll-like receptor (TLR) 2 appears to eventually favor TH2 responses. Hence, GATA3 is induced, and the stimulated T cell produces small quantities of IL-4. With each successive round of T-cell proliferation, epigenetic changes become more established, and the daughter T cells can become

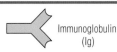
T-cell receptor (TCR)

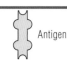
Immunoglobulin (Ig)

Antigen

MCH I

more and more polarized toward a TH2 phenotype. This can occur only if Tregs do not inhibit the polarization. Once a TH2 response is established, high-level IL-4 secretion will stimulate production of IgE by B cells. The IgE produced binds to FcεRI on the surface of mast cells. If antigen cross-links the IgE bound to the FcεRI, mast cells release IL-4. This provides a positive feedback system for the production of more IgE and TH2 cells. IL-4 also inhibits the production of IFN-γ by TH1 T cells. Thus once a T-cell response to an antigen has deviated toward production of TH2 cytokines, positive feedback sustains and enhances the response. In addition, TH2 T cells secrete other cytokines (IL-5, IL-13, eotaxin), which help perpetuate the TH2 response by stimulating the maturation and migration of eosinophils and by switching off TH1 cells (Fig. 27.2).

In summary, APCs make decisions about whether T cells will develop in a TH1, TH17, or TH2 direction, leading to expression of either IL-4 or IFN-γ. During most responses, a mixture of TH1 and TH2 cells are produced, although one type of response will tend to dominate, depending on the triggering infection. TH1 and TH2 cells are able to produce positive feedback for their own type of cells, which could lead to extreme polarization of the immune response. Extreme polarization is normally prevented by Tregs. In the absence of Tregs, an immune response may become overpolarized toward TH2, and allergy may develop.

PREDISPOSITION TO ALLERGY

There are three important facts to consider in the epidemiology of allergy:

- Allergy is very common and affects up to 40% of the population in the developed world.
- Allergy runs in families and appears to have a genetic basis. Twin studies have shown that 80% of the risk of allergy is genetic. Affected family members may have different allergies—such as asthma, hay fever, or eczema—in response to different allergens. It is the *risk* of allergy that is inherited, not the specific allergy.
- The prevalence of allergy has increased in the developed world and is beginning to increase in many parts of the developing world.

Understanding the biologic basis of these epidemiologic facts would help us prevent and treat allergies. The next two sections discuss what is known about genetic and environmental causes of allergy.

Genetics of Allergy

Although allergy clearly has a hereditary component, it has not been possible to find mutations or polymorphisms that occur in everyone affected by allergy. Polymorphisms in several different genes have been implicated, and these probably work together to affect the risk of allergy.

Polymorphisms in the gene for filaggrin are a well-established cause of allergy. Filaggrin is a protein expressed in the keratinocytes of the skin. It has a role in forming the cytoskeleton of these cells, particularly in and around the tight junction between keratinocytes, maintaining the epithelial barrier (Fig. 27.3). In addition, filaggrin is broken down to smaller peptides, which are hygroscopic and act as a natural moisturizing factor (NMF). Finally, NMF helps keep the pH of the skin low, which is thought to help prevent invasion by pathogens.

There is considerable variation in the gene for filaggrin. These variants are regarded as polymorphisms because they occur in more than 1% of the population. These variants are less effective at maintaining the epithelial barrier or moisturizing the skin.

Eotaxin attracts eosinophils and TH2 cells to the site of inflammation

IL-4 stimulates IgE production

TH2

B

TH2

TH1

−

+

IL-4 switches off the TH1 cells

IL-5 stimulates eosinophil maturation

Fig 27.2 Interleukins (ILs) 4 and 5 and eotaxin help sustain the T-helper 2 (TH2) response and suppress the TH1 response. *Ig,* immunoglobulin.

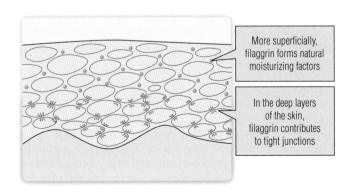

More superficially, filaggrin forms natural moisturizing factors

In the deep layers of the skin, filaggrin contributes to tight junctions

Fig 27.3 Filaggrin helps maintain the cutaneous barrier and moisturize the skin.

 MCH II   Cytokine, chemokine, etc.   Complement (C′)   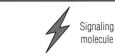 Signaling molecule

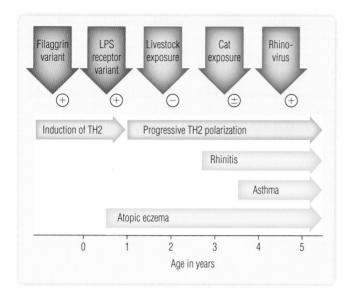

Fig 27.4 A theoretic timeline for how allergies may develop in one individual. Because T-helper 2 (TH2) polarization increases over time, it becomes more difficult to reverse the development of allergies as time passes. Genetic factors are shown in red, and environmental factors are in blue. Note that genetic factors can prevent disease development (eg, livestock exposure builds antibodies) or have both positive and negative effects, probably depending on the genetic makeup and precise timing (eg, exposure to cats early in life vs. later). *LPS,* lipopolysaccharide.

Filaggrin variants are associated with all types of allergy and, for example, are implicated in 50% of cases of severe atopic eczema.

Environmental factors place children who have inherited filaggrin variants at extra risk of developing allergy. For example, exposure of children with filaggrin variants to cats in early childhood increases the risk of developing hay fever (allergic rhinitis caused by grass pollen) in later life. This implies that the filaggrin variants cause systemic changes in immunity so that other organ systems are affected and sensitization to other allergens is increased. Importantly, exposure to cats later in life does not have the same effect; thus the timing of the exposure to the environmental factor is also critical.

Variants in other immune system genes have also been associated with allergy. For example, lipopolysaccharide (LPS) is released from a wide range of organisms. Variants in the CD14 gene (the receptor for LPS) and LPS levels interact to positively or negatively affect the risk of allergies.

Figure 27.4 shows a hypothetical timeline that illustrates how genetic and environmental factors can interact at critical time points to become manifest as allergy.

Environmental Factors and Allergy

The increasing incidence of allergies in the developed world is suggestive of the effects of a changing environmental factor, in particular, increasing urbanization. Studies have shown, for example, that growing up on farms and being exposed to livestock decreases the risk for allergies. This led to the idea that exposure to animals and their excreta and to bacteria in general steered the immune system away from a TH2 pattern and the development of allergies. This thinking was referred to as the

hygiene hypothesis, which posits that the increase in allergies in the developed world is caused by reduced exposure to microorganisms in early life.

The hygiene hypothesis inspired clinical trials that exposed children to harmless microorganisms that have been investigated for their impact on allergy. These have included studies on so called "probiotic" bacteria in milk and live vaccines. Neither of these approaches showed clear benefits in preventing allergy.

However, we now know that the hygiene hypothesis is an oversimplification. For example, infections with some worms, such as schistosomes (Chapter 22), decrease the risk of allergies even though these worms provoke a TH2 response. Allergy is also becoming more common in parts of the world where exposure to infectious microorganisms is still very common, such as in some parts of South America.

Current thinking is that infections can both increase or decrease the subsequent risk of allergy development, depending on the exact timing of exposure and the individual's genotype. In addition, other environmental changes may have contributed to the rise of allergy, such as some types of air pollution and the overabundance of food, causing obesity. Both obesity and airborne pollution are known to trigger inflammation.

As knowledge of epigenetics improves, it is becoming clearer that environmental factors can act in utero or even by exposing the mother (or even the grandmother) before conception. Research into these environmental factors will hopefully lead to the discovery of interventions that can prevent allergy.

■ MEDIATORS OF EARLY PHASE OF ALLERGY

The early phase of allergy is caused by mediators released by mast cells when IgE bound to FcεRI is cross-linked by allergen. Anaphylaxis is the most serious type of allergy and can occur when allergen enters the body from any route. During anaphylaxis, mast cells rapidly synthesize prostaglandins and leukotrienes through the cyclooxygenase and lipoxygenase pathways (Chapter 22). These mediators cause vasodilation and an increase in vascular permeability. In addition, fluid shifts from the vascular to the extravascular space, and a fall in vascular tone occurs. The result of widespread mast cell activation is a dramatic fall in blood pressure, which is characteristic of anaphylaxis. Mast cells in the skin, but not the airway, release histamine, which contributes to swelling and fluid shift.

In other forms of allergy, more localized changes in blood vessels occur that are restricted to the site of allergen entry. For example, in allergic rhinitis, inhaled allergens stimulate mast cells in the nasal mucosa. Subsequent vasodilation and edema in the nose causes nasal stuffiness and sneezing. Leukotrienes (Chapter 22) increase mucus secretion, which causes the discharge characteristic of allergic rhinitis.

Increased mucus secretion in the bronchi also occurs in asthma and contributes to the airflow obstruction. However, in the lungs, leukotrienes cause smooth muscle contraction, which has the most dramatic effects on airflow reduction (Fig. 27.5).

Degranulating mast cells also release enzymes. These activate messenger molecules such as complement and kinins. Mast cell tryptase has a special role in clinical medicine in the diagnosis of anaphylaxis (Box 27.2; see also Box 22.1).

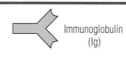 T-cell receptor (TCR)   Immunoglobulin (Ig)   Antigen   MCH I

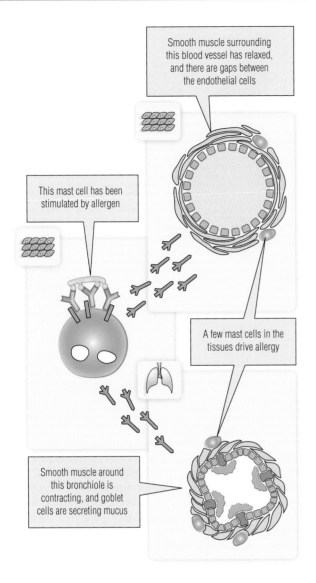

Fig 27.5 Mediators of the early phase of allergy have different consequences depending on the target tissue.

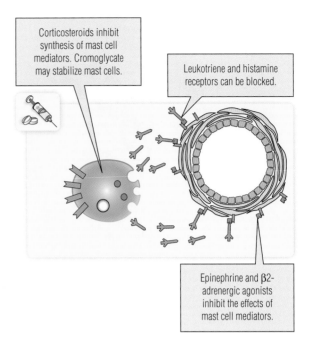

Fig 27.6 Drug treatment for allergy.

response to chemokines. The late phase may last several hours (Fig. 27.6).

In some individuals, this process becomes self-perpetuating as TH2 cells in the bronchial wall secrete cytokines such as IL-4 and attractant chemokines. The result is chronic allergic inflammation in the airways. Mediators released by eosinophils include peroxidase, eosinophil major basic protein, and cationic protein, which all cause direct damage to bronchial tissue. As a result of the chronic allergic inflammation, the bronchial smooth muscle is hypertrophic, and mucus secretion is increased; airflow becomes persistently, rather than intermittently, reduced.

Table 27.1 summarizes the types of symptoms caused by allergy.

TREATMENT

Allergies produce a spectrum of symptoms that range from mild, such as nasal blockage in rhinitis, to life-threatening, as in the case of severe asthma or anaphylaxis. The treatment for allergy is tailored to the individual patient's circumstances and symptoms. General measures in the treatment of allergy include identifying and avoiding possible allergens. This is not always possible when the allergen is widespread in the environment, such as with grass pollen. Other treatments involve the use of drugs or desensitization.

Drug Treatments

Some drugs block the end effects of mediator release; for example, β2-adrenergic agonists, such as salbutamol, mimic the effects of the sympathetic nervous system and work mainly by preventing smooth bronchial muscle contraction in asthma (see Fig. 27.6). Epinephrine (adrenaline) is an important drug and can be lifesaving in anaphylaxis. In anaphylaxis, the blood pressure falls dramatically because fluid shifts out of blood vessels

All of these effects can take place within minutes of exposure to allergen, and symptoms persist while exposure to allergen continues. Even if the person is able to avoid the allergen, late-phase response may occur.

MEDIATORS OF LATE PHASE OF ALLERGY

Type I hypersensitivity reactions are generally characterized by immediate symptoms after exposure to allergens. For example, a patient with asthma who is allergic to cats will develop airway obstruction characterized by wheezing seconds after exposure. The symptoms improve after an hour or so as the immediate response dies down.

Several hours after the acute episode, the airflow in the bronchi may deteriorate again, reflecting the migration of leukocytes—particularly eosinophils—into the bronchi in

 MCH II   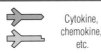 Cytokine, chemokine, etc.   Complement (C′)   Signaling molecule

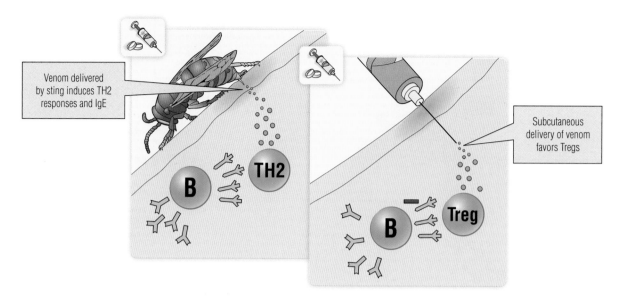

Fig 27.7 Immunotherapy induces regulatory T cells.

and into the tissues when vessel permeability increases. Epinephrine stimulates both α- and β-adrenergic receptors, decreases vascular permeability, increases blood pressure, and reverses airway obstruction.

Antihistamines block specific histamine receptors and have an important role in allergies that affect the skin, nose, and mucus membranes. Antihistamines are much slower acting than epinephrine in the treatment of anaphylaxis and are not very useful in asthma because histamine is not an important allergic mediator released by mast cells in the lung.

Specific receptor antagonists block the effects of leukotrienes. Montelukast, for example, reduces the amount of airway inflammation in asthma.

Corticosteroids are widely used in the prevention of symptoms in patients with allergy. These are discussed in detail in Chapter 31. Corticosteroids can prevent the immediate hypersensitivity reaction, the late phase, and chronic allergic inflammation. To avoid side effects, corticosteroids are often given topically in allergies; for example, inhaled steroids are used in asthma.

Sodium cromoglycate has some effects in preventing allergy attacks. It is thought to work by stabilizing mast cells and reducing degranulation.

Other drugs in development aim to block the TH2 cytokine pathway or prevent IgE binding to the FcεR. Interesting approaches have also been taken to reduce the allergenicity of environmental allergens. For example, one biotechnology company has produced genetically modified cats that do not produce the cat allergen FelD1. These cats do not provoke allergic symptoms in sensitized patients, but at over $1000 per animal, they are not likely to be a popular solution.

Allergen Immunotherapy

Allergen immunotherapy, or desensitization (allergy shots), is a well-established technique that aims to improve allergy symptoms caused by specific allergens. It is most useful when single allergens are involved in the symptoms, and it is often used to prevent anaphylaxis resulting from insect stings or to reduce symptoms from hay fever due to grass pollen allergy. Although treatment starts with very small doses of allergen given by injection, there is a risk for precipitating a full-blown anaphylactic attack. Therefore trained staff must perform the desensitization with access to resuscitation equipment. Over time, the patient is given injections with increasing quantities of allergen until sufficient allergen is being given to dampen the allergic response. Another type of treatment, sublingual immunotherapy, is used to treat hay fever. Patients are given small doses of purified grass pollen under the tongue for several months, again dampening allergy symptoms.

Chapter 18 explained how large doses of bee venom allergen can induce regulatory cells in people who are stung frequently. Immunotherapy injections work in the same way. As the dose builds up, regulatory T cells are induced. These secrete IL-10, which reduces TH2 cell activity and thus reduces IgE secretion (Fig. 27.7). At the same time, specific IgG secretion increases. These regulatory effects are achieved only when a high dose of allergen is delivered.

Sublingual immunotherapy induces regulatory T cells in a slightly different way. The same dose of pollen placed in the nose of someone with pollen allergy would cause severe symptoms. But because the mouth contains few mast cells, doses of grass pollen cannot cause any allergy symptoms when administered orally. The APCs in the mouth and associated lymph nodes tend to induce T-regulatory cells (Tregs) rather than TH2 cells. These Tregs secrete IL-10, which leads to reduced IgE production; and so sublingual exposure to grass pollen eventually leads to reduced allergy symptoms, even when pollen arrives in the nose.

These two types of treatment illustrate how changing the dose (in the case of injection desensitization) or route of delivery (in the case of sublingual desensitization) affects immunologic outcomes.

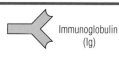 T-cell receptor (TCR)    Immunoglobulin (Ig)   Antigen   MCH I

BOX 27.1 Latex Allergy

A 25-year-old woman developed tongue and lip swelling a few minutes after the beginning of a dental procedure. She has had similar but less dramatic swelling on several occasions immediately after she has eaten fruit salad. She has asthma, and her mother and brother both have allergies.

A skin-prick test is done to investigate the possibility of allergy to latex and fruits. The test results are ready to read in 10 minutes and confirm that she is allergic to latex, banana, avocado, and kiwifruit (Fig. 27.8).

Skin-prick testing is the preferred method for allergy testing. When the antigen introduced by pricking cross-links immunoglobulin E (IgE) on mast cell FcεRI, the rapid release of histamine causes a local flare and a wheal reaction. Skin-prick tests give immediate results, which the patient can see, and they are cheaper and more sensitive than specific IgE testing on blood samples. Skin-prick testing is not possible when patients have taken antihistamines; in these circumstances, measuring levels of specific IgE is most useful. The corresponding figure (Fig. 27.9) shows how skin swelling rapidly develops.

The rubber, banana, avocado, and kiwi plants are botanically related and contain very similar proteins to which the patient is allergic. This is an example of cross-reactivity. If she is exposed to these allergens again, it is possible that she could have much more severe reactions, including anaphylaxis. Patient education is important to ensure that she understands how to avoid related fruits and also latex in the future, such as during medical and dental procedures and in latex condoms.

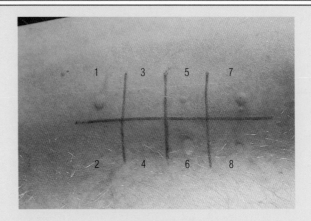

Fig 27.8 Skin-prick testing. To provide a control, a histamine solution is applied at position 1, and saline is applied at position 2. These are pricked through the dermis, and 10 minutes later the histamine has given a positive reaction; this would not have happened had the patient recently taken an antihistamine. The saline has given no reaction, which confirms the patient's skin does not simply react to trauma. House dust mite feces and tree pollen were applied at positions 3 and 4; the patient has not reacted to these. Positions 5, 6, 7, and 8 were occupied by extract of avocado, banana, kiwifruit, and latex suspension. The patient has reacted to all four of these, most strongly to kiwifruit and banana. (Courtesy St. Bartholomew's Hospital, London.)

Continued

 MCH II   Cytokine, chemokine, etc.   Complement (C')   Signaling molecule

BOX 27.1 Latex Allergy—cont'd

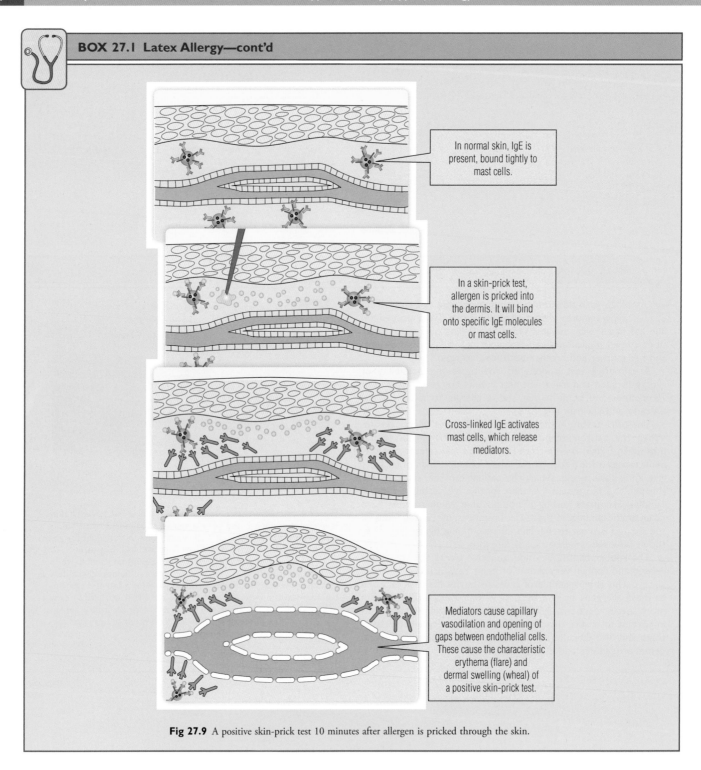

In normal skin, IgE is present, bound tightly to mast cells.

In a skin-prick test, allergen is pricked into the dermis. It will bind onto specific IgE molecules or mast cells.

Cross-linked IgE activates mast cells, which release mediators.

Mediators cause capillary vasodilation and opening of gaps between endothelial cells. These cause the characteristic erythema (flare) and dermal swelling (wheal) of a positive skin-prick test.

Fig 27.9 A positive skin-prick test 10 minutes after allergen is pricked through the skin.

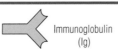 T-cell receptor (TCR)

Immunoglobulin (Ig)

 Antigen

 MCH I

BOX 27.2 Peanut Allergy

A 4-year-old boy has been brought into the emergency department with swelling of the face, generalized itchiness, and drowsiness. The symptoms developed a few minutes after eating a chocolate bar. The emergency department physician finds that he has facial angioedema (Fig. 27.10) and urticaria (Fig. 27.11) and that his blood pressure is low. He is given an intramuscular injection of 150 µg of epinephrine (pediatric dose), and within minutes he begins to recover. His mother explains that he has had minor reactions to nuts in the past, including lip swelling. The boy also has eczema (Fig. 27.12), and his mother thinks that in the past, this has flared up when he has eaten peanuts. She has concluded that he might be allergic to nuts and has tried to eliminate them from the house. The patient has never had any symptoms from milk.

The patient's mother has kept the chocolate bar wrapper, and this confirms that it "'may contain traces of nut." Highly sensitized individuals can react to tiny quantities of allergen that may contaminate harmless foods during processing. Because this patient appears to be very sensitive to nut allergen, the emergency doctor decides not to refer the patient for skin-prick testing. He orders blood samples and arranges for the patient to be seen 2 weeks later in the allergy clinic.

The first blood test shows a high level of mast cell tryptase in the blood. Mast cell tryptase is normally present in the blood at low levels, and its presence at a high level indicates mast cell degranulation occurred prior to the blood sample being taken. Taken along with the history, this confirms that anaphylaxis has taken place (see Box 22.1). The second part of the blood test results are for specific IgE testing. These show no detectable IgE against cow's milk, which is important because this could possibly have been the allergen in the chocolate bar. The second part of the results show this boy is allergic to several species of nut. This reactivity to several nuts is quite common because there is cross-reactivity among the antigens.

An important part of the management of this boy is to reduce the risk for future exposure to nuts, which involves training the boy and his parents to avoid foods that may contain hidden nuts. However, repeated exposure is common, and there is a good chance that this patient may develop life-threatening reactions. He is given an epinephrine intramuscular injector device and is trained in its use in the event of future symptoms. Intramuscular epinephrine is an important part of the treatment of anaphylaxis. Epinephrine reverses vasodilation and closes the gap between endothelial cells. After epinephrine is given, swollen tissues return to normal, and blood pressure is restored.

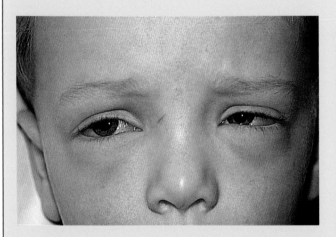

Fig 27.10 This boy has angioedema as a result of exposure to nuts. *IgE,* immunoglobulin E. (Courtesy St. Bartholomew's Hospital, London.)

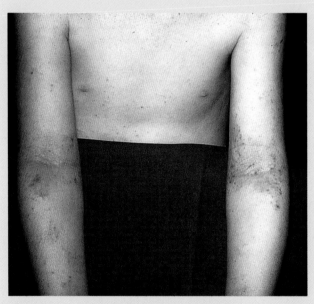

Fig 27.12 Atopic eczema causes a thickened itchy weeping rash, especially affecting the flexures of the knees and the elbows. (Courtesy Bartholomew's Hospital, London.)

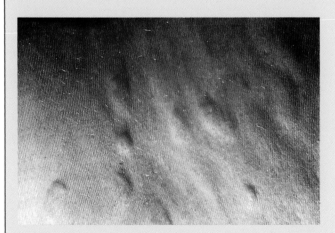

Fig 27.11 Acute urticaria is an itchy rash that can be caused by allergies. When it lasts for more than a few weeks, urticaria rarely has an allergic cause. (Courtesy St. Bartholomew's Hospital, London.)

LEARNING POINTS Can You Now...

1. List the mechanisms of the early and late phases of allergy?
2. Compare the roles of TH1 and TH2 cells from the point of view of cytokines?
3. Describe the immunologic factors that predispose to allergy and explain how these may be increasing allergy at a population level?
4. Describe the techniques used to identify allergens involved in immediate hypersensitivity?
5. Describe anaphylaxis and its immediate treatment?
6. List the modes of action of drugs used to treat allergy?

 T-cell receptor (TCR)

 Immunoglobulin (Ig)

Antigen

 MCH I

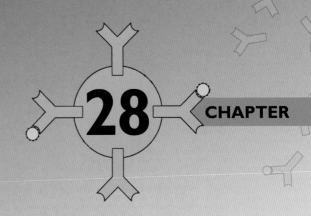

How Autoimmune Disease Develops

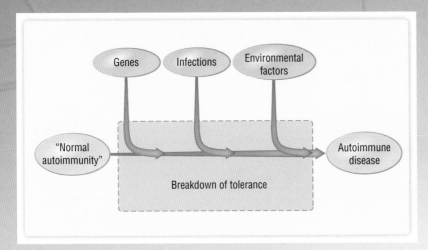

The main part of this chapter discusses how some autoimmunity is a normal finding in healthy individuals, but that more extensive breakdown of tolerance can lead to autoimmune disease. An interplay of genetic factors, infections, and other environmental factors is required for tolerance to break down. The boxes in this chapter describe tests for autoimmunity and the pathogenesis of three autoimmune diseases—type 1 diabetes mellitus (T1DM), celiac disease, and systemic lupus erythematosus (SLE)—in detail. This chapter and Chapters 29 through 31 give more detail on the different hypersensitivity reactions that lead to several important autoimmune diseases.

SOME AUTOIMMUNITY IS NORMAL

Autoimmunity can be defined as adaptive immune responses with specificity for self antigens. *Autoantibodies* are antibodies directed at normal cellular components, referred to as *autoantigens*. Most healthy individuals produce some autoantibodies, although these are usually very low level and low affinity and require sensitive tests for their detection. Higher-affinity autoantibodies detectable with routine clinical tests are also found in some healthy people, especially women and the elderly. For example, low levels of antinuclear cytoplasmic antibodies (ANCAs) are seen in one-fifth of healthy elderly people.

It has been estimated that after random immunoglobulin (Ig) gene recombination, more than half of the emerging B-cell receptors have specificity for self antigen. The checkpoints in B-cell ontogeny (Chapter 14) prevent the majority of B cells from producing autoantibodies. Autoreactive B cells are either deleted or become nonfunctional. In any case, most autoreactive B cells are unable to secrete Ig in the periphery without help from T-helper (TH) cells responding to the same antigen.

This is not the case for B1 cells, which are able to secrete Ig without T-cell help (Chapter 14). B1 cells secrete natural antibodies and are the major source of autoantibodies in healthy individuals. These B cells break some of the rules that normally apply to B cells and do not alter their Ig genes in response to antigen exposure, and they do not undergo somatic hypermutation. Natural antibody produced by B1 cells never improves its fit to any specific antigen. This means that although natural antibodies bind a wide number of antigens with low affinity, they never have high-affinity binding to specific antigens.

Natural antibodies secreted by B1 cells have a number of different activities (Fig. 28.1):
- Natural antibodies bind with low affinity to antigens present on a large variety of bacteria. This activates complement and helps clear invading bacteria rapidly. Thus natural antibodies act like molecules of the innate immune system—they do not rely on genetic recombination, and they are present before an infection starts.
- Natural antibodies cross-react with the inherited A and B antigens of red cells. Unless they have inherited either A or B antigens, individuals make IgM anti-A and anti-B antibodies, even if they have never been exposed to red cells from another

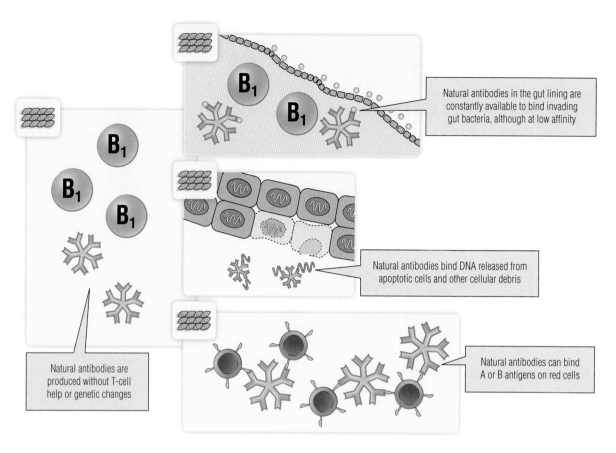

Fig 28.1 Natural antibodies bind a range of antigens with low affinity. Natural antibodies are usually immunoglobulin M pentamers.

person (Chapter 29). Humans also have natural antibodies against sugars expressed on cells of other animal species. These xenogeneic natural antibodies are discussed further in Chapter 34.

- Another consequence of their low specificity is that natural antibodies can also bind to a series of normal cellular constituents, such as nuclear proteins and DNA. This explains why some healthy people have antinuclear antibodies. The autoantigen-binding ability of natural antibodies may be an accidental consequence of cross-reactivity, but these antibodies may have a role, such as clearing up cellular debris.

■ INITIATION OF AUTOIMMUNE DISEASE

Autoimmune disease occurs when autoreactive T cells or autoantibodies cause tissue damage through hypersensitivity reaction types II through IV, defined in Chapter 26. Unlike infectious antigens, autoantigens are almost impossible to clear despite the immune system's best efforts; consequently, once initiated, autoimmune diseases tend to be active for a long time. Autoimmune diseases are common and tend to be chronic diseases that usually last months or years. They can affect any organ system and occur at any age. Understanding how autoimmune diseases arise helps us diagnose, treat, and even prevent these problems.

One possibility is that the natural autoantibodies mentioned above cause autoimmune disease. However, there is evidence that T cells initiate autoimmune disease as follows:

- Even autoimmune diseases caused by IgG-mediated mechanisms (hypersensitivity types II and III) require T-cell help for affinity maturation to produce pathogenic (disease-causing) antibodies.
- Transfer of T cells from an animal with autoimmune disease to a healthy animal can transfer disease.
- Autoimmune diseases are often linked to specific major histocompatibility complex (MHC) genes, which regulate T cells but not B cells.

There is no evidence that the B1 cells, which secrete harmless natural antibodies, can also produce the high-affinity, specific antibodies that can cause autoimmune disease without T-cell help.

For T cells to mediate autoimmune disease, they need to overcome tolerance mechanisms. Before describing how they may do this, a brief reminder is provided regarding how T cells are tolerized to autoantigen.

■ T-CELL TOLERANCE

Tolerance prevents the immune system from responding to specific antigens and was described in Chapter 18. Checkpoints during central and peripheral tolerance have evolved to prevent T cells from mediating autoimmunity. T cells are initially made

 T-cell receptor (TCR)   Immunoglobulin (Ig)   Antigen   MCH I

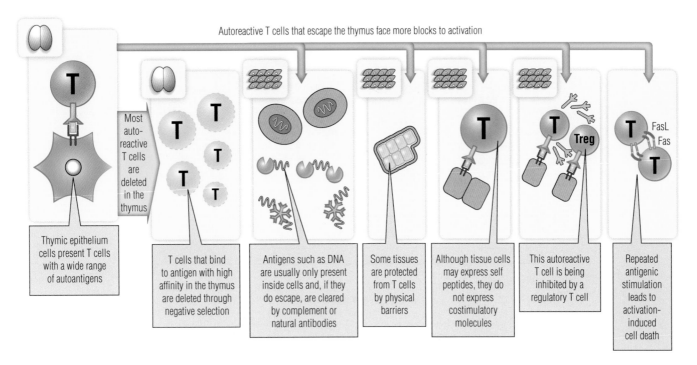

Autoreactive T cells that escape the thymus face more blocks to activation

Most auto-reactive T cells are deleted in the thymus

FasL
Fas

Treg

Thymic epithelium cells present T cells with a wide range of autoantigens

T cells that bind to antigen with high affinity in the thymus are deleted through negative selection

Antigens such as DNA are usually only present inside cells and, if they do escape, are cleared by complement or natural antibodies

Some tissues are protected from T cells by physical barriers

Although tissue cells may express self peptides, they do not express costimulatory molecules

This autoreactive T cell is being inhibited by a regulatory T cell

Repeated antigenic stimulation leads to activation-induced cell death

Fig 28.2 T-cell tolerance. The majority of T cells that recognize autoantigen at high affinity undergo apoptosis in the thymus. Several additional checkpoints are present during peripheral tolerance: sequestration of antigens, absence of costimulatory T-regulatory cells, and activation-induced cell death. These checkpoints prevent T cells from reacting with autoantigens in the periphery. *FasL*, Fas ligand; *Treg*, T-regulatory cell.

tolerant of autoantigens in the thymus; this is central tolerance. Any T cell that binds at high affinity to self peptide in the thymus will be deleted by negative selection in a process referred to as *central tolerance*.

However, it is not possible for every self peptide to be expressed in the thymus, so some autoreactive T cells may escape negative selection. For example, it is unlikely that every possible peptide from a remote, complex organ like the brain is expressed in the thymus; therefore some brain-specific T cells may reach the periphery. For potentially autoreactive T cells that have escaped to the periphery, there are at least three more potential blocks that normally prevent stimulation (Fig. 28.2).

The first way of preventing autoreactive T cells from becoming stimulated is to sequester (hide) the self antigen. Some molecules, such as DNA, are normally hidden inside healthy cells. If they leak out of cells—such as during cell death—they are rapidly cleared by complement or natural antibodies.

In the normal course of events, autoreactive T cells may never encounter specific antigen if it is locked away in an immunologically privileged site. Immunologic privilege can be brought about by physical barriers that prevent access to lymphocytes or antibody. For example, the blood-brain barrier makes the brain a "no go" area for the immune system. Alternatively, there may be molecular devices that prevent immune surveillance of some tissues; testicular cells express Fas, which induces apoptosis in any T cells that manage to enter the testes.

Other autoreactive T cells may enter tissues that express specific antigen, and peripheral tolerance normally prevents these T cells from responding. Tissue cells express MHC class I at all times, and they can be induced to express MHC class II.

However, autoreactive T cells emerging from the thymus also require expression of costimulatory molecules such as CD80 (B7) or CD40. Rather than become stimulated, naive T cells will undergo apoptosis or become anergic when they recognize antigen on nonprofessional antigen-presenting cells (APCs). Anergic cells remain alive but are prevented from responding to antigen.

Autoreactive T cells that have escaped to the periphery can also be prevented from responding by regulatory T cells (Tregs), which appear to be specific for the identical antigen as the T cell they are inhibiting. They inhibit effector T cells by a number of mechanisms, including secretion of inhibitory cytokines such as interleukin 10 (IL-10) and transforming growth factor beta (TGF-β).

Finally, activation-induced cell death (AICD) occurs in T cells that have been repeatedly exposed to the same antigen, typically an autoantigen. These T cells begin to express both Fas and Fas ligand (FasL) and either kill themselves or are killed by neighboring cells.

■ BREAKDOWN OF T-CELL TOLERANCE

Autoimmune diseases tend to run in families. Individuals who have inherited identical genetic predispositions to autoimmunity (eg, identical twins) do not always develop the same autoimmune disease. If they develop autoimmune disease at all, they may do so at different times. This suggests that both genetic and environmental factors are required for autoimmune disease to develop. As for allergy, it is likely that several environmental triggers operating in sequence are required for disease to develop.

 MCH II

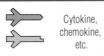 Cytokine, chemokine, etc.

 Complement (C′)

 Signaling molecule

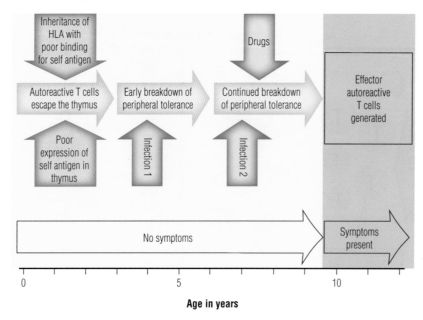

Fig 28.3 A series of different factors may be required to initiate an autoimmune process. The precise nature and timing of the two infections may be critical in determining the type of autoimmunity that results. Genetic factors are shown in pink, and environmental factors are in blue. *HLA,* human leukocyte antigen.

This complexity explains why it has been difficult to unravel the pathogenesis of autoimmune disease (Fig. 28.3). As described in Chapter 35, similar "multihit" mechanisms, combinations of genetic and environmental factors, are required to produce malignancies.

Genetic Factors and Loss of Tolerance

Some rare genetic diseases cause autoimmunity. For example, in autoimmune polyendocrinopathy candidiasis ectodermal dysplasia (APECED) syndrome (Chapter 15), the *AIRE* gene is mutated and central tolerance cannot take place. People with APECED usually experience several autoimmune diseases simultaneously.

However, most autoimmune diseases are relatively common and cannot be explained by rare mutations. For example, T1DM and celiac disease affect about 1:300 and 1:100 people, respectively, depending on the population being studied. This means that common polymorphisms, rather than rare mutations, are implicated in the breakdown of immune tolerance that leads to these diseases.

Some genetic polymorphisms affect how self peptides are expressed in the thymus. For example, insulin is expressed in the normal thymus, where it tolerizes T cells through negative selection. The level of insulin expression in the thymus is genetically determined. Some individuals inherit insulin genes, which are transcribed at lower levels than normal, so less insulin is expressed in the thymus, and insulin-reactive T cells are less likely to be deleted (Fig. 28.4). In addition, inheritance of certain MHC alleles that are less efficient at presenting self peptides to T cells can increase the risk for acquiring autoimmune diseases, including T1DM.

Genetic polymorphisms may also affect peripheral tolerance. For example, hidden ("cryptic") antigens may become exposed to the immune system. For example, DNA released by dying cells is normally removed by molecules such as mannan-binding lectin (MBL) and complement component C1. If DNA cannot be removed by these mechanisms, it may provoke an immune response, which may be the first step in the development of SLE (see Box 28.3).

Environmental Factors and Loss of Tolerance

In some individuals, environmental factors such as exposure to medications and ultraviolet light (see Box 28.3) trigger autoimmunity. However, much more commonly infection acts as an environmental factor in breaking down tolerance.

Peripheral tolerance can break down if tissue cells acquire the ability to present self peptides. This can happen when professional APCs, such as monocytes and macrophages, are recruited to sites of infection. These cells express costimulatory molecules and cytokines that enable naive T cells to respond to self peptides expressed by tissue cells. In this situation, an appropriate inflammatory response to infection spreads to include inappropriate responses to self antigens.

Another possible mechanism that can lead to the breakdown of peripheral tolerance is when an immune response to an infection elicits antibodies or T cells that cross-react with host tissues, called *molecular mimicry.* An example of this is acute rheumatic fever, which can occur rarely following infection with the bacterium β-hemolytic *Streptococcus.* Patients develop a complex of symptoms that include a rash along with heart and nervous system involvement. In these individuals, streptococcal infection induces antibodies that cross-react with heart tissue and trigger type II hypersensitivity. In this instance, streptococcal antigens mimic heart antigen. The infection is able to overcome the tolerance mechanisms that normally prevent the production of autoreactive antibodies because *Streptococcus* activates the innate

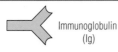 T-cell receptor (TCR)

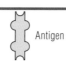 Immunoglobulin (Ig)

 Antigen

MCH I

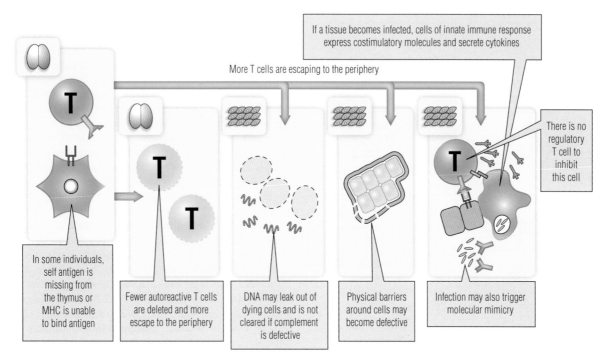

Fig 28.4 How T-cell tolerance breaks down. For autoimmune disease to develop, tolerance needs to break down at several of the points illustrated. *MHC,* major histocompatibility complex.

immune response through its pattern recognition molecules. Rheumatic fever is a transient illness and does *not* cause the chronic disease that is typical of most autoimmune disease. Similar bacteria can cause poststreptococcal glomerulonephritis (Chapter 26) through a very different mechanism.

A handful of other rare infections can trigger short-lived autoimmune disease using molecular mimicry; however, none of the autoimmune diseases persists for more than a few weeks. The current view is that infections may sometimes initiate autoimmune disease using molecular mimicry, but other genetic and environmental factors are required for its maintenance.

Finally, it is also possible that at crucial times, absence of infection can trigger autoimmunity! If a particular strain of mice is kept in microorganism-free conditions, it will develop T1DM. If these mice are exposed to everyday microorganisms, however, they are protected from diabetes. This observation has led to the idea that reduced exposure to microorganisms may be responsible for the increase in prevalence of autoimmune disease in developed countries. This is the hygiene hypothesis, which was discussed in Chapter 27 in relation to allergy. So far, in humans, it has not been possible to identify a microorganism that reduces the risk of autoimmune disease. Table 28.1 summarizes some of the genetic and environmental factors known to trigger autoimmune disease.

■ TESTS FOR AUTOIMMUNE DISEASE

The tests for autoimmune disease rely on detecting evidence of autoantibodies. Chapter 5 described the two main types of tests for antibody specificity. The first is direct immunofluorescence, which is used to find evidence of autoimmune processes in tissues. This is possible only in accessible tissues, such as skin, as

TABLE 28.1 Risk Factors for Autoimmune Disease

	Risk Factor	Associated Disease
Genetic	*AIRE* gene mutations	APECED, multiple autoimmune diseases
	Polymorphisms in the insulin gene	T1DM
	MHC polymorphisms	T1DM, celiac disease, SLE, many other diseases
	MBL, complement C1 polymorphisms	SLE
Environmental	Infection	May trigger T1DM, MS in humans May protect from T1DM in some mice
	Medications	SLE
	Ultraviolet light	SLE
	Gluten in diet	Celiac disease

APECED, *autoimmune polyendocrinopathy candidiasis ectodermal dysplasia (syndrome)*; MBL, *mannan-binding lectin*; MCH, *major histocompatibility complex*; MS, *multiple sclerosis*; SLE, *systemic lupus erythematosus*; T1DM, *type 1 diabetes mellitus.*

in the example described in Box 28.3. The technique of direct immunofluorescence is briefly reviewed in Fig. 28.5.

In most cases, it is much simpler to test a blood sample for autoantibodies. The original autoantibody blood test was indirect immunofluorescence. In this case, the antigen is cells or tissue mounted on a glass slide. The detection system is antihuman IgG conjugated to a fluorescent tag, which is detected in

 MCH II   Cytokine, chemokine, etc.   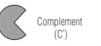 Complement (C′)   Signaling molecule

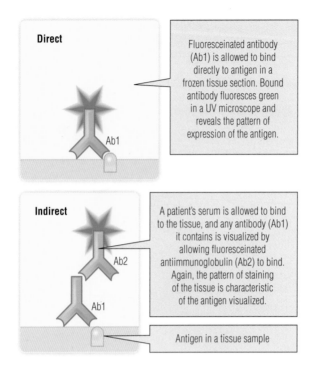

Fig 28.5 illustration labels:

Direct

Fluoresceinated antibody (Ab1) is allowed to bind directly to antigen in a frozen tissue section. Bound antibody fluoresces green in a UV microscope and reveals the pattern of expression of the antigen.

Ab1

Indirect

A patient's serum is allowed to bind to the tissue, and any antibody (Ab1) it contains is visualized by allowing fluoresceinated antiimmunoglobulin (Ab2) to bind. Again, the pattern of staining of the tissue is characteristic of the antigen visualized.

Ab2

Ab1

Antigen in a tissue sample

Fig 28.5 The principles of direct and indirect immunofluorescence. Direct immunofluorescence uses a tissue sample as the clinical material. Indirect immunofluorescence uses a blood sample. *UV*, ultraviolet.

an ultraviolet (UV) microscope (see Fig. 28.5B). Islet cell and endomysial antibodies and antinuclear cytoplasmic antibodies (ANCAs) are used to illustrate indirect immunofluorescence in Boxes 28.1 through 28.3. Newer tests use antigen immobilized on a solid surface, such as the enzyme-linked immunosorbent assay (ELISA) test described in Chapter 5. Antibody in the blood sample is detected by an anti–human IgG antibody conjugated to an enzyme. The enzyme is able to generate either a color change or fluorescence. The amount of color or fluorescence is proportional to the level of autoantibody present in the sample. The advantages of ELISA are that antigens can be purified (in principle giving more specific results), sensitivity is higher to lower levels of antibody, and antibody levels can be quantified.

Although autoantibodies can be helpful in diagnosing autoimmune diseases, one important pitfall must be understood. As explained earlier, some autoantibodies can be found at low levels in perfectly healthy individuals. For example, antinuclear antibodies, which are found at high levels in patients with SLE, can be found at low levels in many normal individuals, particularly women, and more often with increasing age. Other individuals tend to produce autoantibodies transiently following infections, presumably as a result of nonspecific activation of the immune system. These false positives contribute to the low specificity of some of these tests.

BOX 28.1 Type 1 Diabetes Mellitus

A 9-year-old boy has been performing poorly at school for several weeks. He is drinking large amounts of water. His mother is concerned because his older sister was diagnosed as having type 1 diabetes (T1DM) after having the same symptoms 4 years earlier at age 8 years.

The boy has a moderately raised fasting glucose, but no ketones are found in his urine; these findings are not diagnostic of diabetes. His serum is tested by indirect immunofluorescence for autoantibodies and is shown to contain islet cell antibodies (Fig. 28.6), which are highly suggestive of T1DM. He starts taking insulin, and 5 years later he has had no complications of diabetes.

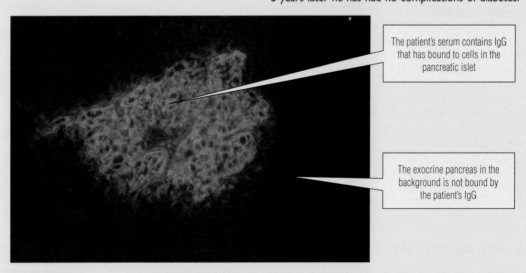

The patient's serum contains IgG that has bound to cells in the pancreatic islet

The exocrine pancreas in the background is not bound by the patient's IgG

Fig. 28.6 Antibodies against pancreatic islet β-cells using indirect immunofluorescence. A section of animal pancreas has been placed on a slide. The patient's serum is incubated on the slide. The patient's immunoglobulin (Ig), which has not bound to the tissue, is washed off. The patient's IgG, which has bound to tissue, is detected with antihuman IgG labeled with a fluorescent dye.

 T-cell receptor (TCR)   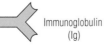 Immunoglobulin (Ig)   Antigen   MCH I

BOX 28.1 Type 1 Diabetes Mellitus—cont'd

The islet cell antibodies seen in T1DM are generally not required for the diagnosis in individuals who have high blood glucose and ketones in the urine. The presence of islet cell antibodies may help make the diagnosis in patients with less clear features, as in this case. In T1DM, pancreatic islet β-cells are damaged by T cells. The islet cell antibodies are a marker of this process and do not have any role in inducing islet cell damage.

T1DM is an example of type IV hypersensitivity. T cells invade the pancreatic islets and specifically destroy the insulin-secreting β-cells. Once autoreactive T cells have entered the pancreatic islets, β-cells are destroyed over a few weeks. There appears to be little chance of regenerating β-cells once they have been destroyed, and patients must start lifelong insulin replacement.

If one identical twin develops T1DM, there is a 50% chance the other twin will as well; this is called the *concordance rate*. The most important genetic factor, which confers about 90% of the genetic risk, is the human leukocyte antigen (HLA) type. In whites, T1DM occurs frequently in people who inherit the HLA allele DQ2. In most HLA-DQ alleles, position 57 in the HLA-DQ β-chain is occupied by an aspartic acid residue. With HLA-DQ2, this position is replaced by another amino acid residue. Figure 28.7 shows how this single amino acid residue change in the β-chain of HLA-DQ2 affects the risk for developing T1DM: A non–aspartic acid residue at position 57 prevents the self peptide lying in the groove. Because the self peptide cannot therefore be presented, T cells specific for the self peptide cannot be deleted in the thymus.

Several other genetic polymorphisms also affect the risk for diabetes. For example, polymorphisms near the insulin gene affect insulin expression in the thymus. Individuals who inherit a polymorphism that leads to lower levels of insulin secretion in the thymus have an increased risk for diabetes. This presumably happens because low expression allows insulin-reactive T cells to reach the periphery.

Even in identical twins, the risk for concordance with diabetes is only 50%; therefore environmental factors must be important. One possible environmental factor is infection. In theory, different infections at different times may increase or decrease the risk of T1DM. For example, viral infections may cause low-grade inflammation in the pancreatic islets. The inflammatory signals attract innate immune system cells, which express costimulatory molecules and secrete cytokines. These allow tissue antigens to be presented to autoreactive T cells. However, although T1DM is a common autoimmune disease, no single infection has been identified that consistently acts as a trigger. Currently, most data support enteroviruses as possible triggers, especially a particular type of enterovirus called *coxsackievirus*.

Furthermore, the prevalence of T1DM is increasing at about 3% per annum at a time when childhood infections are decreasing in intensity in the developed world. This has led some researchers

to suggest that it may be absence of infection at specific ages that triggers T1DM. This type of thinking is supported by the evidence of diabetes being common in some strains of mice when they are not exposed to microorganisms. This is analogous to the hygiene hypothesis proposed to explain the increase in allergy prevalence in genetically predisposed individuals (Chapter 27). It may be that in "hygienic" circumstances, regulatory T cells are not generated, and autoreactive T cells are not prevented from destroying pancreatic islet β-cells.

Figure 28.8 illustrates these views about T1DM pathogenesis. In this kind of model, the precise timing of infections may be more important than whether an infection takes place.

T1DM is common and can reduce life expectancy considerably. Much research is being carried out on how to prevent T1DM. When one child is a family has been affected, it is possible to periodically screen the other siblings for islet cell antibodies. In children who develop islet cell antibodies, immunosuppressive drugs such as cyclosporine (Chapter 11) can delay the onset of diabetes for up to 1 year. These drugs work by inhibiting T cells, but soon after the drugs are stopped—and they are too toxic to be used for long periods of time—the disease becomes apparent. Other approaches have attempted to induce tolerance to pancreatic islet β-cells, but these have proven unsuccessful so far. If it becomes clear which infections, if any, trigger T1DM, vaccine strategies may be helpful.

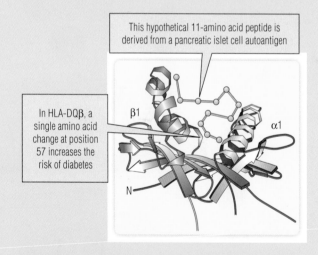

Fig 28.7 Current thinking is that human leukocyte antigen DQ2 has reduced binding for a pancreatic islet cell antigen. Consequently, T cells that recognize islet cell antigen cannot be deleted in the thymus, and the potential for autoimmunity is increased.

Continued

 MCH II   Cytokine, chemokine, etc.   Complement (C′)   Signaling molecule

BOX 28.1 Type I Diabetes Mellitus—cont'd

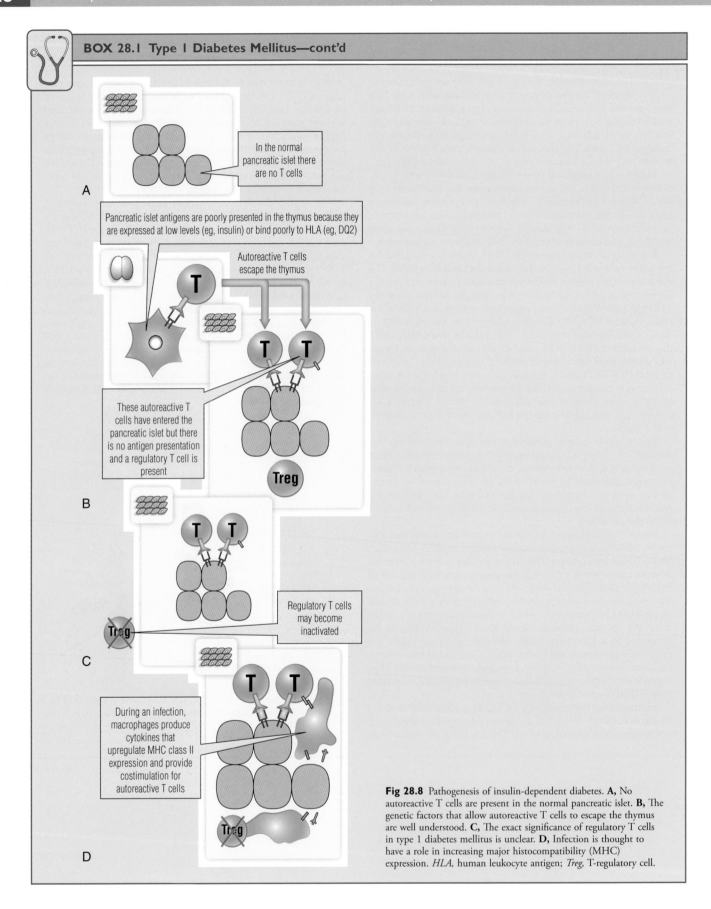

In the normal pancreatic islet there are no T cells

Pancreatic islet antigens are poorly presented in the thymus because they are expressed at low levels (eg, insulin) or bind poorly to HLA (eg, DQ2)

Autoreactive T cells escape the thymus

These autoreactive T cells have entered the pancreatic islet but there is no antigen presentation and a regulatory T cell is present

Regulatory T cells may become inactivated

During an infection, macrophages produce cytokines that upregulate MHC class II expression and provide costimulation for autoreactive T cells

Fig 28.8 Pathogenesis of insulin-dependent diabetes. **A,** No autoreactive T cells are present in the normal pancreatic islet. **B,** The genetic factors that allow autoreactive T cells to escape the thymus are well understood. **C,** The exact significance of regulatory T cells in type 1 diabetes mellitus is unclear. **D,** Infection is thought to have a role in increasing major histocompatibility (MHC) expression. *HLA,* human leukocyte antigen; *Treg,* T-regulatory cell.

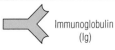 T-cell receptor (TCR)

 Immunoglobulin (Ig)

 Antigen

MCH I

BOX 28.2 Celiac Disease

The younger sister of the diabetic patient discussed in Box 28.1 develops diarrhea and weight loss. She is shown to have mild malabsorption. Her serum is tested by indirect immunofluorescence and is found to contain immunoglobulin A (IgA) autoantibodies against endomysium (Fig. 28.9). Enzyme-linked immunosorbent assay (ELISA) testing shows antibodies against tissue transglutaminase (tTG). In a child of this age, these blood tests are considered diagnostic of celiac disease. The patient is started on a gluten-free diet, and her symptoms improve dramatically. The endomysial antibodies are no longer present 6 months later.

Celiac disease is the most common cause of small bowel disease in the developed world and causes a spectrum of clinical problems that range from mild anemia to severe malnutrition. Celiac disease is an autoimmune disease in which lymphocytes and macrophages infiltrate the jejunum; it is therefore a type IV delayed hypersensitivity reaction against an exogenous antigen, a polypeptide called *gliadin,* and an autoantigen, tTG.

Wheat, rye, and barley contain a protein called *gluten,* which in turn contains gliadin. When gliadin is removed from the diet, the symptoms of celiac disease and jejunal histology improve.

tTG is an enzyme that converts the amino acid glutamine to glutamic acid. It can irreversibly bind to substrate peptides. Antibodies to endomysium (see Fig. 28.9) are an indirect way of detecting antibodies to tTG.

Identical twins have a high concordance rate (75%) for celiac disease. Most patients with this disease have inherited the human leukocyte antigen (HLA) DQ2 allele. In celiac disease, jejunal T cells recognize gliadin peptides bound to HLA-DQ2 (Fig. 28.10). However, pockets on the side of the peptide-binding groove on HLA-DQ2 only bind charged amino acids; gliadin will not bind unless glutamine residues have been converted to glutamic acid by tTG. As a result of binding to gliadin, tTG itself becomes a target of autoantibodies (Fig. 28.11).

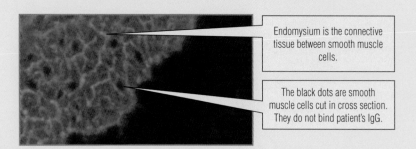

Endomysium is the connective tissue between smooth muscle cells.

The black dots are smooth muscle cells cut in cross section. They do not bind patient's IgG.

Fig 28.9 Patients with celiac disease have autoantibodies against endomysium, connective tissue surrounding bundles of smooth muscle fibers. In this indirect immunofluorescence test, a section of animal tissue has been placed on a slide. This is incubated with patient serum, and the immunoglobulin G (IgG) is detected with a fluorescent anti-IgG antibody. Endomysium is a good source of tissue transglutaminase, the autoantigen in celiac disease.

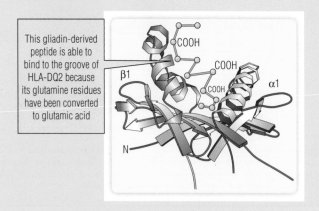

This gliadin-derived peptide is able to bind to the groove of HLA-DQ2 because its glutamine residues have been converted to glutamic acid

COOH

COOH

COOH

β1

α1

N

Fig 28.10 Gliadin peptides bound to human leukocyte antigen (HLA) DQ2.

Continued

 MCH II

 Cytokine, chemokine, etc.

 Complement (C′)

 Signaling molecule

BOX 28.2 Celiac Disease—cont'd

In endomysium, the connective tissue between smooth muscle cells, tTG is present at high quantities. Endomysial antibody testing using indirect immunofluorescence performs as well as ELISA for tTG in testing for celiac disease.

Members of the same family will often develop type 1 diabetes mellitus (T1DM) and celiac disease. Family members may also be at higher risk for developing autoimmune thyroid or adrenal disease or gastritis. These diseases frequently coexist in the same individuals and are called *organ-specific autoimmune diseases*.

The HLA genes are all closely situated on chromosome 6, and they tend to be inherited as a block, called a *haplotype* (Chapter 8). One relatively common haplotype consists of HLA alleles B8, DR3, and DQ2. It is the inheritance of this haplotype that explains why organ-specific autoimmune disease occurs in families. The HLA-DQ2 allele increases the risk for T1DM and celiac disease. It is not clear which genes in the major histocompatibility complex (MHC) are associated with the other organ-specific autoimmune diseases, and many genes are possible candidates (see Table 8.2). Different family members tend to have different autoimmune diseases, presumably because slightly different environmental factors trigger each disease.

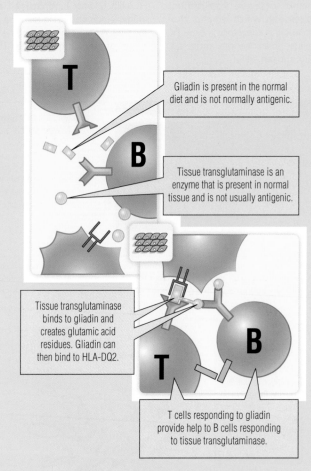

Gliadin is present in the normal diet and is not normally antigenic.

Tissue transglutaminase is an enzyme that is present in normal tissue and is not usually antigenic.

Tissue transglutaminase binds to gliadin and creates glutamic acid residues. Gliadin can then bind to HLA-DQ2.

T cells responding to gliadin provide help to B cells responding to tissue transglutaminase.

Fig 28.11 The pathogenesis of celiac disease. Jejunal damage in celiac disease is mediated by T cells responding to deaminated gliadin bound to human leukocyte antigen (HLA) DQ2. These T cells produce cytokines, such as interferon-γ, which may damage villi. The pathogenic role of the antibodies produced against gliadin and tissue transglutaminase is unclear, although both antibodies are useful diagnostically.

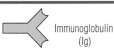 T-cell receptor (TCR)

 Immunoglobulin (Ig)

Antigen

MCH I

BOX 28.3 Systemic Lupus Erythematosus

A young woman develops a rash in a sun-exposed area—her face (Fig. 28.12A). She has also developed painful lesions in the pulps of her toes (Fig. 28.12B). A skin biopsy is taken for direct immunofluorescence and shows her skin contains deposits of immunoglobulin G (IgG) and complement (Fig. 28.13). She was also found to have some abnormalities on blood testing that included an antinuclear cytoplasmic antibody (ANCA) screening done by indirect immunofluorescence (Fig. 28.14) and an anti-DNA antibody assay (by enzyme-linked immunosorbent assay [ELISA]). These findings are strongly suggestive of systemic lupus erythematosus (SLE). Note that the DNA antibodies found in the blood sample do *not* bind nuclei in vivo. This is because the IgG antibodies form immune complexes with DNA that has been released from cells. (This case history is continued in Chapter 29.)

SLE is an autoimmune disease mediated by immune complexes; that is, it is a type III hypersensitivity. The hypersensitivity reaction in SLE is mediated by antibodies against DNA and other nuclear components, such as ribonucleoproteins.

A detailed description of how SLE causes disease appears in Chapter 29. This chapter is concerned with how high levels of antibodies against DNA and ribonucleoproteins are generated. Although SLE is an antibody-mediated disease, the key step in its pathogenesis is the loss of T-cell tolerance to DNA.

Genes play an important role in the pathogenesis of SLE; the concordance rate for SLE in identical twins is approximately 60%. SLE is more frequent in individuals who inherit the human leukocyte antigen (HLA) allele DR2. In addition, polymorphisms in the genes for debris-clearing proteins are also important.

Some proteins of the innate immune system are involved in clearing up cellular debris. For example, mannan-binding lectin (MBL) and complement component C1q can recognize and bind fragments of DNA that are released during cell death (Fig. 28.15). This is thought to happen when neutrophils undergo neutrophil extracellular trap (NET) formation. These fragments are then cleared, perhaps through phagocytosis. Patients with low levels of C1q or MBL are at higher risk for SLE, presumably because DNA produced as a result of cell death is able to trigger production of anti-DNA antibodies. Some drugs also interfere with the clearance of DNA by inhibition of methyltransferase enzymes. In predisposed individuals, these drugs can trigger the production of anti-DNA antibodies. Hydralazine and procainamide are two drugs that can induce SLE, possibly through this mechanism.

Toll-like receptor (TLR) 9, expressed on B cells and dendritic cells, has a physiologic role in recognizing bacteria by binding unmethylated cytosine and guanine (CpG) motifs. Normally, recognition of bacterial CpG DNA motifs leads to increased immunoglobulin secretion by B cells or interferon (IFN) secretion by dendritic cells. In patients with SLE, immune complexes that contain DNA are capable of stimulating TLR-9. This leads to increased secretion of type 1 IFNs and may provide additional stimulation for B cells to perpetuate the secretion of anti-DNA antibodies (see Fig. 28.15). Infections may promote the process by increasing the apoptosis of cells and triggering additional secretion of type 1 IFNs.

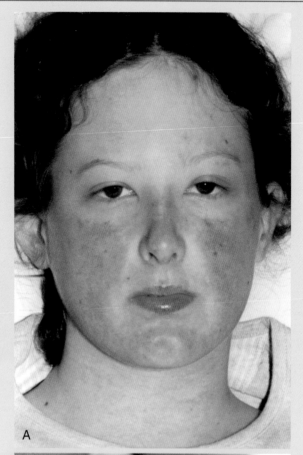

A

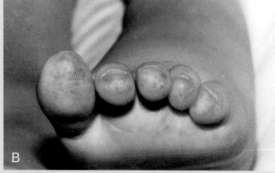

B

Fig 28.12 A, This woman has a facial rash typical of systemic lupus erythematosus. **B,** The lesions on her toes reflect underlying vasculitis, blood vessel inflammation.

Continued

 MCH II

 Cytokine, chemokine, etc.

 Complement (C')

 Signaling molecule

BOX 28.3 Systemic Lupus Erythematosus—cont'd

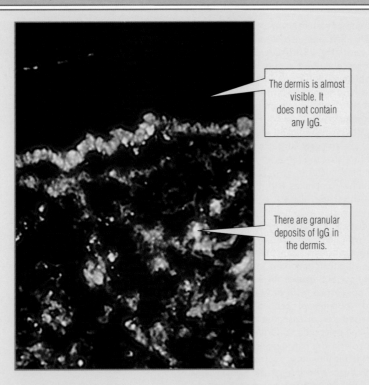

The dermis is almost visible. It does not contain any IgG.

There are granular deposits of IgG in the dermis.

Fig 28.13 A section from a fresh skin biopsy is incubated with anti–human immunoglobulin G (IgG) tagged with a fluorescent label. When viewed under an ultraviolet light microscope, IgG in the tissue produces green fluorescence. How these deposits are formed is discussed in Chapter 30. (Courtesy Dr. R. Cerio, Royal London Hospital, London, United Kingdom.)

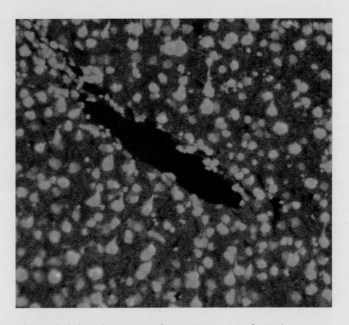

Fig 28.14 Antinuclear antibody by indirect immunofluorescence. A piece of animal tissue is mounted on a slide, and the patient's immunoglobulin G is bound to nuclei in the tissue.

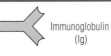 T-cell receptor (TCR)

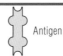 Immunoglobulin (Ig)

 Antigen

MCH I

BOX 28.3 Systemic Lupus Erythematosus—cont'd

Two additional factors affect the development of SLE. In general, autoimmune diseases are more common in women; SLE, however, is an extreme example—it affects women 20 times more frequently than men. The higher incidence of autoimmunity in women is probably related to higher levels of the sex hormone estrogen. SLE can sometimes develop shortly after starting estrogen-containing contraceptive pills, and it often gets worse during pregnancy, when estrogen levels are high. Estrogen has the physiologic effect of increasing antibody production, and it may thus increase autoantibody secretion. Some autoimmune diseases (eg, type 1 diabetes) affect men and women equally. These autoimmune diseases tend to be caused by T cells rather than antibody.

Exposure to ultraviolet (UV) light has a role in triggering SLE, and sun-exposed skin is often affected by a characteristic rash.

It is not yet clear how UV light has these effects. One possible mechanism is that it induces apoptosis in cells in the skin. An alternative is that UV light–induced skin damage triggers the release of proinflammatory cytokines, such as tumor necrosis factor (TNF) or type 1 IFNs, which either costimulate B cells or add to local tissue damage. Figure 28.16 illustrates the series of events that may be required to trigger SLE.

Low levels of ANCA are present in many healthy individuals. It is known that ANCA levels can increase several years before the development of SLE symptoms. In addition, the production of antibodies specifically against double-stranded DNA commences. The factors that switch patients from symptom-free to symptomatic SLE are not well documented but probably include infections, exposure to UV light, and estrogens.

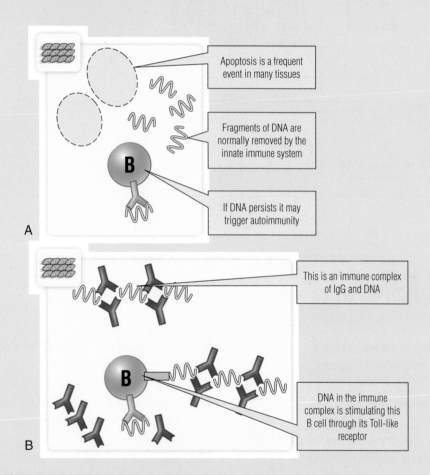

Fig 28.15 A, Impaired clearance of DNA may initially prime production of anti-DNA antibodies. **B,** Immune complexes that contain DNA may then stimulate Toll-like receptors and perpetuate antibody secretion. *Ig,* immunoglobulin.

Continued

 MCH II   Cytokine, chemokine, etc.   Complement (C′)   Signaling molecule

BOX 28.3 Systemic Lupus Erythematosus—cont'd

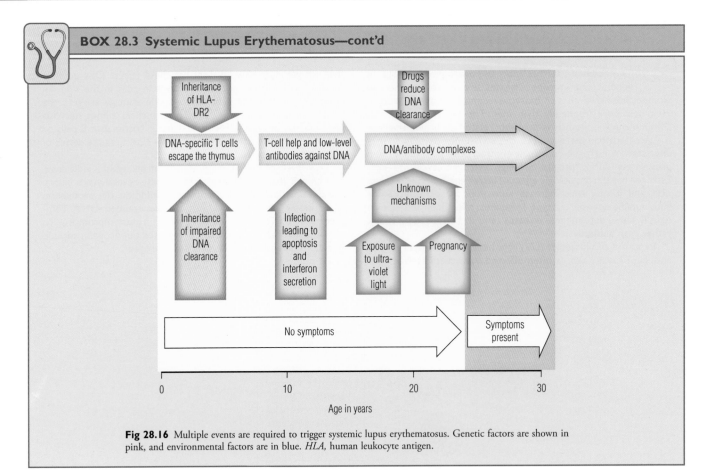

Fig 28.16 Multiple events are required to trigger systemic lupus erythematosus. Genetic factors are shown in pink, and environmental factors are in blue. *HLA,* human leukocyte antigen.

LEARNING POINTS Can You Now...

1. List what evidence there is for autoimmunity in normal, healthy individuals?
2. Describe the origin and function of natural antibodies?
3. Describe how the immune system tolerates most autoantigens and how tolerance can break down?
4. Describe how immunofluorescence tests and ELISAs are used to detect autoantibodies?

5. Contrast direct and indirect immunofluorescence?
6. List three blood tests for autoantibodies?
7. Explain why autoantibodies can have low specificity in the diagnosis of autoimmune disease?
8. Using the examples of type 1 diabetes, celiac disease, and systemic lupus erythematosus, describe how genes and environmental factors work together to cause autoimmune disease?

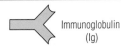 T-cell receptor (TCR)   Immunoglobulin (Ig)   Antigen   MCH I

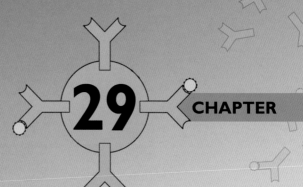

Antibody-Mediated Hypersensitivity (Type II)

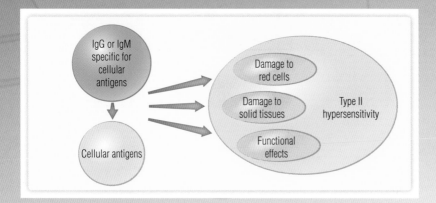

Type II hypersensitivity reactions are a consequence of immunoglobulin G (IgG) or IgM binding to the surface of cells. Antibody binding frequently damages red blood cells, either through activation of complement or because the antibodies opsonize the target erythrocytes. This is referred to as *immune-mediated hemolysis*. Antibody binding may also damage solid tissues, where the antigen may be cellular or part of the extracellular matrix (eg, basement membrane). Less often, antibodies may modify the function of cells by binding to receptors for hormones, which is illustrated in autoimmune thyroid disease. Hyperacute graft rejection is also a version of type II hypersensitivity, which is discussed in Chapter 34.

▇ IMMUNE-MEDIATED HEMOLYSIS

Red Blood Cell Antigens

Red blood cells express a variety of antigen systems. The rhesus and ABO antigen systems contain alleles inherited in a mendelian fashion (Fig. 29.1). The genetics and immunology of the clinically important rhesus and ABO systems differ.

The rhesus blood group system consists of three loci—C, D, and E—of which D is the most important. Most individuals express a D locus antigen and are therefore rhesus positive. About one in six people are homozygous for a null D allele; they express no D antigen and are therefore rhesus negative. D is a conventional protein antigen, and rhesus-negative individuals make IgG anti-D after exposure to the antigen (see Fig. 29.1A).

The A and B blood group antigens are oligosaccharide molecules produced on the surface of red cells. These sugars are inherited in a codominant fashion: an individual can inherit the A antigen (blood group A), the B antigen (blood group B), both A and B (blood group AB), or a null allele (blood group O).

The A and B antigens are similar to oligosaccharide expressed on bacteria. Natural antibodies produced by B1 cells recognize A and B (Chapter 14). Thus anti-A and anti-B are IgM natural antibodies, physiologically produced as a defense against bacteria and capable of cross-reacting with A or B red cell antigens. Hence, individuals who are blood group O and have inherited neither A nor B antigen will produce IgM against A and B from birth, regardless of whether they have been exposed to these antigens. Individuals who have inherited A antigen but not B antigen produce anti-B only, and so forth (see Fig. 29.1B).

Other red cell antigens are nonallelic; the same molecule is expressed by everyone. For example, the I antigen is expressed by adults on the surface of red cells. I behaves as a regular self antigen and should not normally elicit anti-I antibodies (see Fig. 29.1C).

Antigens of the ABO and rhesus systems are *alloantigens*—they differ from person to person. The antibodies produced against these antigens can cause type II hypersensitivity when cells are transferred from one individual to another, such as in blood transfusion or during pregnancy.

Antigens of the rhesus and I systems can also act as autoantigens. They can cause type II hypersensitivity when they become targets of autoimmunity.

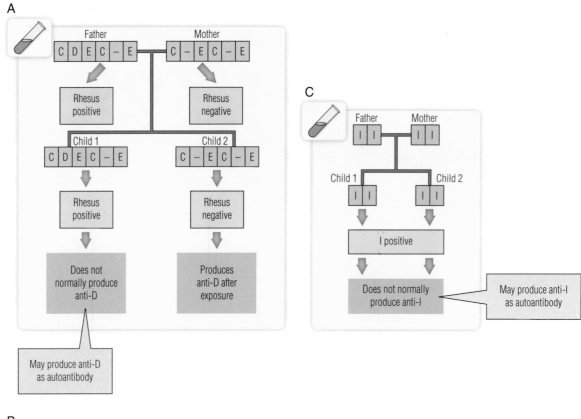

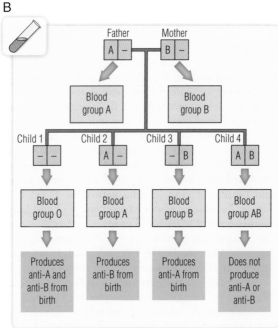

Fig 29.1 Genes *(orange)*, antigens *(yellow)*, and alloantibodies *(blue)* involved in the blood group systems. Alloantibodies are produced spontaneously against A and B and after exposure to D. As shown, D and I may become targets for autoantigens.

 T-cell receptor (TCR)

 Immunoglobulin (Ig)

Antigen

 MCH I

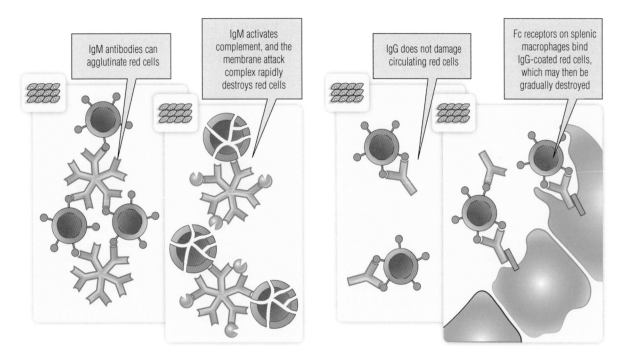

Fig 29.2 Mechanisms of immune hemolysis. Immunoglobulin M (IgM) antibodies are more dangerous than IgG antibodies in immune hemolysis.

Anti–Red Cell Antibodies

IgM antibodies against red cell antigens are produced as natural antibodies against A and B or as autoantibodies against I in some types of autoimmune hemolytic anemia (AIHA). IgM antibodies are highly effective at activating complement and rapidly cause damage through activation of the membrane attack complex (Fig. 29.2).

IgG antibodies are produced against rhesus antigens, either as a response to allogeneic stimulation (see Box 29.1) or in some types of AIHA. IgG is not very effective in activating complement and does not cause hemolysis in the circulation. Instead, IgG-coated red cells are recognized by Fc receptors on resident macrophages in the liver and spleen. The IgG-coated red cells are then destroyed by phagocytosis.

Types of Immune-Mediated Hemolysis

Alloimmune Hemolysis

The rhesus antigens behave like conventional antigen—exposure is required to produce IgG antibody. This most frequently occurs in pregnancy when IgG antibodies against rhesus antigens cross the placenta and cause hemolytic disease of the newborn. As described in Box 29-1, these IgG antibodies cause fairly gradual destruction of red cells. This is because the IgG-coated red cells are only slowly recognized by macrophages in the spleen, which have Fc receptors for IgG.

Incompatibility in the ABO system is the most common cause of serious blood transfusion reactions. For example, an A-positive individual who requires a transfusion possesses natural antibodies against B-positive cells. If B-positive cells are inadvertently transfused, they will be rapidly hemolyzed in the circulation. The hypersensitivity reaction can take place within

seconds of the donor cells entering the recipient. IgM reactions are very fast because pentameric IgM is able to efficiently activate complement. This is because each IgM molecule is able to aggregate antigen more effectively and because of the greater numbers of Fc components, which activate the early classic complement cascade.

Units of blood for transfusion contain mainly red cells and very little antibody-containing plasma. The recipient's antibodies and the donor's red cell antigens must be checked for compatibility prior to transfusion. In most routine clinical situations, considerable precautions are taken to ensure patients receive the correct type of blood. Mismatched transfusions should be 100% preventable, but every year, a handful of deaths are caused by transfusion errors (see Box 29.2). In emergencies, when the laboratory does not have time to determine the recipient's blood group, O cells—which have neither A nor B antigens—can be used for transfusion into any type of recipient.

Autoimmune Hemolysis

Autoimmune hemolytic anemia can be triggered by infections or drugs (see Box 26.2), or it can be part of generalized autoimmune diseases such as systemic lupus erythematosus (SLE; Chapter 30). Autoantibodies can also be produced by malignant clones of B cells in diseases such as chronic lymphocytic leukemia or lymphoma. However, most cases of AIHA are not explained. Red cell antigens can become targets for IgG and IgM autoantibodies.

The most common type of AIHA is caused by IgG autoantibodies against rhesus antigens. The antibody-coated red cells are only slowly removed by the spleen, and the onset of anemia is gradual.

The I antigen is generally the target when IgM antibodies cause AIHA. Much more rapid and dangerous intravascular

 MCH II   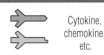 Cytokine, chemokine, etc.   Complement (C′)   Signaling molecule

hemolysis occurs as a result of complement activation. Another feature of IgM antibodies is that they often bind red cells best at temperatures below 37°C. These cold hemagglutinins can cause red cells to aggregate in vessels in the hands and feet, which may cause ischemic damage. Similar alloimmune and autoimmune processes can affect platelets and neutrophils.

Type II Autoimmune Hypersensitivity Against Solid Tissue

Autoantibodies can also attack and damage components of solid tissues. For example, in Goodpasture syndrome, IgG autoantibodies bind a glycoprotein in the basement membrane of the lung and glomeruli. Anti–basement membrane antibody activates complement, which can trigger an inflammatory response. Goodpasture syndrome can be diagnosed by finding antibodies to glomerular basement membrane in patient's serum on indirect immunofluorescence (Fig. 29.3). In a variety of other comparable conditions, IgG antibodies bind to other cells or to tissue components. For example, in the blistering skin condition pemphigus, antibodies bind on the intercellular cement protein desmoglein. In myasthenia gravis, IgG binds to the acetylcholine receptor in skeletal muscle, causing widespread weakness. A characteristic that this group of diseases shares with AIHA is that the diagnosis can be made by detecting the autoantibody in blood samples. Treatment is aimed at removing or blocking the autoantibody.

TYPE II HYPERSENSITIVITY AND ANTIBODIES THAT AFFECT CELL FUNCTION

In other situations, antibodies bind to cells and affect their function. These antibodies can simply stimulate the target organ function without causing much target organ damage, such as in Graves disease.

Graves Disease

Graves disease is the most common cause of hyperthyroidism, often affecting young women (see Box 29.3) with a family history. Graves disease is linked to the human leukocyte antigen (HLA) allele DR3. In Graves disease the thyroid is stimulated by an autoantibody that binds onto the thyroid-stimulating hormone (TSH) receptor (Fig. 29.4). The anti-TSH receptor antibody mimics the effects of the hormone. Graves disease is thus a special kind of type II hypersensitivity. In pregnant women with Graves disease, IgG thyroid-stimulating antibody can cross the placenta and cause transient neonatal hyperthyroidism. Graves disease is associated with exophthalmos (protruding eyes) resulting from T cells infiltrating the orbit of the eye. Exophthalmos is thought to be caused by an orbital antigen that cross-reacts with a thyroid antigen.

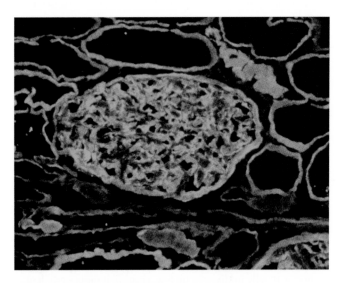

Fig 29.3 Indirect immunofluorescence has been used to detect autoantibodies in this patient with Goodpasture syndrome. Kidney tissue is used as the target antigen for this test. Linear staining is seen along the glomerular basement membrane, which appears to be "lit up" compared with the renal tubules in the background.

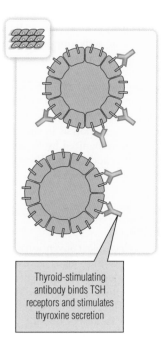

Thyroid-stimulating antibody binds TSH receptors and stimulates thyroxine secretion

Fig 29.4 Graves disease. The autoantibodies against the thyroid-stimulating hormone (TSH) receptor mimic the effects of the hormone.

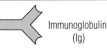 T-cell receptor (TCR)   Immunoglobulin (Ig) Antigen   MCH I

BOX 29.1 Hemolytic Disease of the Newborn

A woman presents to the antenatal clinic in week 29 of her pregnancy. She is a refugee from a developing country. She has one healthy child who was born without complications. Over the next few weeks the pregnancy runs smoothly, but the woman is found to be rhesus blood group negative. Further tests show that she has antibodies to the rhesus D antigen. At 34 weeks of pregnancy, an ultrasound scan shows signs of fetal distress. Labor is induced, and a baby girl is born. The baby is profoundly anemic. A Coombs test on the baby's blood is positive, confirming the diagnosis of hemolytic disease of the newborn (Fig. 29.5).

If a rhesus-negative woman carries a rhesus-positive fetus, she will produce antibodies if fetal cells leak into the maternal circulation. This can occur during pregnancy and especially during labor (Fig. 29.6). Rhesus antigens act as conventional antigens; immunoglobulin G (IgG) antibody levels therefore increase with each successive pregnancy with a rhesus-positive child. The IgG antibodies produced cross the placenta and bind fetal red cells, which are then destroyed in the fetal spleen and liver.

The treatment for hemolytic disease of the newborn is exchange transfusion, a technique that replaces fetal red cells with donor rhesus-negative cells. Hemolytic disease of the newborn is entirely preventable through the use of anti-D antibody injections (Fig. 29.7). Anti-A or anti-B antibodies only very rarely cause hemolytic disease of the newborn because IgM natural antibodies are not actively transported across the placenta.

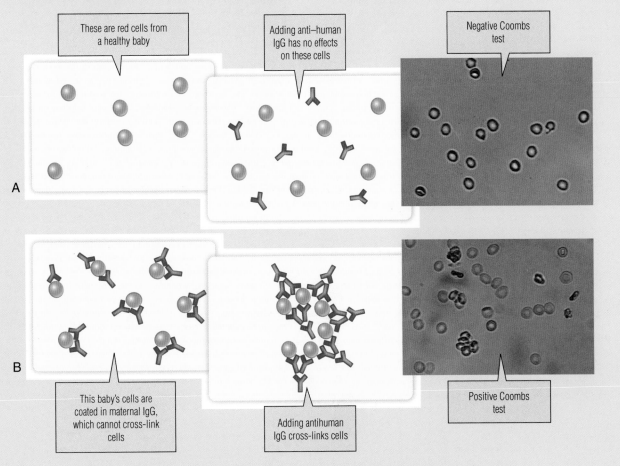

Fig 29.5 The Coombs test detects cells coated with antibody. In a healthy child (**A**), addition of anti–human immunoglobulin G (IgG) has no effects, whereas in a child with hemolytic disease of the newborn (**B**), anti–human IgG cross-links red cells, leading to agglutination.

Continued

 MCH II   Cytokine, chemokine, etc.   Complement (C′)   Signaling molecule

BOX 29.1 Hemolytic Disease of the Newborn—cont'd

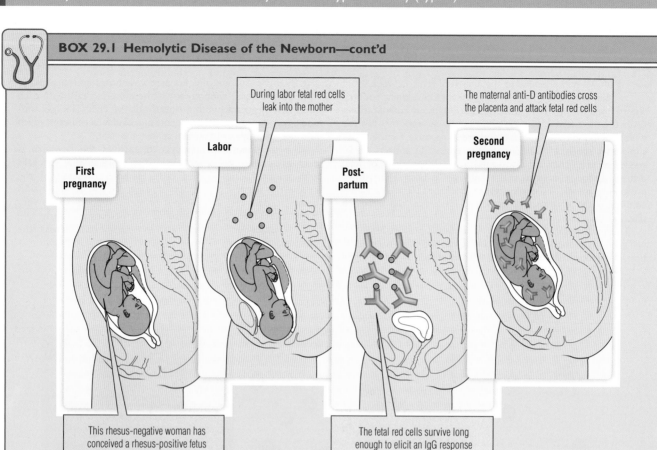

During labor fetal red cells leak into the mother

The maternal anti-D antibodies cross the placenta and attack fetal red cells

Labor

First pregnancy

Post-partum

Second pregnancy

This rhesus-negative woman has conceived a rhesus-positive fetus

The fetal red cells survive long enough to elicit an IgG response

Fig 29.6 Hemolytic disease of the newborn.

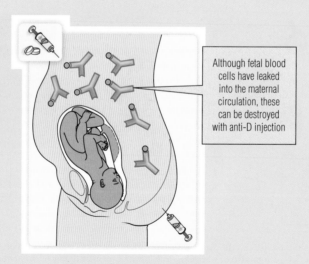

Although fetal blood cells have leaked into the maternal circulation, these can be destroyed with anti-D injection

Fig 29.7 Anti-D antibody should be given to rhesus-negative women pregnant with a rhesus-positive child. Anti-D destroys rhesus-positive fetal cells in the maternal bloodstream before the mother has an opportunity to make her own anti-D, which can affect the next pregnancy. Anti-D is a type of passive immunotherapy that can prevent hemolytic disease of the newborn when used appropriately.

T-cell receptor (TCR)

Immunoglobulin (Ig)

Antigen

 MCH I

BOX 29.2 Blood Transfusion Reaction

A 48-year-old man has undergone open heart surgery. He lost a considerable amount of blood while on bypass, and his surgeon has ordered a blood transfusion of 3 units of red cells. The patient's blood group was checked before the operation and is known to be type A. Several units of blood have been prepared for him. The first unit of blood does not cause any problems. The second unit of blood is started at 4:25 PM. At 4:30 PM the patient complains of widespread pain and difficulty breathing. His blood pressure has fallen, and he has developed a temperature of 39.6°C.

When the transfusion is stopped, the clinician notes that the unit of blood had been prepared for another patient with a similar name. This unit of blood is AB. Steps are taken to resuscitate the patient, and he gradually improves.

Because his blood group was A, he had preexisting ("natural") immunoglobulin M (IgM) antibodies against the B blood group. The moment the AB red cells began to enter the patient's blood, they would have reacted with the antibodies, activated complement, and triggered the membrane attack complex. Hemolysis would have started within seconds. Complement is activated via the classical pathway, leading to production of large quantities of the anaphylatoxins C3a and C5a (Chapter 20). These in turn activate the innate immune system, and systemic inflammatory response syndrome (SIRS) ensues (Chapter 21).

Many serious transfusion reactions are caused by ABO incompatibility; all of these are entirely preventable by careful management of blood transfusions.

BOX 29.3 Graves Disease

A 62-year-old woman complains of increasing anxiety and restlessness. Her doctor notices that she has an enlarged thyroid gland and a fast pulse, both signs of hyperthyroidism. She also has exophthalmos (Fig. 28.8). Blood tests show that her thyroid gland is overactive and she has autoantibodies to thyroid peroxidase and the thyroid-stimulating hormone receptor, all diagnostic of Graves disease. She is treated with antithyroid drugs and her symptoms improve.

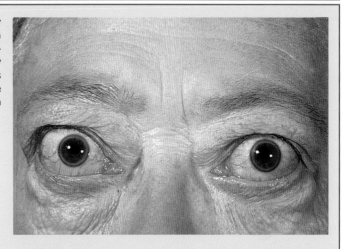

Fig 29.8 This patient with Graves disease has exophthalmos (protruding eyes) because of swelling of the orbital soft tissue. (Courtesy St. Bartholomew's Hospital, London.)

LEARNING POINTS Can You Now...

1. List the antigens involved in autoimmune and alloimmune hemolysis?
2. Explain how IgG and IgM antibodies can cause hemolysis?
3. Describe the genetics of the rhesus and ABO blood groups?
4. Explain how autoantibodies cause the symptoms of Graves disease?
5. List which tests are used to diagnose these autoimmune diseases?
6. List preventive actions and treatments for type II hypersensitivity diseases?

 MCH II   Cytokine, chemokine, etc.   Complement (C')   Signaling molecule

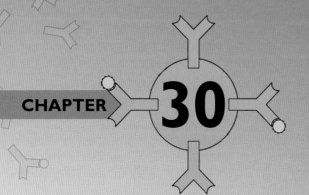

CHAPTER 30

Immune Complex Disease (Type III Hypersensitivity)

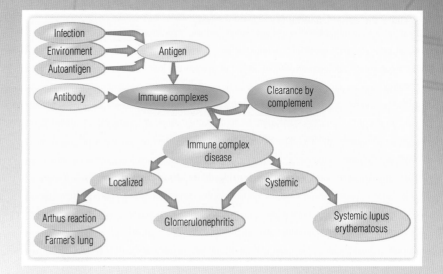

This chapter discusses how immune complexes can form in certain circumstances when antibodies combine with antigen. The antigens can be derived from infection, innocuous environmental substances, or autoantigen. Immune complexes are usually cleared by the complement system, but when this does not happen, immune complex diseases may arise. Farmer's lung and the Arthus reaction are examples of *local immune complex disease*. Poststreptococcal glomerulonephritis is an example of *circulating immune complex disease* and is described in Chapter 26. This chapter examines another *systemic immune complex disease,* systemic lupus erythematosus (SLE), in more depth.

Immune complexes are lattices of antigen and antibody; they may be localized to the site of antigen production or may circulate in the blood. They are produced as part of the normal immune response and are usually cleared by mechanisms that involve complement, as described later. Immune complexes cause disease in a number of situations.

ANTIGENS IN IMMUNE COMPLEXES

Antigens that can form immune complexes must be polyvalent; that is, each antigen molecule must be able to bind more than one antibody molecule. For immune complexes to develop,

antigen must be present long enough to elicit an antibody response. Immune complexes usually form when antigen is in slight excess of antibody (Fig. 30.1). Immune complexes may form when antigen is produced from one of three sources: (1) infectious antigens, (2) innocuous environmental antigens, and (3) autoantigens.

Infectious Antigens

Most infections are short lived and are controlled by the immune response. Even in such rapidly controlled infections, immune complexes may cause hypersensitivity, such as after streptococcal infection (Chapter 26). Infections such as hepatitis B are not always controlled and can cause sustained high levels of antigen in blood (*antigenemia*), resulting in more chronic immune complex disease.

Innocuous Environmental Antigens

Harmless environmental antigens can elicit an immunoglobulin G (IgG) response if they are small enough to enter the tissues. A good example is fungal spores, which cause the localized immune complex disease known as *farmer's lung* (Box 30.1).

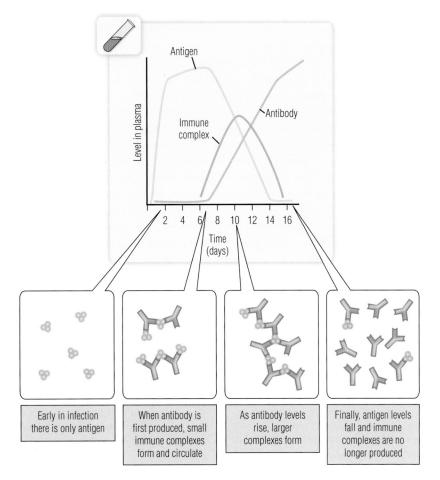

Fig 30.1 The largest immune complexes form at a time during infection when antibody levels slightly exceed antigen levels.

Drugs are also environmental antigens and sometimes cause localized immune complexes, such as the *Arthus reaction* (Box 30.2).

Drugs can also cause circulating immune complexes. This leads to a disorder referred to as *serum sickness*. The name was coined in the period before antibiotics were available, when patients with infections were given immune horse serum. Nowadays, serum sickness most often happens as a result of the use of mouse monoclonal antibodies to treat cancer or autoimmune disease (Chapter 36). Repeated exposure leads to production of antimouse antibodies and circulating immune complexes. Serum sickness then causes fever, rash, and joint pain. This problem can be overcome by genetically manipulating the mouse antibodies to humanize them.

Autoantigens

Autoantigens can only cause immune complex disease in the presence of autoantibodies. DNA is an antigen in SLE (see Box 30.3). SLE is the most prevalent immune complex disease. DNA is released into the circulation when cells die, especially if innate immune system mechanisms usually responsible for clearing DNA are defective (Chapter 28). DNA that is not rapidly cleared can elicit an antibody response.

■ ANTIBODIES IN IMMUNE COMPLEXES

Immune complexes will form only when the ratio between antigen and antibody is exactly right. At low levels of antibody, each antigen molecule binds several immunoglobulin molecules (see Fig. 30.1). When antibody and antigen levels are approximately equal, or antibody levels are slightly in excess, large complexes can form. When antibody exceeds antigen, small complexes form.

During an infection, this means that immune complexes will be produced very transiently at the point where antibody levels are increasing. Immune complexes rarely become persistent during infections and do so only when the infection cannot be cleared by antibodies (e.g., hepatitis virus infections).

■ CLEARANCE OF IMMUNE COMPLEXES

Immune complexes can form in normal individuals when antibodies are produced during infections. These complexes must be cleared or they will cause disease through the mechanisms described later. Two mechanisms involving complement can clear immune complexes (Chapter 20).

 MCH II

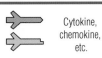 Cytokine, chemokine, etc.

 Complement (C′)

 Signaling molecule

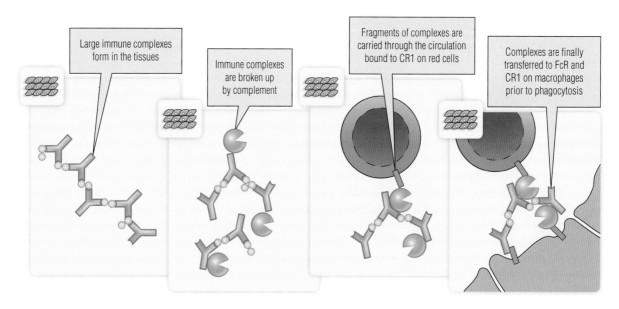

Fig 30.2 Clearance of immune complexes. Red blood cells are not damaged when immune complexes are transferred to macrophages. *CR1,* complement receptor 1; *FcR,* Fc receptor.

Complement Breaks Down Large Soluble Complexes

Immune complexes of antigen and immunoglobulin contain high numbers of immunoglobulin Fc in close proximity, which activates complement through the classical pathway (Fig. 30.2). Small molecular components, especially activated C3, are produced through activation of the complement pathway. These molecules insert themselves into and break up the lattice of the immune complex.

Complement Receptor 1 Transfers Complexes to Phagocytes

Red blood cells transfer circulating immune complexes from tissues and blood to the phagocytes of the liver and spleen. Red cells express complement receptor 1 (CR1), the receptor for activated C3. Immune complexes bind to the complement receptor CR1 on red cells, which then circulate through the liver and spleen. In the liver and spleen, receptors take up the immune complexes and in doing so stimulate the macrophages to phagocytose them (see Fig. 30.2). This mechanism is highly efficient and can entirely remove immune complexes from the circulation in a few minutes. Furthermore, because the spleen is home to a large population of B cells, antigens originally present in the periphery are rapidly presented to B cells to boost antibody production.

Failure of Clearance

These immune complex clearance mechanisms can be saturated in situations where there is excessive, ongoing production of immune complexes—for example, in antigenemia resulting from chronic infection. Some individuals lack complement and, because the mechanisms described cannot function, are predisposed to immune complex disease (see Box 20.2).

■ MECHANISMS OF INFLAMMATION IN IMMUNE COMPLEX DISEASE

Immune complexes that are not cleared rapidly cause damage by activating components of the innate immune system (Fig. 30.3).

Immune complexes activate complement. Although this process helps to clear complexes, low-molecular-weight anaphylatoxins are produced, which increase permeability of blood vessels and are chemotactic for leukocytes.

Complexes bind to and activate cells such as neutrophils, mast cells, and platelets. Neutrophils and mast cells release proteolytic enzymes, which damage blood vessels and initiate inflammation. Activated platelets bind to the endothelium and form thrombi.

If antigen is present predominantly at one site, immune complexes cause localized damage—for example, the Arthus reaction (see Box 30.2) and farmer's lung (see Box 30.1). Small complexes produced when antigen is in excess enter the circulation and form circulating immune complexes. Circulating complexes cause damage to blood vessels that range from inflammation of the vessel walls to occlusion of the vessel and ischemic damage. Immune complex disease is one cause of vessel inflammation (vasculitis). Circulating immune complexes cause damage at specific sites, especially the joints, skin, and kidney. Immune complexes can become deposited in joints and cause synovitis, which causes pain and swelling.

■ IMMUNE COMPLEX DISEASE IN THE KIDNEY

Involvement of the kidney in type III hypersensitivity is a common cause of renal failure. The kidney is often affected because blood pressure in the glomerulus is four times higher than that in the systemic circulation. High blood pressure

 T-cell receptor (TCR)   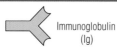 Immunoglobulin (Ig)   Antigen   MCH I

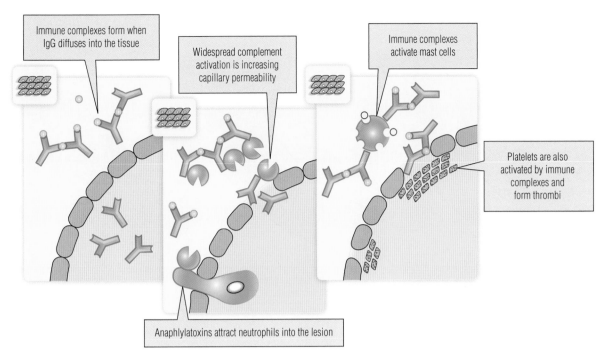

Fig 30.3 Immune complexes cause damage by activating the innate immune system. *Ig,* immunoglobulin.

increases immune complex deposition in vessel walls. Glomerular cells also express the complement receptor CR1, which may predispose to immune complex deposition at this site. Synovial cells also express CR1, which may explain why joints are also often involved in circulating immune complex disease.

Immune complex disease in the kidney can result in two clinically defined syndromes: *nephrotic syndrome,* in which protein leaks into the urine and there is gradual-onset renal failure, and *nephritis,* in which there is rapid-onset renal failure, blood and protein in the urine, and hypertension. Both types of disease are produced by inflammation in the glomeruli (glomerulonephritis).

In the nephrotic syndrome, immune complexes are deposited in the glomerular basement membrane where they activate complement (Fig. 30.4). This usually causes subtle damage to the basement membrane, which allows proteins to leak into the urine. In nephritis, by comparison, there is a cellular infiltrate in addition to complement activation. Neutrophils are attracted into the glomeruli, and the resulting inflammation causes blood and protein to leak into the urine, impairing the ability of the kidney to excrete toxic metabolites. Which type of glomerular lesion is produced depends on several factors, including the size of immune complexes, the rate at which they are produced, and the duration of immune complex production.

In poststreptococcal glomerulonephritis (see Box 26.3), the renal disease is dramatic but short lived because infection is brought under control by the immune response. When drugs cause immune complex–mediated kidney disease, stopping the drug improves kidney function. In SLE, the immune complexes contain autoantigens, and therefore the renal disease has gradual onset but is not self-limiting (Box 30.3).

Immune complexes are not the only immunologic cause of glomerulonephritis. Renal damage can also occur in Goodpasture syndrome (Chapter 29) and when immunoglobulin light chains damage the kidney in multiple myeloma (Chapter 35).

Laboratory tests are crucial in the investigation of nephritis and the nephrotic syndrome. Indirect immunofluorescence is used to find antibodies implicated in immune complex disease (e.g., anti-DNA antibodies) or other types of autoantibody (antiglomerular basement membrane antibody). Sometimes it is necessary to perform direct immunofluorescence on a renal biopsy specimen to determine what type of process is causing damage.

■ TREATMENT OF IMMUNE COMPLEX DISEASE

Antigen avoidance is possible in some cases of type III hypersensitivity—for example, farmer's lung or some drugs and vaccines. In the case of autoantigens, however (e.g., DNA), avoidance is clearly not possible.

In autoimmune causes of immune complex disease, corticosteroids block some of the damage caused by effector cells, such as neutrophils. Cyclophosphamide is an alkylating agent that impairs DNA synthesis and prevents rapid proliferation of cells such as lymphocytes. Although cyclophosphamide has some effects on T cells, its main benefit is in reducing B-cell proliferation and hence autoantibody levels. Cyclophosphamide is often used in severe SLE.

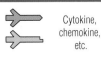 MCH II   Cytokine, chemokine, etc.   Complement (C′)   Signaling molecule

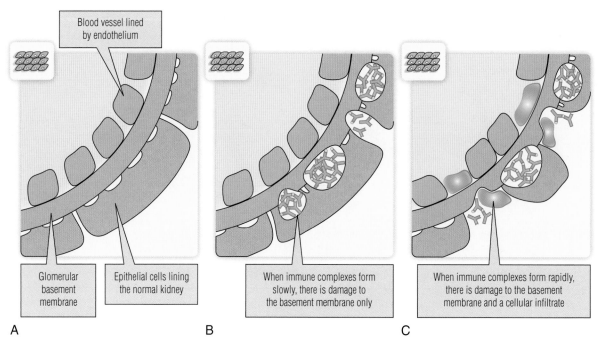

A B C

Fig 30.4 Nephrotic syndrome. **A,** Normal glomerulus. **B,** Slow complex formation, such as in hepatitis B virus infection. **C,** Rapid complex formation, such as after streptococcal infection.

In figure A:
- Blood vessel lined by endothelium
- Glomerular basement membrane
- Epithelial cells lining the normal kidney

In figure B:
- When immune complexes form slowly, there is damage to the basement membrane only

In figure C:
- When immune complexes form rapidly, there is damage to the basement membrane and a cellular infiltrate

---

BOX 30.1 Farmer's Lung

A 23-year-old farmer complains of breathlessness, cough, malaise, and fever on several occasions after feeding his cattle. The symptoms develop several hours after exposure to hay and last about 2 days. A blood sample shows he has immunoglobulin G (IgG) antibodies against mold extract. In addition, his symptoms are reproduced 5 hours after deliberate challenge with mold spores, confirming a diagnosis of farmer's lung. He is instructed to breathe through a filter mask when handling hay, and his symptoms do not recur.

Patients with farmer's lung produce IgG antibodies against proteins in mold spores. Immune complexes form in the lungs after exposure to spores. Over several hours, these immune complexes trigger inflammation in the alveoli (Fig. 30.5). The process is different from IgE-mediated hypersensitivity, which produces immediate symptoms on exposure to antigen and does not produce fever or symptoms outside the lungs.

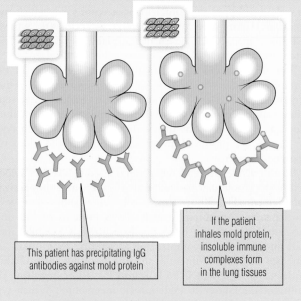

This patient has precipitating IgG antibodies against mold protein

If the patient inhales mold protein, insoluble immune complexes form in the lung tissues

Fig 30.5 Farmer's lung. *IgG,* immunoglobulin G.

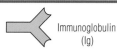 T-cell receptor (TCR)

Immunoglobulin (Ig)

 Antigen

 MCH I

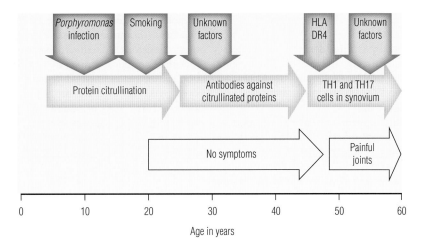

Fig 31.2 How rheumatoid arthritis (RA) may arise. Red indicates genetic factors, and blue shows environmental factors. Note that the triggers for anti–cyclic citrullinated peptide (CCP) antibodies and localization of pathology to the synovium are unknown. *HLA,* human leukocyte antigen.

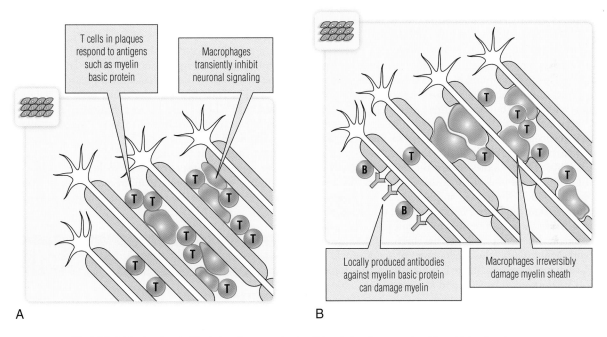

Fig 31.3 Multiple sclerosis. The lesions in acute relapsing (**A**) and chronic progressive (**B**) multiple sclerosis are different.

settles, the disability improves. Between attacks, there is usually good recovery of function, at least early in the disease. The chronic disability that usually occurs later in MS is the result of another process, axonal loss. Although demyelinated nerve cells can remyelinate to some extent, axon loss from the nerve cell is irreversible.

Although T cells are thought to initiate much of the damage in MS, there are also B cells in the CNS that secrete antibodies against a wide variety of brain components, including myelin basic protein. These antibodies may participate in inflammation and also provide a marker of antibody production in the CNS, which can sometimes help make a diagnosis of MS.

Treatment of Delayed Hypersensitivity Reactions

In delayed hypersensitivity, it is sometimes possible to avoid the relevant environmental antigens. For example, some types of contact dermatitis are improved by avoiding exposure to nickel. In celiac disease, avoiding dietary gluten improves symptoms and reduces levels of antiendomysium antibodies. In these examples, an *exogenous antigen* is driving an autoimmune disease. Where the cause is an *endogenous antigen,* treatment is more complex. Options currently used are antiinflammatory drugs—which mainly have effects on effectors of delayed hypersensitivity, especially macrophages—and immunosuppressive drugs, which have effects on T cells.

 MCH II

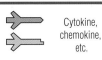 Cytokine, chemokine, etc.

 Complement (C′)

 Signaling molecule

Antiinflammatory Drugs

Antiinflammatory drugs work by cutting down the mediators released during inflammation, usually by cells of the innate system. For example, nonsteroidal antiinflammatory drugs—such as aspirin, ibuprofen, and indomethacin—inhibit arachidonic acid metabolism (Chapter 22).

Endogenous corticosteroids suppress the immune response during physiologic stress. Corticosteroids are often used as immunosuppressive drugs during the treatment of autoimmunity and allergy and after transplantation. Their effects are mediated by affecting gene transcription when used at low to moderate doses. Corticosteroids bind specific receptors that transport them to the nucleus and are responsible for binding to regulatory gene sequences. At higher doses they affect cell signaling directly.

Although corticosteroids are thought to affect the transcription of 1% of all genes in a wide range of cells, their dominant therapeutic effects are on phagocytes. Effects on lymphocytes may be largely a result of poor antigen processing and costimulation provided by phagocytes.

The side effects of corticosteroids are well known. From the immunologic point of view, immunosuppression is a particular concern, and it may result in reactivation of infections normally controlled by macrophages, such as tuberculosis.

Corticosteroids have some effects in MS, but only at high intravenous doses. Corticosteroids probably work in MS by reducing the actions of macrophages (Box 31.2). Corticosteroids are of some value in RA but are too toxic for long-term use.

Newer approaches introduced in the past 20 years exploit the increasing knowledge of cells and molecules in inflammation. For example, drugs that block TNF, IL-6, the costimulatory molecule CD80, and antibodies against B cells are all now routinely used in RA. These biologic drugs have been very effective, and for the first time RA patients can go into lasting remission and avoid irreversible disability. However, special problems with biologics occur that will be discussed in Chapter 36.

Recombinant interferon (IFN)-β has been used in some patients with MS; it delays the development of acute attacks of nervous system inflammation. There is some evidence to suggest that IFN-β has long-term benefits and can prevent the chronic disability associated with demyelination.

As discussed in Chapter 20, type I interferons (IFN-α and IFN-β) have potent antiviral effects and weaker immunostimulatory effects, increasing antigen presentation and activating natural killer cells. It is therefore surprising that IFN-β is effective in MS, in which antiinflammatory effects would be expected to be more beneficial. One possibility is that IFN-β reduces the migration of T cells across the blood-brain barrier. This illustrates the pleomorphism of cytokines; that is, that any one cytokine can have multiple effects on many different cell types. More recently, other potent antiinflammatory and immunosuppressive drugs have been found to be more effective in MS.

Immunosuppressive Drugs

Immunosuppressive drugs inhibit the specific immune response that drives delayed hypersensitivity and are most relevant in autoimmune delayed hypersensitivity, when antigen cannot be avoided. Immunosuppressive drugs are discussed in Chapter 34 because they are most often used in transplant recipients. The benefits of immunosuppressive drugs must be balanced against their dangerous side effects, particularly the increased the risk for infection. For example, in T1DM, pancreatic islet cell function can be maintained while patients receive immunosuppressive drugs. However, the drugs would have to be given for life, and the side effects are unacceptable; insulin replacement is a safer option. Immunosuppressive drugs have not been widely tested in MS.

Immunologically Mediated Drug Reactions

Drug reactions are common and affect up to 15% of hospital patients. The majority of reactions are predictable and are directly related to the pharmacologic effects of the drug. For example, a patient given an incorrectly high dose of a sedative drug will sleep longer than expected. Other side effects are less predictable and are described as being *idiosyncratic*. Some of these reactions may occur when a patient lacks an enzyme that is responsible for metabolizing a drug. For example, a patient who has low levels of the appropriate metabolizing enzyme will experience excessive sleepiness, even after the correct dose of sedative.

Idiosyncratic drug reactions also commonly have an immunologic basis. Some of these effects are mediated by the innate immune system. For example, morphine can stimulate mast cell degranulation, leading to histamine release and the development of the itchy rash urticaria. Reactions can also involve the adaptive system, and they can cause any type of hypersensitivity (Table 31.1). These reactions occur only after a patient has previously been exposed to a drug so that antibodies or reactive T cells can develop.

It is important to diagnose the cause of these reactions because repeat exposure can lead to life-threatening reactions. Laboratory tests can provide indirect evidence of immunologic hypersensitivity. For example, elevated blood mast cell tryptase

TABLE 31.1 Immunologically Mediated Drug Reactions

Hypersensitivity Type	Reaction	Useful Test
I	Anaphylaxis	Specific IgE test (Chapters 27 and 28) Skin prick testing
II	Drug-induced hemolysis	Coombs test (Chapter 29)
III: Localized	Arthus reaction to vaccines	Antibody levels (Chapter 30)
III: Circulating complexes	Serum sickness with monoclonal antibodies	
IV	Contact dermatitis to antibiotic-containing cream	Patch testing (Chapter 26)

Ig, *immunoglobulin.*

 T-cell receptor (TCR)

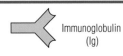 Immunoglobulin (Ig)

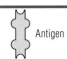 Antigen

 MCH I

levels suggest mast cell involvement through innate mechanisms or type I hypersensitivity. An allergist will try to confirm the presence of specific IgE against the drugs, either by skin testing or blood testing (Chapter 27).

You have already read some clinical examples of hypersensitivity reactions to drugs (Box 22.1, anesthetic allergy; Box 26.2, penicillin-induced hemolysis) and examples of iatrogenic reactions (Box 27.1, latex allergy; Box 29.2, blood transfusion reactions). Do you now feel confident that you could ask the right questions to prevent these reactions from happening?

Review of Hypersensitivity Reactions

The Gell and Coombs classification of hypersensitivity (Chapter 26) is an oversimplification, and many diseases overlap the different types. For example:

- Asthma is generally classified as an allergic disorder causing immediate symptoms mediated by IgE. However, the late phases of the type I reactions in asthma and atopic dermatitis are characterized by T-cell infiltrates more typical of type IV reactions.
- Although celiac disease and RA are both type IV reactions, autoantibodies (anti–tissue transglutaminase and anti-CCPs) play an important role.

Nonetheless, understanding the different types of hypersensitivity guides the diagnosis and treatment of these important conditions. For example, all allergies are best diagnosed by identifying specific IgE by blood or skin tests. These tests would not be used for any other type of hypersensitivity. Table 31.2 summarizes the hypersensitivity reactions described in the last six chapters. None of these conditions is rare, so clinicians should be familiar with them.

TABLE 31.2 Summary of Hypersensitivity Reactions

Type of Hypersensitivity	Antigen Type	Name of Disease	Antigen	Innate Immune System Involvement	B-cell Involvement	T-cell Involvement
Type I allergy	Harmless environmental substance	Hay fever Peanut allergy Latex allergy	Grass pollen Peanut allergen Latex protein	Mast cells and mast cell mediators	IgE	TH2 cells
Antibody-mediated type II	Alloantigen	Blood transfusion reaction	ABO	Complement	IgM	NA (T-independent antigen)
	Alloantigen	Hemolytic disease of the newborn	Rhesus antigen	Macrophages	IgG	TH1 (minor role)
	Harmless environmental substance	Drug-induced hemolysis	Penicillin	Macrophages	IgG	TH1 (minor role)
	Autoantigen	Graves disease	TSH receptor	NA	IgG	TH1 (minor role)
Immune complex–mediated type III	Harmless environmental substance	Farmer's lung	Mold spores	Complement, neutrophils	IgG	TH1 (minor role)
	Pathogen	Poststreptococcal glomerulonephritis	*Streptococcus*			
	Autoantigen	SLE	DNA			
Type IV delayed	Autoantigen	Rheumatoid arthritis	Citrullinated peptides	Neutrophils	Anti-CCP, rheumatoid factor	TH1 and TH17 cells
		Multiple sclerosis	Myelin	Macrophages	Antibody production in the CNS	TH1 and TH17 cells
		Type I diabetes	Pancreatic islet cells	Macrophages	Antibodies against pancreatic islet	TH1 cells
	Autoantigen plus food	Celiac disease	tTG plus gliadin	Macrophages	Antibodies against tTG	TH1 cells
	Harmless environmental substance	Contact dermatitis	Weeds	Dendritic cells	NA	TH1

ABO, the ABO blood groups; CCP, cyclic citrullinated peptide; CNS, central nervous system; Ig, immunoglobulin; NA, not applicable; SLE, systemic lupus erythematosus; TH, T helper; TSH, thyroid-stimulating hormone; tTG, tissue transglutaminase.

 MCH II

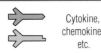 Cytokine, chemokine, etc.

 Complement (C')

 Signaling molecule

BOX 31.1 Rheumatoid Arthritis

A 50-year-old man complains of a 6-month history of pain in his hands, wrists, and feet. The pain is worse in the morning, when his joints are stiff for an hour or so. The metacarpophalangeal and proximal interphalangeal joints in both of his hands are swollen and tender (Fig. 31.4). He also has reduced movement in his wrists and elbows. Blood tests show he is having an acute-phase response with an elevated sedimentation rate and elevated levels of C-reactive protein. A radiograph of his hands shows erosions typical of rheumatoid arthritis (Fig. 31.5). His blood also contains anti–cyclic citrullinated peptide (CCP) antibodies and rheumatoid factor (immunoglobulin M [IgM] anti-IgG autoantibodies). Taken together, the clinical features, radiographs, and blood tests are diagnostic of rheumatoid arthritis.

The patient is started on a nonsteroidal antiinflammatory drug and feels somewhat better, and his pain and stiffness have decreased. However, 1 year later examination shows more joint involvement, and a radiograph shows progression of the changes. Once he is started on a monoclonal antibody against tumor necrosis factor (TNF), his symptoms improve considerably. However, he then develops a complication of the anti-TNF (see Box 24.2).

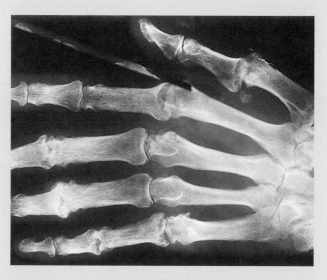

Fig 31.4 Swelling of the metacarpophalangeal and proximal interphalangeal joints is characteristic of rheumatoid arthritis. (Courtesy St. Bartholomew's Hospital, London.)

Fig 31.5 A radiograph showing erosions—areas of "bitten out" bone along the joint margins of the metacarpophalangeal joints—in rheumatoid arthritis. (Courtesy St. Bartholomew's Hospital, London.)

BOX 31.2 Multiple Sclerosis

A 22-year-old woman complains of visual impairment in her left eye. On two occasions, 4 years and 1 year earlier, she had noticed numbness and tingling in both legs for several weeks. She did not see a doctor about these symptoms. On both occasions she became pregnant and the symptoms improved. About 2 months ago, she had some unsteadiness on her feet. These symptoms also improved after 2 weeks or so, and again she did not seek medical advice.

On examination, she has signs of optic neuritis in her left eye. A magnetic resonance imaging (MRI) brain scan is performed, which shows many lesions in the white matter (Fig. 31.6). The diffuse, asymmetric lesions are consistent with the patchy inflammation seen in multiple sclerosis (MS). She also has a lumbar puncture, and examination of her cerebrospinal fluid (CSF) shows oligoclonal bands (Fig. 31.7) consistent with active inflammation in the central nervous system.

The history of different types of neurologic symptoms over time in this patient is typical of MS, and symptoms often improve during pregnancy, possibly because estrogens inhibit the activity of T-helper 1 (TH1) cells. Together, the clinical examination, MRI, and CSF findings are diagnostic of MS. Over the next few weeks, the patient's vision improves on high-dose corticosteroid treatment.

 T-cell receptor (TCR)

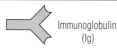 Immunoglobulin (Ig)

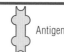 Antigen

 MCH I

BOX 31.2 Multiple Sclerosis—cont'd

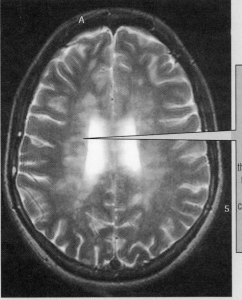

There are patchy lesions in this patient's MRI brain scan that are consistent with demyelinating plaques. Note how these are sited around the lateral ventricles (bright bodies in center of scan). These give the scan an asymmetric appearance.

Fig 31.6 A magnetic resonance imaging (MRI) scan showing plaques of demyelination in the brain. (Courtesy Dr. J. Evanson, Royal London Hospital, London.)

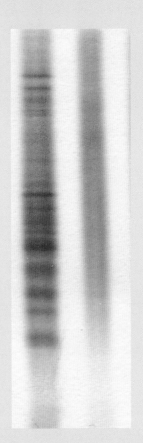

Fig 31.7 High-resolution electrophoresis of cerebrospinal fluid (CSF; strip on left) and serum (strip on right) stained for immunoglobulin G (IgG) antibody. The CSF shows 20 or so bands, each corresponding to IgG antibody produced by a small population of different B cells resident in the central nervous system (CNS). The same oligoclonal B-cell populations are not present outside the CNS, and thus there are no bands in the serum sample. (Courtesy Prof. H. Willison, University of Glasgow.)

LEARNING POINTS   Can You Now ...

1. Recall how delayed hypersensitivity reactions rely on the cytokine network?
2. Describe the pathogenesis, diagnosis, and treatment of multiple sclerosis and rheumatoid arthritis?
3. Describe the benefits and limitations of corticosteroids in delayed hypersensitivity?

4. Describe the clinical implications of cytokine redundancy and pleomorphism in antiinflammatory treatments?
5. Describe how the Gell and Coombs classifications of hypersensitivity are used to diagnose and treat a wide range of disorders?

 MCH II   Cytokine, chemokine, etc.   Complement (C′)   Signaling molecule

CHAPTER 32

Primary Immunodeficiency

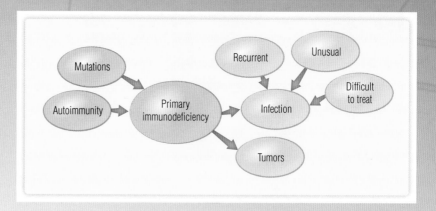

Primary immunodeficiencies are disorders in which part of the immune system is either missing or functioning abnormally. In primary immunodeficiency, the defect arises because of a problem with the immune system itself; it is not secondary to other disease processes, toxins, or drugs. These secondary immunodeficiencies are the topic of Chapter 33.

More than 100 primary immunodeficiencies have been discovered, the majority of which are caused by mutations. Several of these individual disorders have been described in previous chapters, and it may be useful to review these sections at this stage. A smaller number of primary immunodeficiencies are caused by autoimmunity.

Primary immunodeficiency predisposes to infections and tumors. This chapter explains how different types of infections can suggest the presence and severity of different types of immune deficiency. You will also read how primary immunodeficiency is diagnosed and treated.

▮ INFECTIONS PROVIDE CLUES TO THE TYPE OF IMMUNODEFICIENCY

In early life, immunity to common pathogens has not yet developed. It is therefore normal for a young child to have three or four upper respiratory tract infections over the winter. However, it would be unusual for a child to have continuous, recurrent upper respiratory tract infections or to experience bouts of pneumonia. Healthy adults also experience infections from time to time. From the age of about 20 to 60 years, most healthy people

will experience two or three infections each year. The majority of these improve without any medical intervention.

However, repeated, unusual, or difficult-to-treat infections are an important sign of immunodeficiency, which should be considered in anyone who requires multiple courses of antibiotics or is hospitalized for infections. The type of infection gives clues to the cause and degree of immunodeficiency (Fig. 32.1).

Repeated infection with encapsulated bacteria is a sign of defective antibody production because antibody is a key player in the eradication of extracellular bacteria. Antibodies, immunoglobulin G (IgG), and IgA are the main defense against respiratory tract infection, and antibody deficiency leads to recurrent respiratory infection caused by pneumococcus or *Haemophilus* spp., which leads to irreversible damage to the bronchi, or bronchiectasis. However, infections with staphylococci, gram-negative bacteria, and fungi are more characteristic of a reduced number or abnormal function of phagocytes. For unknown reasons, some complement defects predispose to meningitis caused by *Neisseria meningitidis* (see Chapter 20).

T cells and macrophages have a particular role in recognizing and eradicating intracellular infection. Defects in T cells or macrophages predispose to infection with intracellular organisms such as protozoa, viruses, and intracellular bacteria, including mycobacteria (see Fig. 32.1). Reactivation of latent herpesvirus infection is particularly linked to T-cell immunodeficiency. Recurrent attacks of cold sores (herpes simplex) or shingles (herpes varicella zoster) may suggest mild immunodeficiency. Recurrent *Candida* infection is suggestive of defects in the TH17

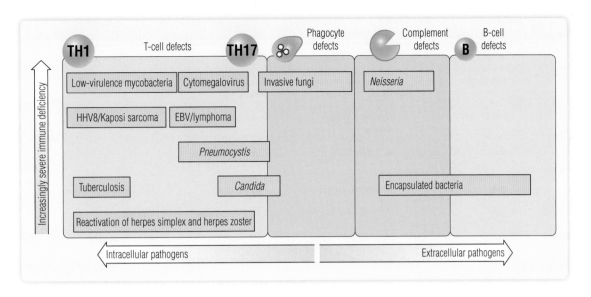

Fig 32.1 The type of opportunist infection present also gives clues to the degree and cause of immunodeficiency. For example, mycobacteria indicate defects in T-cell immunity, whereas extracellular encapsulated bacteria indicate defects in antibody or complement. Note also that the severity of the immune deficiency is also reflected in the type of infection. *Candida* can cause infection in very mild immune deficiency, and even sometimes in healthy people, whereas invasive fungal infections nearly always indicate severe immune deficiency. Herpes simplex and cytomegalovirus are both herpesvirus family members, but only cytomegalovirus infection indicates severe immune deficiency. *EBV*, Epstein-Barr virus; *HHV*, human herpesvirus.

pathway. Herpesvirus-induced tumors, notably Kaposi sarcoma (human herpesvirus 8 [HHV8]), and non-Hodgkin lymphoma (Epstein-Barr virus [EBV]) are characteristic of T-cell dysfunction. These are discussed further in Chapter 35.

The severity of T-cell immunodeficiency is also reflected in patterns of mycobacterial infection (see Fig. 32.1). *Mycobacterium tuberculosis* is a virulent organism that causes lung infection in immunocompetent people. In mild T-cell immunodeficiency, the same organism is able to invade the body outside the lungs. More severe immunodeficiency predisposes to widespread infection with mycobacteria of low virulence normally found in the environment (e.g., *M. avium intracellulare* complex).

■ CAUSES OF PRIMARY IMMUNODEFICIENCY

The causes of primary immunodeficiencies can be classified as:
- *Mutations:* These are rare and can affect any part of the immune system and cause severe disease.
- *Polymorphisms:* These are common traits that affect any part of the immune system and cause a moderate increased risk for infection.
- *Polygenic disorders:* These relatively common disorders affect mainly antibodies. Some of these polygenic conditions may be caused by autoimmunity.

Many of these conditions have been discussed in earlier chapters and are summarized in Table 32.1 and Figure 32.2.

Mutations and Immunodeficiency

More than 100 mutations leading to immune deficiency are known. This book has described a dozen or so important

mutations in genes for the adaptive immune system that cause immunodeficiency. Many mutations result in *severe combined immunodeficiency* (SCID), which refers to a group of disorders that affect both T and B cells. The different types of SCID represent the most severe type of primary immunodeficiency and can be caused by cytokine γ-chain receptor defects and *RAG* mutations. SCID is severe because both T and B cells are affected. Infants with SCID die in the first few months of life unless treatment is given. Some of these disorders are autosomally inherited (eg, *RAG* deficiency; see Box 7.1), and there may be a family history of consanguinity (marriage of related individuals). Other types of SCID are X-linked SCID (eg, γ-chain deficiency; see Box 12.2) and the hyper-IgM syndrome (see Box 16.2), and there may be a history of early deaths in maternal uncles. The DiGeorge syndrome (see Box 15.1) is caused by a large part of chromosome 22 being translocated to other chromosomes, which is not inherited.

Polymorphisms and Immunodeficiency

Genetic polymorphisms are alleles (different forms) of the same gene occurring at a single locus in at least 1% of the population. Eye color is a good example of genetic polymorphism. Human leukocyte antigen (HLA) alleles are polymorphic and affect the outcome of infections, including hepatitis B and HIV (see Box 3.1). Individuals with HLA alleles that are unable to bind viral peptides have a worse outcome. Polymorphisms of chemokines and their receptors associated with risk of HIV are discussed in Chapter 33.

Mannan-binding lectin (MBL) is a collagen-like protein that binds sugars in bacterial cell walls and activates the classic complement pathway (Chapter 20). Polymorphisms in MBL and

 MCH II

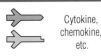 Cytokine, chemokine, etc.

 Complement (C′)

 Signaling molecule

TABLE 32.1   Causes of Primary Immunodeficiency

Genetics	Cell or Pathway	Name of Disorder	Defect	Main Type of Infection	Chapter
Monogenic	T and B cells	Autosomal recessive SCID	Recombinase (*RAG*) mutations	All pathogens	7
Monogenic	T and B cells	Wiskott-Aldrich syndrome	Actin cytoskeleton		32
Monogenic	T and NK cells reduced, B cells not functional	X-linked SCID	Cytokine receptor common γ chain		12
Monogenic	T cells	DiGeorge syndrome	Absent thymus	Intracellular pathogens	15
Autoantibodies	T cells	Anti–IL-17	TH17 responses	*Candida*	32
Autoantibodies	T cells	Anti–IFN-γ	TH1 responses	Mycobacteria	32
Monogenic	B cells	Hyper-IgM syndrome	Mutations in CD154	Pneumococcus and *Haemophilus*	16
Monogenic	B cells	X-linked antibody deficiency	Mutations in *BTK*		11
Polygenic	B cells	Common variable immunodeficiency	Not known		32
Polygenic	B cells	IgA deficiency	Not known		32
Polygenic	B cells	Specific antibody deficiency	Not known		32
Monogenic	Antigen presentation	TAP defects	Impaired antigen processing	All pathogens	10
Polymorphisms	Antigen presentation	HLA	Antigen presentation	Viruses	3
Monogenic	Complement	Complement deficiency	Membrane attack complex	Bacteria, especially *Neisseria*	20
Polymorphisms	Complement cascade	Mannan-binding lectin	Complement cascade	Many pathogens	32
Monogenic	Phagocytes	Chronic granulomatous disease	Oxidative burst	Staphylococci and invasive fungi	21

Note how different primary immunodeficiency disorders lead to different types of infections. SCID, which predisposes to all types of infections, is the most dangerous type of primary immunodeficiency.

HLA, human leukocyte antigen; IFN, interferon; Ig, immunoglobulin; IL, interleukin; NK, natural killer; SCID, severe combined immune deficiency; TAP, transporter associated with antigen presentation; TH, T helper.

complement affect the risk for infections (Fig. 32.3). The effects of polymorphisms on individuals are small and may only be discovered in studies on populations.

Polymorphisms persist in different frequencies in different populations affected by prevalent infections. The best known example lies outside the immune system. The hemoglobin S polymorphism (sickle cell anemia) protects against malaria and is more common in populations living in, or with origin in, malarious zones.

Polygenic Disorders

Polygenic disorders are caused by the interaction of several genes, with a contribution from environmental factors. *Common variable immunodeficiency* (CVID), IgA deficiency, and specific antibody deficiency are relatively common polygenic disorders that affect mainly antibody production. *IgA deficiency* affects about 1 in 600 people, although why infections are seen only in about one-third of patients is unclear. Celiac disease (Chapter 28) is more common in patients with IgA deficiency.

CVID (see Box 32.1) occurs in about 1 in 20,000 young people and affects men and women equally. CVID is the most common primary immunodeficiency requiring treatment. Patients have low levels of total IgG, although other findings—such as levels of IgA and IgM and numbers of B and T cells—are variable. CVID is a convenient label for what will probably emerge as a heterogeneous group of diseases. CVID causes recurrent bouts of infection of the respiratory tract, starting in early adult life. Infections that involve the gut, skin, and nervous system also occur. Autoimmunity is common in CVID and

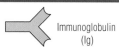
T-cell receptor (TCR)

Immunoglobulin (Ig)

Antigen

MCH I

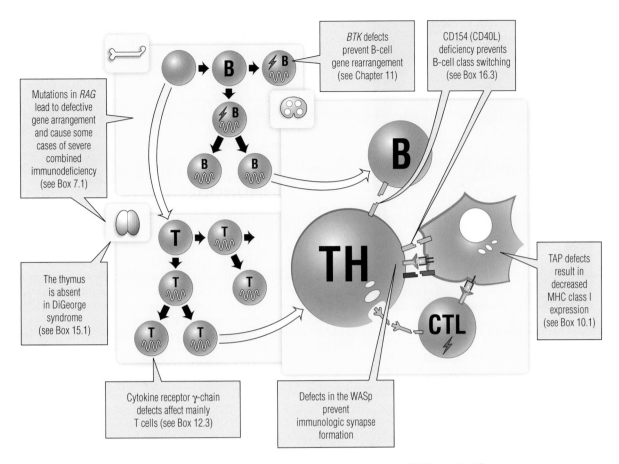

Fig 32.2 Disorders with mainly T-cell defects—such as DiGeorge syndrome, ZAP-70, and Jak defects—present soon after birth with infections with intracellular pathogens. B-cell disorders, such as X-linked agammaglobulinemia, present at around 6 months of age, when maternal antibody levels have fallen. *BTK,* Bruton's tyrosine kinase; *CTL,* cytotoxic T lymphocytes; *MHC,* major histocompatibility complex; *TAP,* transporter associated with antigen presentation; *WASp,* Wiskott-Aldrich syndrome protein.

frequently includes pernicious anemia and thyroid disease, arthritis, and immune thrombocytopenia.

A genetic component exists to CVID, and many patients have either a history of other affected family members or of consanguinity, which suggests autosomal-recessive inheritance. However, the late onset of CVID suggests that unidentified environmental factors play a key role.

Patients with *specific antibody deficiency* have a tendency to develop recurrent infections with pneumococcus or *Haemophilus* spp. despite normal total IgG, and they do not respond to polysaccharide antigens and have poor titers of antibodies to pneumococcal antigens even after vaccination. Specific antibody deficiency is often seen transiently during infancy and permanently after splenectomy (see Box 13.1), but it does exist as a disease entity in its own right.

Some other primary immunodeficiencies are caused by autoimmunity. For example, patients with autoimmune polyendocrinopathy candidiasis ectodermal dysplasia (APECED; Box 15.2) frequently experience severe recurrent *Candida* infection, as the name of the condition suggests. Patients with APECED have a defect in central tolerance and experience many types of autoimmunity. Some patients with APECED produce autoantibodies against interleukin 17 (IL-17), which results in impaired responses to *Candida*.

Other individuals who have no genetic defects produce antibodies against interferon (IFN)-γ. These individuals experience recurrent problems with mycobacterial infection, as would be expected from the important role of IFN-γ in controlling this group of organisms (Chapter 23). For unknown reasons, this condition appears to mainly affect individuals of Southeast Asian origin.

■ SCREENING FOR SEVERE COMBINED IMMUNE DEFICIENCY

Infants born with SCID will die if not treated by stem cell transplantation. Although stem cell transplant can cure SCID, it has to be done quickly. If it is performed very soon after birth, 90% infants survive; if it is delayed for a few months, only 50% infants survive the transplant procedure. For these reasons, many countries screen for SCID in newborns so that SCID cases can be diagnosed and treated early.

SCID screening can be done on the dried blood spots (Guthrie spots) used for other screening tests. The screening test looks for the presence of T-cell excision circles (TRECs) created when the T-cell receptor (TCR) gene segments undergo gene rearrangement in the thymus. The unused TCR gene segments from each recombination step are removed from the genome

 MCH II    Cytokine, chemokine, etc.   Complement (C′)   Signaling molecule

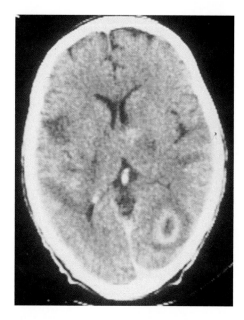

Fig 32.3 This patient has inherited polymorphisms in the genes that encode complement C2 and C4 and mannan-binding lectin. These reduce the activity of the complement cascade and predispose the patient to unusual infections. The ring-enhancing lesion seen in the cerebral cortex in this computed tomographic brain scan is typical of a brain abscess. (Courtesy St. Bartholomew's Hospital, London.)

and are placed in an excision circle (Fig. 32.4). The DNA in the excision circle survives in one daughter cell and is not reproduced during mitosis. The TRECs are diluted out during subsequent mitoses. For this reason, good numbers of TRECs in blood are a marker of the production of T cells in the thymus. Low numbers or absent TRECS suggest T cells are *not* being produced for whatever reason. Screening with TRECs can detect cases of SCID and other disorders in which T-cell numbers are reduced.

■ DIAGNOSIS OF PRIMARY IMMUNODEFICIENCY

Because children with SCID have defective T cells and B cells, they develop infections in the first few weeks of life. Children with SCID often have unusual or recurrent infection, failure to thrive, diarrhea, unusual rashes, a family history of neonatal death or consanguinity, and a very low total lymphocyte count (less than 1×10^9/L [10^6/mL]). In such infants with suspected T-cell immunodeficiency, lymphocyte numbers should be measured by flow cytometry (Chapter 5).

Antibody deficiency presents later in life because babies are born with maternal immunoglobulin transferred across the placenta. This protects the infant for the first few months of life. Some forms of antibody deficiency, such as CVID, do

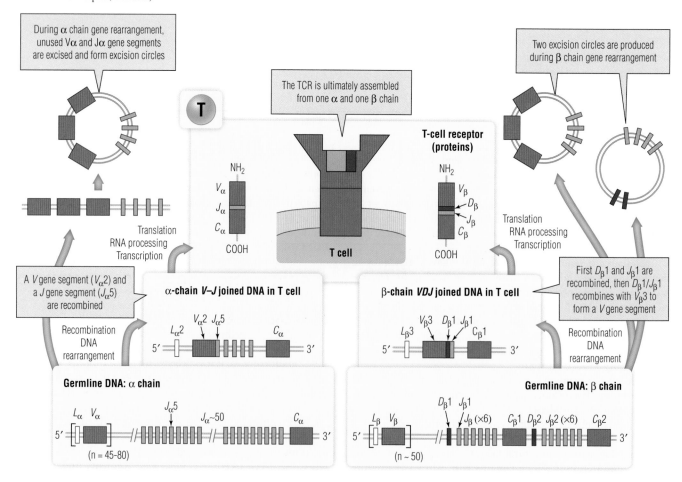

Fig 32.4 T-cell receptor (TCR) excision circles are produced once only during T-cell development.

 T-cell receptor (TCR)

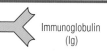 Immunoglobulin (Ig)

 Antigen

 MCH I

not present until adulthood. The most common indication for testing for antibody deficiency is chronic or recurrent bacterial respiratory infection. IgG, IgA, and IgM should be measured. In patients with low levels of immunoglobulins, causes of secondary immunodeficiency—such as protein loss from the gut or kidneys—should be excluded. If total Igs are normal, specific antibodies against *Haemophilus* spp. and pneumococcus should be measured. If these tests are all normal, it is important to check to ensure no problems are apparent with complement or neutrophil function, such as chronic granulomatous disease (CGD; Chapter 21), before concluding that no immunodeficiency is present.

■ TREATMENT

The aim of treatment is to prevent infection. In cases of mild immunodeficiency, such as specific antibody deficiency, prophylactic antibiotics may be adequate.

In more severe antibody deficiency, immunoglobulin replacement therapy is required. Administration of immunoglobulin is a type of passive immunotherapy (Chapter 4; see Box 4.2). Antibodies against a wide range of pathogens are needed; therefore Ig pooled from several thousand normal donors is used. Ig replacement can be given intravenously or subcutaneously. Replacement therapy is different from high-dose Ig replacement therapy, which is immunosuppressive.

Plasma donors are screened for HIV and for hepatitis B and C antibodies. Manufacturing processes to purify IgG destroys many pathogens, but further steps, such as pasteurization (heating to 56°C) or adding detergents, are usually taken to reduce the risk for hepatitis C carriage. If SCID is suspected and HIV infection has been excluded, the infant should be referred to a specialty center where the diagnosis will be confirmed and definitive treatment given (often stem cell transplantation [SCT]). Until this can be done, simple steps are taken to avoid serious infection. These include avoiding live vaccines (eg, measles, mumps, rubella, polio) and using prophylaxis against opportunist infections such as *Pneumocystis jiroveci* pneumonia.

In SCID and most T-cell deficiencies, SCT may be required. SCT is discussed more fully in Chapter 34. SCT is most successful if it can be done within a few weeks of birth, before the infant has developed any infections. If this is possible, SCT carries a 90% success rate and is curative. When SCT is not an option, usually because no suitable donors are available, gene therapy may be attempted in patients with T-cell defects.

Gene Therapy

Gene therapy uses recombinant technology to correct the genetic defect in the patient's own stem cells, which can then reconstitute the immune system. It has been used in some patients with SCID for whom no suitable stem cell donor was available. Gene therapy has so far not been successful in other inherited diseases.

For gene therapy to be successful, several criteria must be met:

1. *The genetic mutation for each patient must be identified, and there must be evidence that correcting the mutation will improve his or her condition.* A child who already had been diagnosed with X-linked SCID (Chapter 12) underwent a second spontaneous mutation in which the defect in the common γ-chain reverted in a single lymphoid precursor cell. This reversion enabled the cell to proliferate and partially restore the lymphocyte population in this child. This proved that correcting a mutation in SCID can be helpful. For gene therapy to work, the gene must be delivered to the cell safely. It is possible to recover stem cells from the blood of an SCID patient, and these are transfected with the normal gene. Viral constructs are often used to deliver the normal gene (Fig. 32.5). With this method, about 500 stem cells are transfected.

2. *The transfected gene must confer a proliferation or survival advantage.* In X-linked SCID, the mutation is in the common γ-chain, which forms part of the receptor for T-cell growth factors (IL-2, IL-7). Cells in which the receptor is functioning are able to proliferate and survive. From the original 500 cells delivered, 12 cycles of division generates 1 million daughter T-cell precursors, each with different T-cell receptors. These cells are enough to reconstitute all the different T-cell populations.

3. Gene therapy must not cause malignancy. If a gene with an active promoter is inserted next to an oncogene, the latter may become constitutively active and cause cancer. This is known as *insertional mutagenesis,* and it remains a major cause for concern. Five of the original 20 patients who received gene therapy for X-linked SCID developed a lymphoid malignancy because the enhancer for the common γ-chain inserted itself next to the oncogene *LMO2.* The *LMO2* gene was then transcribed under the influence of this enhancer. In subsequent experiments, a "suicide gene" has been included into the gene construct. The suicide gene can be switched on if a malignancy develops.

Gene therapy has been tried in other primary immunodeficiencies, such as CGD (Chapter 21). This is a disease in which normal numbers of neutrophils are produced, but the neutrophils are unable to undergo the oxidative burst normally used to kill pathogens. Although it was possible to show that the mutation was corrected in some stem cells and that some normal neutrophils were produced, the project was not a long-term success. After the initial few weeks, very few normal neutrophils were produced. This is probably because the neutrophil precursors with a corrected mutation did not have a proliferation or survival advantage over uncorrected neutrophils. The neutrophils with the corrected gene could not take over the marrow.

Cystic fibrosis is the most common genetic disease. The mutation is in the *CFTR* gene, which is normally expressed in epithelial cells in the airways, gut, liver, and pancreas. Although the abnormal gene has been identified for many years and retroviral constructs with the corrected gene have been produced, it has proven very difficult to transfect these target cells. Part of the problem is that unlike hematopoietic stem cells, it is not easy to access the cells from, for example, the respiratory tract for gene transfection. In addition, if the normal gene were to be successfully transfected and expressed, there would remain a significant theoretic problem: Would the immune system recognize the *CFTR* gene product as a "foreign" protein and mount an immune response? For these reasons, gene therapy is most likely to be unsuccessful, for the near future at least, in SCID.

 MCH II

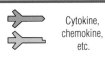 Cytokine, chemokine, etc.

 Complement (C′)

 Signaling molecule

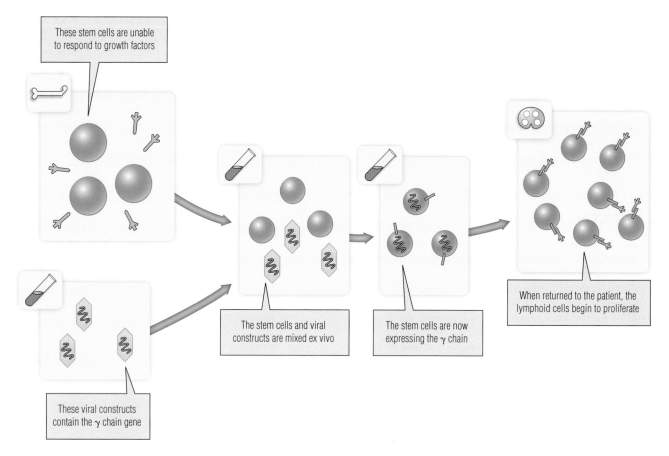

Fig 32.5 There are two reasons gene therapy was successful in X-linked severe combined immune deficiency (SCID): first, it was relatively simple to access stem cells; second, cells transfected with a common γ chain were able to proliferate.

BOX 32.1 A Delayed Diagnosis

A 25-year-old woman has been referred with daily sputum production and worsening shortness of breath. She had recurrent chest infections as a college student, and she was unable to complete her studies. Over the past 3 years, her chest symptoms have become continuous. She has chronic sinusitis and has had three (unsuccessful) sinus drainage operations. She is a nonsmoker with an unremarkable family history.

On examination, she has clinical signs of bronchiectasis, which is confirmed on computed tomography of her lungs (Fig. 32.6). Bronchiectasis is irreversible damage to the airways caused by repeated bouts of infection. *Haemophilus* bacteria are present in her sputum. Her immunologic investigations are shown in Table 32.2.

Causes of secondary immunodeficiency were excluded. She is given a test vaccination with a vaccine containing pneumococcal polysaccharide. Further testing shows that she does not respond to the vaccine, and she now meets diagnostic criteria for common variable immunodeficiency (CVID). Her symptoms improved on intravenous immunoglobulin, and she has subsequently graduated.

CVID often develops in the late teens and early twenties. Once immunoglobulin is started, the frequency and severity of respiratory infections diminish. However, when the diagnosis is delayed, as in this case, irreversible complications may have already developed. Checking immunoglobulin levels in patients with recurrent or unusual infections can prevent the development of this scenario.

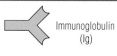 T-cell receptor (TCR)   Immunoglobulin (Ig)   Antigen   MCH I

BOX 32.1 A Delayed Diagnosis—cont'd

TABLE 32.2 Immunologic Investigations in a Patient With Common Variable Immunodeficiency

Component	Patient Values	Normal Range
Immunoglobulin G (g/L)	0.2	7.0–18.0
Immunoglobulin A (g/L)	0.1	0.8–4.0
Immunoglobulin M (g/L)	0.2	0.4–2.5
CD3⁺ T cells (cells × 10⁶/L)	420	820–2100
CD19⁺ B cells (cells × 10⁶/L)	230	760–4200

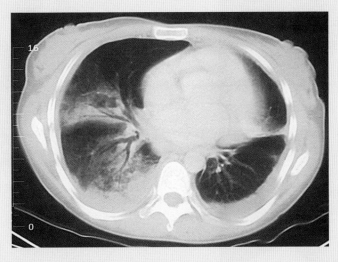

Fig 32.6 This lung scan shows bronchiectasis and patchy pneumonia in a woman with common variable immunodeficiency. In the right lung, the bronchi are visible because of the consolidation in the surrounding lungs. The bronchi are somewhat dilated, and their lumens are not smooth. (Courtesy St. Bartholomew's Hospital, London.)

BOX 32.2 Wiskott-Aldrich Syndrome

The patient in Figures 32.7 and 32.8 presented as a young child with bruising and bleeding, which were found to be due to a reduction in the number of circulating platelets. He also had severe eczema and unusual viral infections. In Figure 32.7, multiple warty lesions can be seen on his face; these are molluscum contagiosum, caused by a member of the poxvirus family. In children with normal immune systems, molluscum contagiosum causes a transient infection, usually with only one or two lesions, which are cleared within a few weeks by cytotoxic T lymphocytes. The unusually extensive and persistent infection seen in this patient is typical of an opportunist infection.

The patient also had a type of malignancy known as B-cell lymphoma. As discussed in Chapter 35, lymphoma in patients with immune deficiencies is often caused by the Epstein-Barr virus (EBV).

The patient's clinical characteristics—low platelet count, eczema, infection, and malignancy—led his pediatrician to suspect Wiskott-Aldrich syndrome, a primary immunodeficiency. A DNA sample was obtained from the patient, and the Wiskott-Aldrich syndrome protein (WASp) gene was sequenced. The patient's Wiskott-Aldrich syndrome gene (*WAS*) was found to contain a mutation, confirming the diagnosis.

Wiskott-Aldrich syndrome is an X-linked disorder, but this particular family had no history of affected male relatives; this patient's mutation was thought to have occurred de novo.

The patient's lymphoma was brought under control, and he underwent stem cell transplantation (Chapter 34). Two years later, he leads a normal life (see Fig. 32.8).

Continued

 MCH II   Cytokine, chemokine, etc.   Complement (C')   Signaling molecule

BOX 32.2 Wiskott-Aldrich Syndrome—cont'd

WASp regulates the actin cytoskeleton. In ways that are not well understood, defects in WASp prevent the normal development of platelets. How WASp defects affect the immune system is much more clearly understood. After normal T-cell activation, ZAP-70 (Chapter 11) activates WASp molecules, which leads to changes in the cytoskeleton that appear to culminate in the formation of an immunologic synapse (Chapter 16) and, in cytotoxic T lymphocytes, delivery of perforin and granzyme into target cells (Fig. 32.9). With defects in these T-cell functions, it should come as no surprise that intracellular viral pathogens cannot be cleared in patients with Wiskott-Aldrich syndrome. In addition, these patients have defects in B-cell and dendritic cell function, which result in impaired antibody production.

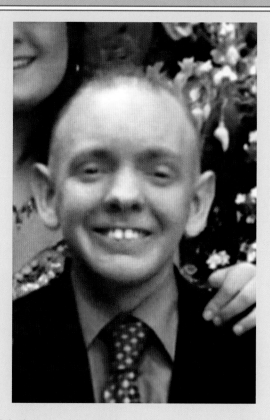

Fig 32.8 The patient from Figure 32.7 is shown 2 years after stem cell transplantation.

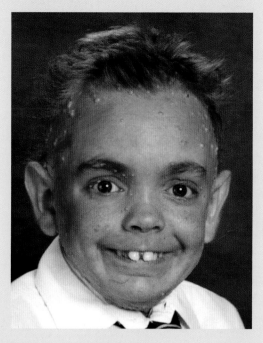

Fig 32.7 A patient with Wiskott-Aldrich syndrome. The lesions on his face are molluscum contagiosum.

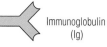 T-cell receptor (TCR)   Immunoglobulin (Ig)   Antigen   MCH I

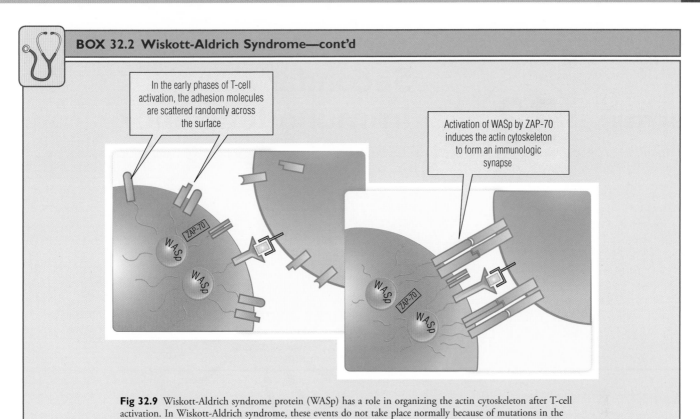

BOX 32.2 Wiskott-Aldrich Syndrome—cont'd

In the early phases of T-cell activation, the adhesion molecules are scattered randomly across the surface

Activation of WASp by ZAP-70 induces the actin cytoskeleton to form an immunologic synapse

Fig 32.9 Wiskott-Aldrich syndrome protein (WASp) has a role in organizing the actin cytoskeleton after T-cell activation. In Wiskott-Aldrich syndrome, these events do not take place normally because of mutations in the *WAS* gene.

LEARNING POINTS Can You Now...

1. List the clinical features that would make you suspect primary immunodeficiency?
2. Construct lists of the types of infections that affect patients with T- and B-cell disorders?
3. List the primary immunodeficiencies caused by mutations, polymorphisms, and polygenic factors?
4. Write bullet points on gene therapy?

 MCH II

 Cytokine, chemokine, etc.

 Complement (C′)

 Signaling molecule

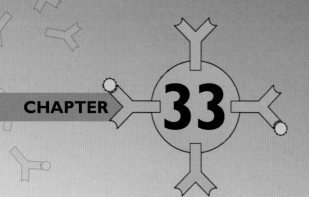

CHAPTER 33

Secondary Immunodeficiency

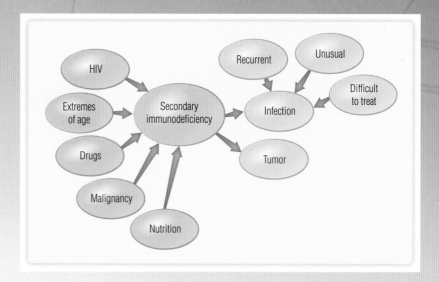

This chapter describes several secondary immunodeficiencies. Of these, HIV is the most important because it is common and causes severe immunodeficiency. Secondary immunodeficiency causes the same infections and tumors as primary immunodeficiency. The exact type of infection depends on what part of the immune system the secondary immunodeficiency affects.

■ HIV INFECTION

More than 40 million people are currently infected with HIV. Each year, 2 million more people are infected, 10% of whom are children. Each year, 1.2 million people die of HIV infection. Clinicians need to understand the natural history of HIV disease and how HIV interacts with the immune system, which lays the foundation of understanding how anti-HIV drugs work, how to monitor HIV infection, and why vaccines have been difficult to develop.

Entry of HIV Into Host Cells

HIV is a simple virus (Fig 33.1A). Its genome contains only three genes, although through RNA splicing and peptide processing it encodes about nine different proteins. HIV is a retrovirus, and its RNA genome is reverse transcribed into a DNA template in host cells. The genome, along with some enzymes, is surrounded by an envelope that consists of two glycoproteins, gp120 and gp41, used to bind and enter host cells (see Fig. 33.1B–E):

1. Initially, gp120 binds CD4 molecules. HIV binds the long, flexible CD4 molecule easily, but this interaction does not bring the virus close to the host cell surface. The presence of CD4 on cells is a prerequisite for HIV, which therefore only infects CD4$^+$ T cells, monocytes and monocyte-derived macrophages, and dendritic cells (see Fig. 33.1B).
2. gp120 then binds to one of several chemokine receptors (see Fig. 33.1C), usually CCR5.
3. Chemokine receptors have short extracellular domains (Chapter 24), and binding draws gp120 closer to the host cell. Binding to a chemokine receptor also induces a change in the gp41 molecule, which normally has a structure similar to a closed zipper. When gp120 binds to a chemokine receptor, gp41 unzips and penetrates the cell membrane (see Fig. 33.1D).
4. The final step is that gp41 zips back up to its original length, effectively fusing the virus envelope and the cell membrane. (see Fig. 33.1E)

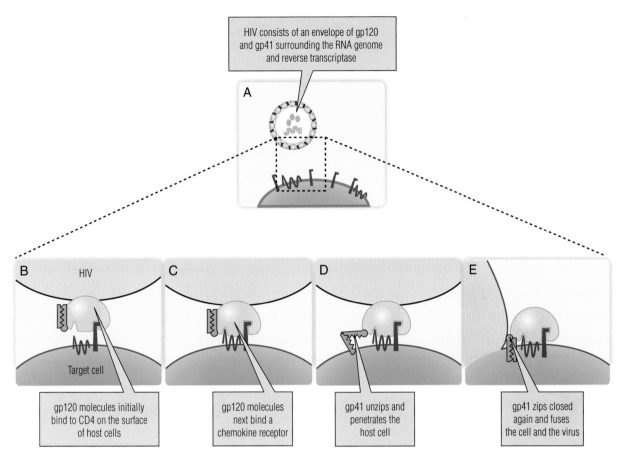

HIV consists of an envelope of gp120 and gp41 surrounding the RNA genome and reverse transcriptase

A

B

HIV

Target cell

gp120 molecules initially bind to CD4 on the surface of host cells

C

gp120 molecules next bind a chemokine receptor

D

gp41 unzips and penetrates the host cell

E

gp41 zips closed again and fuses the cell and the virus

Fig 33.1 HIV uses CD4 and chemokine receptors to infect host cells. B through E are close-up views of HIV interacting with a target cell. *gp,* glycoprotein.

Reverse Transcription of the HIV Genome

The enzyme reverse transcriptase enters host cells along with the RNA genome. Reverse transcriptase uses the RNA genome to make a double-stranded DNA transcript, which inserts itself into the host genome (Fig. 33.2A, B). Reverse transcriptase is an error-prone enzyme, and up to 1 in 10,000 bases mutate during the process. Furthermore, HIV has no mechanism for correcting these mutations. This means that one in three HIV life cycles leads to a virus that contains a new mutation.

Because of this high mutation rate, within a few weeks of infection with a single HIV virus many different strains of virus are detectable in most patients.

HIV Latency and Transcription

Once inserted into the host genome, the three HIV genes behave exactly like host genes. Most of the time the genes are silent and are not transcribed. This is referred to as *viral latency;* in the majority of infected cells, the virus remains latent. These latently infected cells, particularly macrophages, provide a reservoir of infection because in the absence of replication, no HIV peptides are expressed and infected cells are not recognized by the immune system.

However, if the host cell becomes activated, transcription will commence. In infected T cells, HIV genes are regulated in the same way as immune response genes. For example, the transcription factors nuclear factor (NF)-κB and NF-AT (Chapter 11), generated during T-cell activation, also promote transcription of HIV genes. New viral RNA is formed, and HIV precursor proteins are synthesized. A protease encoded by HIV cleaves the precursor proteins, forming a new virus (see Fig. 33.2C, D).

High levels of viral replication destroy host cells, referred to as *viral cytopathic effects,* but this is only one of the ways that HIV damages CD4⁺ T cells.

Immune Responses to HIV

Innate Immune Response

Plasmacytoid dendritic cells of the innate immune system secrete type I interferons in response to HIV (Fig. 33.3A). Although these cells are capable of inhibiting HIV replication in vitro, their function is often impaired in infected patients.

Antibody Response

Infected individuals produce high levels of antibodies against HIV. These form the basis of the HIV test, usually an enzyme-linked immunosorbent assay (ELISA). However, these antibodies usually recognize epitopes of gp120 or gp41 that are not involved in CD4 or chemokine receptor binding and do not prevent infection. The parts of gp120 that bind CD4 and chemokine receptors are hidden deep in the molecule and are

 MCH II

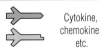 Cytokine, chemokine, etc.

 Complement (C′)

 Signaling molecule

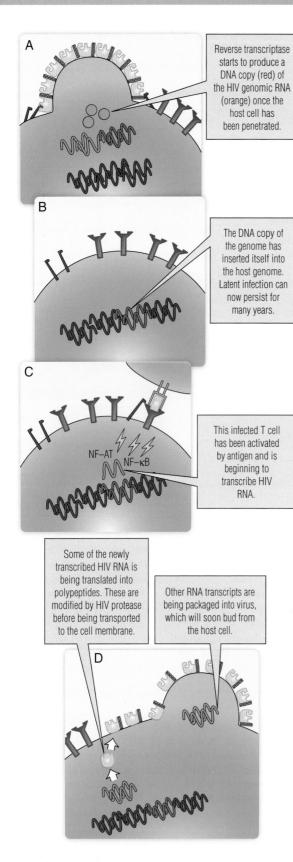

A — Reverse transcriptase starts to produce a DNA copy (red) of the HIV genomic RNA (orange) once the host cell has been penetrated.

B — The DNA copy of the genome has inserted itself into the host genome. Latent infection can now persist for many years.

C — NF-AT NF-κB — This infected T cell has been activated by antigen and is beginning to transcribe HIV RNA.

D — Some of the newly transcribed HIV RNA is being translated into polypeptides. These are modified by HIV protease before being transported to the cell membrane.

Other RNA transcripts are being packaged into virus, which will soon bud from the host cell.

Fig 33.2 Reverse transcription is an error-prone process. It enables HIV to mutate its antigenic structure, its affinity for different chemokine receptors, and its susceptibility to antiretroviral drugs.

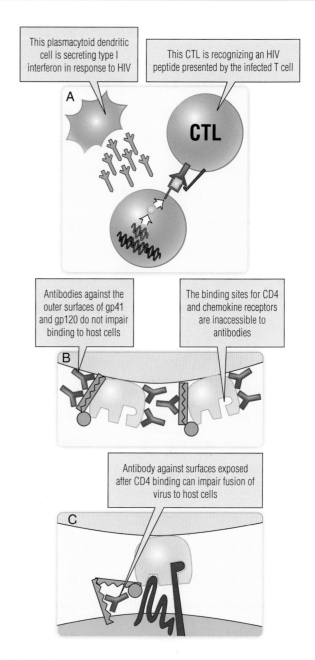

This plasmacytoid dendritic cell is secreting type I interferon in response to HIV

This CTL is recognizing an HIV peptide presented by the infected T cell

CTL

Antibodies against the outer surfaces of gp41 and gp120 do not impair binding to host cells

The binding sites for CD4 and chemokine receptors are inaccessible to antibodies

Antibody against surfaces exposed after CD4 binding can impair fusion of virus to host cells

Fig 33.3 Although there are innate (type I interferon) and adaptive (cytotoxic T lymphocyte [CTL] and antibody) immune system responses to HIV, these rarely keep apace of mutations in HIV. *gp*, glycoprotein.

inaccessible to antibody (see Fig. 33.3B). For these reasons, antibodies are not usually able to prevent infection of T cells.

Cytotoxic T-Lymphocyte Response

Cytotoxic T lymphocytes (CTLs) have the most important role in HIV infection and are able to kill cells that actively express and display HIV peptides (see Fig. 33.3A). Thus CTLs cannot kill cells in which infection remains latent. HIV is also able to overcome the CTL response by mutation in that previously generated CTLs cannot recognize cells that express mutated HIV peptides.

An infected individual typically produces at least 10^5 new viruses each day. One in three will carry a new mutation;

 T-cell receptor (TCR)

 Immunoglobulin (Ig)

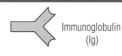 Antigen

 MCH I

therefore CTL and antibody have to contend with at least 3×10^4 new viral strains each day. Both immunoglobulin G (IgG) antibody production and CTLs require help from CD4+ T cells. However, HIV infects and kills or damages CD4+ T cells; therefore the immune system is less able to produce new CTL or antibody responses.

In summary, HIV is able to evade the immune system in three ways: (1) by hiding important epitopes of gp120, (2) by high rates of mutation, and (3) by lying dormant in infected macrophages.

How HIV Kills Infected Cells

Over time, HIV kills infected T cells. This is partly because the virus has a cytopathic effect against T cells. Infected T cells may also be killed because they are targets of CTL. Finally, the widespread activation of the immune system induces apoptosis of CD4+ T cells. Chapter 18 described how persistent activation of T cells can induce apoptosis, such as in activation-induced cell death (AIDC). In HIV infection, immune activation is driven by the HIV infection itself, as well as by some of the consequences of HIV infection, such as infection with opportunist organisms (see below).

Clinical Features of HIV Infection

Some newly infected patients have rashes, malaise, or a fever. This stage is referred to as *HIV seroconversion illness* because it occurs at about the time antibodies to HIV appear.

Over the next few weeks, the mechanisms described above bring viral replication under control. A lower level of viral replication then continues in lymph nodes, and a steady state of virus production and CD4+ T-cell death is matched by an equivalent rate of CD4+ T-cell production. During this phase, patients have no symptoms, although lymphadenopathy may be found. This asymptomatic stage of HIV infection may persist for several years.

During asymptomatic infection, up to 10^9 virions are produced each day, many of which contain mutated antigenic peptides. Viral replication is measured by viral load testing. In most individuals, HIV eventually escapes from antibody and CTL control. As a result of increased T-cell death, the CD4 count (the number of circulating CD4+ T cells) begins to fall.

As the number of CD4+ T cells declines, patients become susceptible to infections. HIV affects both T-helper 1 (TH1) and TH17 cells, so risk of infection with both intracellular organisms (eg, mycobacteria, viruses) and extracellular organisms (eg, *Candida, Pneumocystis jiroveci*) is increased. Initially, HIV infection predisposes to virulent organisms such as *Candida albicans* (see Box 16.4) and *Mycobacterium tuberculosis*. After further falls in the CD4 count, the patient becomes susceptible to opportunist organisms such as *Pneumocystis* (Fig. 33.4). Finally, when little residual immune response remains, organisms such as low-virulence mycobacteria and cytomegalovirus (CMV) cause infections. Tumors such as non-Hodgkin lymphoma and Kaposi sarcoma also occur.

Factors That Affect Outcome

The rate of disease progression varies considerably from person to person and is affected by genetic factors. For example, a polymorphism in the CCR5 chemokine receptor reduces the ability of HIV to bind to and fuse with mucosal macrophages, dendritic cells, and T cells. Individuals who are homozygous for this polymorphism have a decreased risk for becoming infected with HIV after sexual exposure and have a delayed rate of disease progression if they do become infected, such as by blood transfusion. Polymorphisms in CCR5 do not cause any harmful effects on the immune system.

CTL responses to HIV vary among patients. For example, enhanced CTL responses protect some female sex workers against HIV for up to 12 years despite repeated unprotected intercourse. The ability to produce CTLs against HIV may be determined by human leukocyte antigen (HLA) polymorphisms in two important ways: first, the ability of different HLA alleles to bind HIV peptides and present them to CTLs may vary; second, individuals who are homozygous for all HLA alleles effectively have half as many different HLA molecules available for HIV peptide presentation as individuals who are heterozygous at all alleles. People who are heterozygous at all HLA alleles tend to have better outcomes after HIV infection (see Box 3.1).

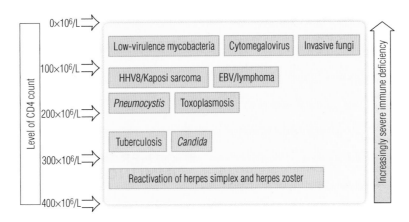

Fig 33.4 Different opportunistic infections occur after HIV has caused different levels of immunodeficiency. For example, infection with low-virulence mycobacteria requires much more severe immunodeficiency than tuberculosis. *EBV*, Epstein-Barr virus; *HHV*, human herpesvirus.

 MCH II

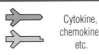 Cytokine, chemokine, etc.

 Complement (C′)

 Signaling molecule

Vaccines

To date, no vaccines have proven consistently successful against HIV infection. Many attempts at developing HIV vaccines focused on eliciting antibodies against gp120, and it was hoped that immunoglobulin G (IgG) against epitopes on gp120 and gp41 molecules that are exposed only during HIV binding and entry (see Fig. 33.3C) might inhibit HIV infection. There were also hopes that IgA antibodies against HIV present in genital secretions would be protective. Even though both IgG and IgA anti-HIV antibodies have been produced in clinical trials of vaccines, so far these have not been found to be protective against HIV infection.

Strong CTL responses are also known to be important in protecting from HIV infection, as discussed earlier. However, to elicit these, vaccines would need to deliver antigen to the cytoplasm so that peptides from this vaccine are eventually expressed on major histocompatibility complex (MHC) class I molecules. This has been achieved in some experiments with live recombinant vaccines constructed from canarypox and containing HIV genes. These vaccines can produce strong CTL responses.

The overwhelming problem for any vaccine is the vast antigenic variation seen in viral samples obtained from different geographic sites because of rapid HIV mutation. A vaccine that induces killing of HIV from one individual will not necessarily induce killing of virus from someone else. For these reasons, even though vaccines have induced CTL responses, they also have so far failed to protect from HIV infection in clinical trials.

Treatments for HIV Infection

Highly active antiretroviral therapy (HAART) has dramatically changed the prognosis in HIV infection. HAART consists of combinations of antiretroviral drugs. Four classes of drug are currently licensed (Fig. 33.5):

- *Reverse-transcriptase inhibitors* are generally nucleoside analogues that are incorporated into the DNA transcript. These drugs then terminate the synthesis of the DNA strand because reverse transcriptase is unable to correct errors (see Fig. 33.5B).
- *Integrase inhibitors* prevent the viral DNA strand from being integrated into the host genome (see Fig 33.5B).
- *Protease inhibitors* inhibit the enzyme responsible for generating HIV structural proteins (see Fig. 33.5C).
- *Fusion inhibitors* bound to gp41 prevent it from contacting and initiating fusion with the host cell (see Fig. 33.5A).

If only one drug is given at a time, HIV rapidly mutates and becomes resistant. For this reason, HIV antiretroviral drugs must be given in combination, usually as three drugs, to reduce the risk for the emergence of resistant strains. After initiation of successful HAART, the viral load should fall, and the CD4$^+$ T-cell count should recover. Immune recovery is associated with reduced numbers of opportunist infections and improved outcomes. HAART has made HIV infection a chronic, manageable illness. However, because latent virus can persist in long-lived cells, current treatments cannot cure HIV infection.

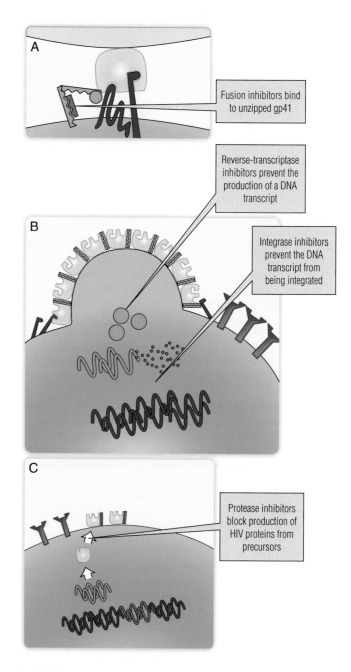

Fig 33.5 The four major classes of antiretroviral therapy are *fusion inhibitors* (two drugs licensed), *reverse-transcriptase inhibitors* (about 20 drugs licensed), *integrase inhibitors* (one drug), and *protease inhibitors* (10 drugs licensed).

Labels in figure:
- Fusion inhibitors bind to unzipped gp41
- Reverse-transcriptase inhibitors prevent the production of a DNA transcript
- Integrase inhibitors prevent the DNA transcript from being integrated
- Protease inhibitors block production of HIV proteins from precursors

■ OTHER SECONDARY IMMUNODEFICIENCIES

A variety of other factors can cause secondary immunodeficiency. These factors often operate together. This can happen very easily during hospital admissions, when patients are exposed to stress, drugs, and possibly inadequate nutrition.

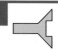 T-cell receptor (TCR)

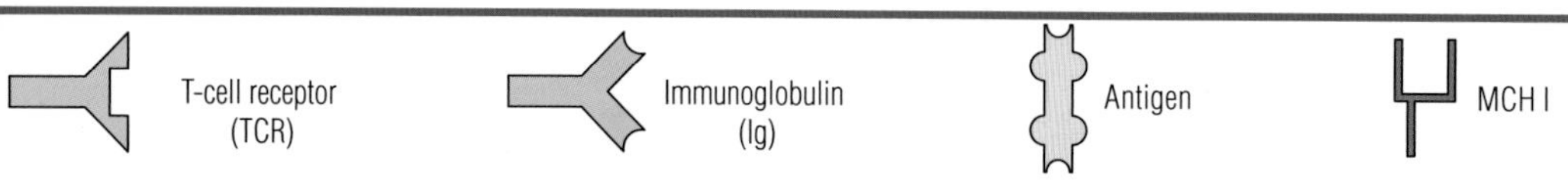

 Immunoglobulin (Ig)

 Antigen

 MCH I

Extremes of Age

Immune System in the First Year of Life

Throughout the first year of life, the specific immune system remains immature. Although neonates have high numbers of T cells, these are all naive and therefore do not respond well to antigen (Chapter 17).

Fetal antibody synthesis begins at 20 weeks, but adult levels of IgG are not reached until about 5 years. For the first few months of life, infants are reliant on maternal IgG. Pregnant women produce increased Igs under the effects of estrogens. IgG is transported across the placenta by specialized Fc receptors in the last 10 weeks of pregnancy. IgA in breast milk is an additional source of protection in early life and protects against lung and gastrointestinal infection. Bottle-fed infants are 60 times more likely to develop pneumonia in the first 3 months of life.

Premature babies face the greatest problems with infection because they have had less time to receive maternal Ig during the late stages of pregnancy. Immaturity of innate mechanisms such as lung surfactant (Chapter 20) can increase the risk of respiratory infection.

Many infants develop low levels of antibody during the first year of life. Transient hypogammaglobulinemia of infancy is caused by a delay in maturation of Ig synthesis at a time when maternal antibody levels are falling.

The Aging Immune System

The elderly suffer more infections than younger patients. The mild immune deficiency that occurs with aging mainly affects T cells, and T-cell memory appears to be lost more rapidly than B-cell memory (see Fig. 25.4). However, it is also more difficult for the immune system to generate more memory T cells, which are what fail in the elderly (Fig. 33.6).

The thymus shrinks by about 3% a year throughout middle age, and there is a corresponding fall in the thymic production of naive T cells. Because fewer T cells emerge from the thymus in later life, proliferation of T cells in the periphery is mainly responsible for maintaining adequate T-cell numbers in adults. However, a biologic clock limits the number of occasions T cells can replicate. Each time a cell divides, there is a stepwise shortening of telomeric DNA. When telomere length is considerably shortened, cells can no longer divide. This replicative senescence affects T cells after about 40 divisions.

A third factor that affects T cells in old age is CMV, a herpesvirus family member that drives increasing numbers of T cells. In the elderly, the T-cell response becomes highly oligoclonal, with disproportionate numbers of T cells having CMV specificity. These cells leave little room in the immune system for other specificities. Consequences of impaired T-cell numbers and function in old age include poor response to vaccines, increased infections, and a possible increased risk for malignancy.

However, B-cell function in the elderly is not decreased. As described in Chapter 25, memory for preexisting antibody responses to effective vaccines may last for up to 50 or 60 years. Aged B cells may show signs of a lifetime of exposure to microorganisms. Immunoglobulin synthesis is increased, and outgrowth of B-cell clones may lead to the presence of monoclonal immunoglobulin in the blood or B-cell malignancy (Chapter

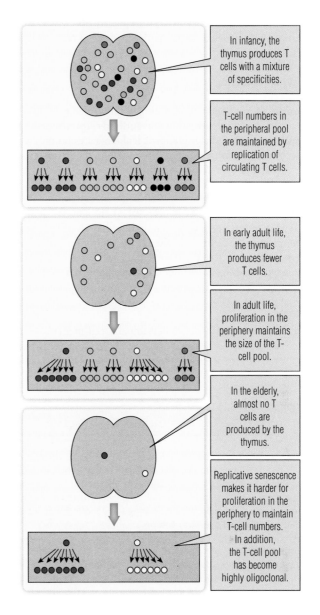

Fig 33.6 Why the number of T cells declines in later life.

35). Autoantibodies are also more common in the elderly but are not usually associated with disease.

Miscellaneous Factors

Drugs

Drugs are a common cause of secondary immunodeficiency, and eliminating the offending drug usually improves the immune response. Patients often develop neutropenia during cytotoxic therapy for malignancy (see Box 21.1).

Damage to T and B cells is an expected side effect of corticosteroids, cytotoxic drugs, and the immunosuppressive regimens used in autoimmune disease and transplant rejection prophylaxis. Patients starting these drugs need to be aware that they are prone to opportunistic infections. Other drugs can

 MCH II

 Cytokine, chemokine, etc.

 Complement (C')

 Signaling molecule

cause antibody deficiency as an unexpected side effect. Among the most notorious are anticonvulsants used to treat epilepsy.

B-Cell Malignancy

Myeloma and chronic lymphocytic leukemia are malignancies of B cells (Chapter 35). Although both may produce large amounts of monoclonal immunoglobulin (paraprotein), they are associated with low levels of antibody against pathogens. Myeloma and chronic lymphocytic leukemia are common causes of secondary immunodeficiency in the elderly. Thymoma is a rare tumor that can cause immunodeficiency.

Kidney and Gut Disease

In nephrotic syndrome (Chapter 30), there may be significant renal protein loss and a reduction in blood levels of IgG and IgA with normal IgM. Igs can also be lost via the gut in severe diarrheal diseases. Renal failure and diabetes also cause secondary phagocyte defects, although the mechanism by which they do this is unknown.

Nutrition

Zinc and magnesium deficiency impairs cell-mediated immunity, particularly TH1-pattern cytokine secretion. This type of deficiency in micronutrients occurs in a wide range of situations, such as in postoperative patients. Although vitamins are required by the immune system, especially vitamins A and E, their role is less significant than mineral nutrients.

Physiologic Stress

Stress has potent effects on the adaptive immune system. Lymphocytes have receptors for both epinephrine (adrenaline) and corticosteroids. These hormones are secreted in response to stress: epinephrine mediates rapid-onset, short-term effects, and corticosteroids mediate longer-term effects. Physiologic stress, such as endurance training, can therefore inhibit immune responses to infection.

Infections

Infections can also cause immunodeficiency. Malaria and congenital rubella may cause antibody deficiency, and measles is well known for causing defects in cell-mediated immunity—sometimes enough to reactivate tuberculosis. Many of these factors operate together in acutely ill patients (see Box 33.2).

BOX 33.1 Monitoring HIV Infection

A 29-year-old woman is seen in a general medical clinic for lumps in her neck. She has no other symptoms, notably no fever or sweats. She had two normal pregnancies in her early twenties and an episode of pelvic inflammatory disease (caused by *Chlamydia* infection) at age 26. She is a single parent, and her children are both healthy.

On examination, she is found to have generalized lymphadenopathy affecting her cervical, axillary, and inguinal nodes. Such generalized lymphadenopathy is not a feature of cancer or localized infection. However, HIV can cause generalized lymphadenopathy, and the patient gives consent for an HIV antibody test, which is positive. Further testing shows a reduced CD4 count (310×10^6/L; normal is above 500×10^6/L), and her viral load is 2×10^5/mL. Despite her lack of symptoms, these results are consistent with moderately advanced HIV infection. She is very concerned about her children, but when her antenatal records are checked, they confirm that her screening HIV test was negative during both pregnancies.

Because the first count could have been lowered by psychological stress, the CD4 count is repeated and is found to be 290×10^6/L. She agrees to begin highly active antiretroviral therapy (HAART) and is prescribed a combination of three different reverse-transcriptase inhibitors. She tolerates these well, and her viral load falls rapidly with a more gradual improvement in her CD4 counts (Fig. 33.7).

Patients with HIV infection require immunologic (CD4 count) and virologic (viral load) monitoring. Different levels of CD4 cell counts are associated with risks for different opportunistic infections. For example, patients with CD4 counts below 200×10^6/L have a high risk for *Pneumocystis jiroveci* pneumonia (PJP) and should receive preventive medication (prophylaxis). Viral-load tests measure HIV viremia and reflect long-term risk for disease progression. Viral load and CD4 counts are used to determine the use of antiretroviral treatment. This patient had a very high viral load and evidence of significant CD4+ T-cell depletion.

CD4 cell counts are taken by flow cytometry (see Fig. 5.7) and are affected by hormones. For example, because corticosteroid secretion has a diurnal pattern, so do CD4 counts—they are the lowest in the morning. Corticosteroid secretion in response to acute and chronic stress will suppress CD4 counts. In addition, CD4 counts are affected by estrogen levels and therefore vary at different stages of the menstrual cycle. These factors need to be taken into account when monitoring CD4 counts.

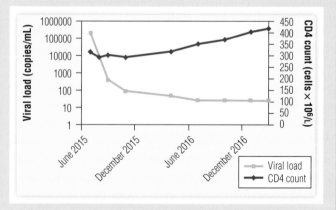

Fig 33.7 The effects of highly active antiretroviral therapy (HAART) on HIV viral load and CD4 count. The viral load falls rapidly after its replicative cycle is blocked. The CD4 count takes much longer to recover.

  T-cell receptor (TCR) 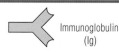 Immunoglobulin (Ig) Antigen MCH I

BOX 33.2 Secondary Immunodeficiency in Acute Illness

A previously healthy 30-year-old man was admitted after a motor vehicle collision. He is unconscious and has signs of cerebral edema. The patient is intubated, and a central venous line and urinary catheter are inserted. He is given high-dose corticosteroids in an attempt to reduce cerebral edema. After a series of convulsions, the anticonvulsant phenytoin is given intravenously (Fig. 33.8).

Two weeks later, the patient is recovering from his neurologic episode when he develops pneumonia (Fig. 33.9). In addition to physiologic stress and poor nutrition, this patient has had his innate barriers penetrated at three different sites and is then exposed to two drugs that impair the immune system. It is no surprise his defenses against infection are lowered.

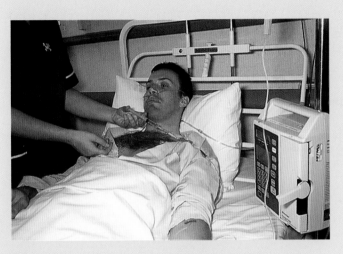

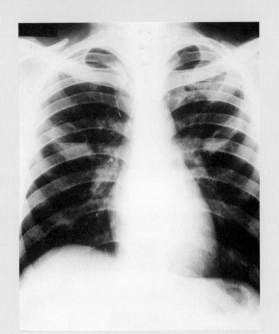

Fig 33.8 When an acutely ill patient is admitted to the hospital, many factors interact to cause immunodeficiency. This is made worse when physical barriers are breached by cannulas and intravenous lines and because of the wide range of pathogens found inside hospitals. (Courtesy St. Bartholomew's Hospital, London.)

Fig 33.9 A chest radiograph showing abscesses typical of staphylococcal pneumonia. This avoidable, life-threatening infection is a consequence of multiple factors in this patient. (Courtesy St. Bartholomew's Hospital, London.)

LEARNING POINTS Can You Now...

1. List the cells affected by HIV infection and briefly describe their functions and roles in HIV infection?
2. Diagram the life cycle of HIV?
3. List how mutations benefit the HIV virus?
4. Describe how you would monitor a patient with HIV infection?
5. List host factors that affect the course of HIV infection?
6. Make a list of the challenges to be overcome in the development of a safe HIV vaccine that is able to offer good protection from infection?
7. Explain which factors interact to predispose hospital patients to infection?

 MCH II   Cytokine, chemokine, etc.   Complement (C')   Signaling molecule

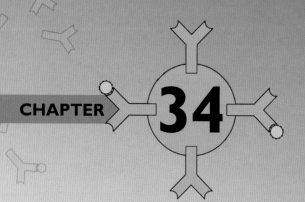
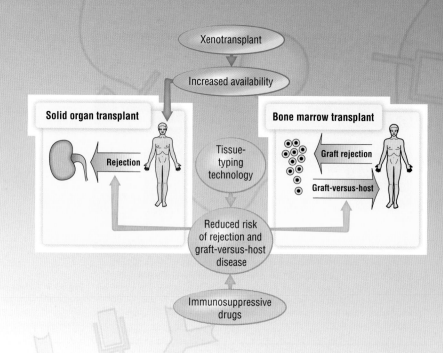

This chapter discusses the biology of transplantation and how graft rejection can complicate both solid organ and stem cell transplantation (SCT). Also discussed are how graft-versus-host disease (GVHD) is an additional complication in SCT, as well as how tissue-typing techniques and immunosuppressive drugs are used to reduce the risk of these complications. Finally, some of the problems that need to be overcome for xenotransplantation to become an effective alternative are reviewed.

TRANSPLANTATION TERMINOLOGY

The following terms were first introduced in Chapter 8:
- *Rejection* refers to damage done by the immune system to a transplanted organ.
- *Autologous transplant* refers to tissue returning to the same individual after a period outside the body, usually in a frozen state.
- *Syngeneic transplant* refers to transplant between identical twins; there is usually no problem with graft rejection.

- *Allogeneic transplant* takes place between genetically nonidentical members of the same species; there is always a risk of rejection.
- *Cadaveric transplantation* uses organs from a dead donor.
- *Xenogeneic transplant* takes place between different species and carries the highest risk of rejection.

SOLID ORGAN TRANSPLANTATION

When Transplantation Is Indicated

Transplantation may be an option when a variety of solid organs stop functioning. Several criteria must be met before transplantation:
- There must be good evidence that the damage is irreversible or that alternative treatments are not applicable.
- The disease must not recur; for example, renal transplant is contraindicated in patients with Goodpasture syndrome who have antiglomerular basement membrane antibodies (Chapter 29).

- The chances of rejection must be minimized:
  - The donor and recipient must be ABO compatible.
  - The recipient must not have antidonor human leukocyte antigen (HLA) antibodies.
  - The donor should be selected with a close as possible HLA match to the recipient.
  - The patient must take immunosuppressive treatment.

The main problem with all solid organ transplants is the risk for rejection, which is illustrated by renal transplant, the most common type of solid organ transplant. As shown in Table 34.1, procedures vary for different organs. For example, because the cornea is not vascularized and is rarely exposed to the recipient immune system, corneal transplant recipients do not have to take immunosuppressive drugs. For reasons that are not well understood, liver transplantation can be done between HLA-mismatched donors and recipients. Heart transplantation is almost always done when severe heart failure has developed rapidly and the patient will die without a transplant. There is not always time to wait for an HLA-matched donor for heart transplantation; the first heart that becomes available is often transplanted, and the recipient is treated with the most potent immunosuppressive drugs.

Mechanisms of Rejection

Hyperacute Rejection

Hyperacute rejection takes place within hours of transplantation and is caused by preformed antibodies binding to either ABO blood group or HLA class I antigens on the graft (Fig. 34.1A). The recipient may have formed anti-HLA class I antibodies after exposure to allogeneic lymphocytes during pregnancy, blood transfusion, or a previous transplant. Antibody binding triggers a type II hypersensitivity reaction, and the graft is destroyed by vascular thrombosis. Hyperacute rejection can be prevented through careful ABO and HLA cross-matching and is now quite rare.

Acute Rejection

Acute rejection is a type IV (cell-mediated) delayed hypersensitivity reaction and therefore takes place within days, and sometimes weeks, of transplantation. Acute rejection takes several days to develop because donor dendritic cells must first stimulate an allogeneic response in a local lymph node for responding T cells to proliferate and migrate into the donor kidney.

Acute rejection takes place if there is HLA incompatibility. Recipient T cells can respond to donor peptides presented by recipient major histocompatibility complex (MHC) or to donor MHC molecules (see Fig. 34.1). Although attempting to minimize any HLA mismatch of the donor and recipient can reduce acute rejection, the shortage of donor kidneys often means that a partially mismatched kidney is used. The survival of the kidney is related to the degree of mismatching, especially at the HLA-DR loci (Fig. 34.2).

Alternatively, the recipient may respond to *minor histocompatibility antigens* presented by donor or recipient cells (see Box 34.1). *Minor antigens* are proteins that have different amino acid sequences in the donor and recipient; they are encoded by genes situated outside the HLA. Minor histocompatibility antigen mismatches are not detected by standard tissue-typing techniques. The term *minor antigens* may be misleading in terms of importance; even when an HLA-matched, living related donor is found, these antigens can cause graft rejection in up to one-third of transplants.

Acute rejection is more likely to develop if the donated kidney has been damaged. For example, if the kidney is not immediately placed on ice, it will be damaged by hypoxia. The damage-associated molecular patterns (DAMPs) induced by hypoxia are detected by pattern recognition molecules,

TABLE 34.1 Transplantation Procedures for Various Organs*

Organ	Characteristics	Type of Donor	Procedures per Million per Year	Graft Survival (%)
Cornea	Immunosuppression is not required because the cornea does not become vascularized.	Cadaveric	20	>90
Liver	Used for alcoholic liver disease, primary biliary cirrhosis, and virus-induced cirrhosis; outcome is not affected by degree of HLA matching.	Live or cadaveric	10	>60
Kidney	Live-related donor kidneys are often used; graft survival is optimized by HLA match, and immunosuppression is required.	Live or cadaveric	50	>80
Pancreas	Pancreas is usually transplanted along with kidneys in diabetic patients with renal failure. Separated islet cells have also been infused into the vena cava.	Cadaveric	3	~50
Heart	Used for coronary artery disease, cardiomyopathy, and some congenital heart disease; HLA matching is not always possible, and potent immunosuppression is required.	Cadaveric	10	>80
Stem cells	Used in malignancy, hematologic conditions, and some primary immunodeficiency; best results are achieved when there is a match of HLA-A, -B, -C, and DR.	Live	100	≤80

*Transplantation of a variety of tissues is now possible. Examples proceed from the most immunologically simple to more complex types of transplantation. Stem cell transplantation is the most complex because graft-versus-host disease can occur in addition to graft rejection.
HLA, human leukocyte antigen.

 MCH II   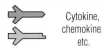 Cytokine, chemokine, etc.   Complement (C')   Signaling molecule

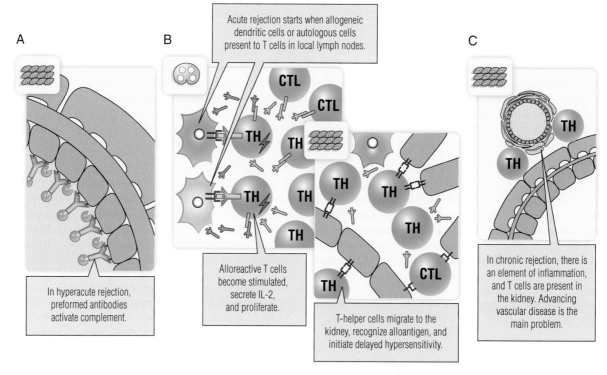

Fig 34.1 Mechanisms of renal transplant rejection. Hyperacute (**A**) and acute (**B**) solid organ graft rejection involves different mechanisms. The mechanism of chronic rejection (**C**) is not clear. *CTL,* cytotoxic T lymphocyte; *IL,* interleukin; *TH,* T-helper cell.

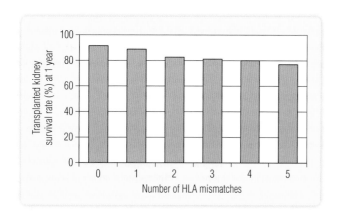

Fig 34.2 Survival rate is worse after transplantation with human leukocyte antigen (HLA) mismatches. Even for mismatched kidneys, immunosuppressive drugs can prevent rejection.

which in turn stimulate the production of danger signals (Chapter 19).

Chronic Rejection

Chronic rejection takes place months or years after transplant. An element of allogeneic reaction is often mediated by T cells in chronic rejection, which can result in repeated acute rejection. In some cases, chronic rejection may be caused by recurrence of preexisting autoimmune disease. In other cases, no direct evidence of damage caused by the adaptive immune system is apparent.

Tolerance

Tolerance can be defined as a state of unresponsiveness to molecules the immune system has the capacity to recognize and attack (Chapter 18). In the context of transplantation, this means that there is no response to alloantigens present on the transplanted tissue, but responses to pathogens are not affected. However, tolerance of transplanted solid organs has not been achieved artificially in humans.

Immunosuppressive drugs prevent rejection if given at the time of transplantation, but once the drugs are stopped, rejection still takes place. Immunosuppressive drugs also lack the specificity of true tolerance and thus prevent immune responses to infectious agents. Opportunist infections are a major limit to the use of potent immunosuppressive drugs.

▉ STEM CELL TRANSPLANTATION

Hematopoietic stem cells are used to restore myeloid and lymphoid cells in some clinical situations. In autologous SCT, marrow is removed, frozen, and reinfused after potent chemotherapy has been given. Autologous transplants carry minimal immunologic risk. Allogeneic SCT is a much riskier procedure than most solid organ transplants. Even with well-matched donors and in the best of circumstances, the mortality rate can be as high as 20% (see Box 34.2). The additional risks are due to GVHD. Because of the high risks, allogeneic SCT is carried out only in certain dire situations when no other treatment is available, such as the following:

• In hematologic malignancy (SCT is used after initial treatment if there is a high chance for relapse; it is preceded by

  T-cell receptor (TCR)   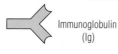 Immunoglobulin (Ig)    Antigen   MCH I

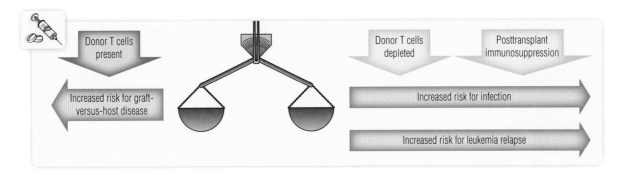

Fig 34.3 T-cell depletion has complex effects on stem cell transplantation. The decision on whether to deplete T cells rests on the degree of donor matching and the condition being treated.

potent chemotherapy and irradiation to eradicate residual tumor cells.)

- When myeloid cell production is reduced or notably abnormal, such as in aplastic anemia
- In primary immunodeficiencies such as severe combined immunodeficiency (SCID)

Source of Stem Cells

After transplantation, myeloid cells are regenerated from hematopoietic stem cells. These can be obtained from a number of sources:

- Bone marrow is the usual source of stem cells. Harvesting requires aspiration of a considerable amount of donor marrow under general anesthetic.
- Peripheral blood stem cells are usually harvested after treating the donor with colony-stimulating factors to increase the numbers of circulating stem cells.
- Cord blood contains a large number of stem cells, which can be frozen before use. An advantage of cord blood is that the immature lymphocytes are less likely to cause GVHD (discussed later). Cord blood yields only enough stem cells to transplant into children or small adults.

Conditioning

Conditioning consists of high-dose chemotherapy or radiotherapy, which destroys the recipient's own stem cells and allows donor stem cells to engraft. Apart from creating a physical space in the bone marrow for the donor marrow cells to engraft, it reduces the risk of the recipient immune system rejecting the allogeneic (donor) stem cells.

Graft-Versus-Host Disease

GVHD occurs when donor T cells respond to allogeneic recipient antigens. It occurs when there are mismatches in major or minor histocompatibility antigens. All patients who receive SCT are given immunosuppressive drugs to prevent GVHD, even if the donor and the recipient are HLA identical. This maneuver in itself has risks for infection. Acute GVHD occurs up to 4 weeks after SCT. Involvement of skin, gut, liver, and lungs is widespread; when severe, acute GVHD carries a 70%

mortality. Chronic GVHD occurs later and affects the skin and liver.

Removing mature T cells from the source of the stem cells using immunologic techniques reduces the risk for GVHD. T-cell depletion, however, increases the risk for graft rejection.

Donor T cells are also capable of reacting against recipient tumor cells, especially when there is a degree of HLA mismatch and mild GVHD is taking place. This beneficial graft-versus-leukemia effect is lost after T-cell depletion of stem cell preparations (Fig. 34.3).

■ TISSUE-TYPING TECHNIQUES

Before most allogeneic transplants, it is desirable to ensure that the donor and recipient have as closely matched as possible HLA alleles. It is also important to ensure that the donor has no antibodies against recipient cells, tested for using the crossmatch procedure. Collectively, these tests carried out before allogeneic transplantation are referred to as *tissue typing* and are used to identify donor-recipient pairs with the lowest risk for complications.

Human Leukocyte Antigen Typing

A patient who is being considered for a transplant is tissue typed to identify HLA alleles. Over several million years, more than 500 different HLA alleles have evolved in humans. Specialized molecular biology techniques are required to precisely define any individual's HLA type (Fig. 34.4A). If he or she has suitable siblings, a family search may be made for a living related donor. However, any one sibling has only a one-in-four chance of being HLA identical. If an identical sibling is found, he or she can act as a donor. Otherwise, patients who require solid organ transplants, such as kidneys, go on a waiting list registry for a cadaveric organ (see Fig. 34.4B). When an organ becomes available, the donor is HLA typed, and a search is made in tissue-typing registries for a suitable recipient (see Fig. 34.4C). Even when organ registries extend across many states or nations, it is possible to wait many months before a well-matched organ becomes available.

Registries are also used for patients who require SCT. In this case, registries consist of volunteers who have agreed to be potential donors and have been HLA typed. Even when these registries

 MCH II   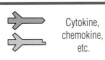 Cytokine, chemokine, etc.   Complement (C′)   Signaling molecule

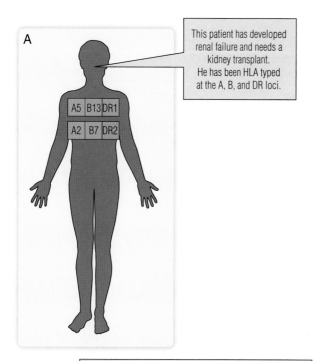

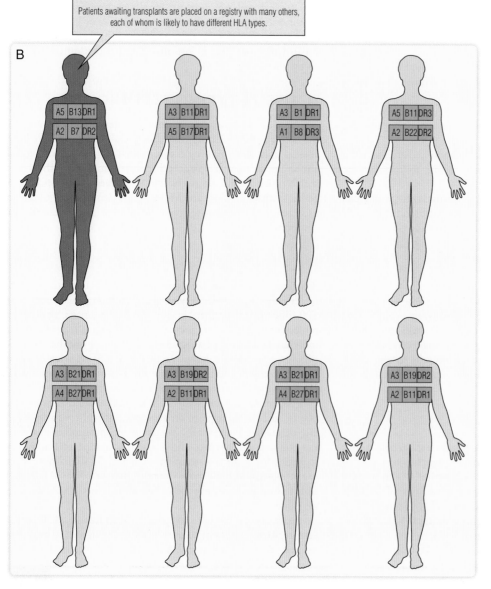

Fig 34.4 Patients who require kidney transplants are human leukocyte antigen (HLA) typed (**A**) and then placed on a registry (**B**). If a brain-dead donor becomes available, such as after a motor vehicle accident, the family is asked to grant consent for organ donation.

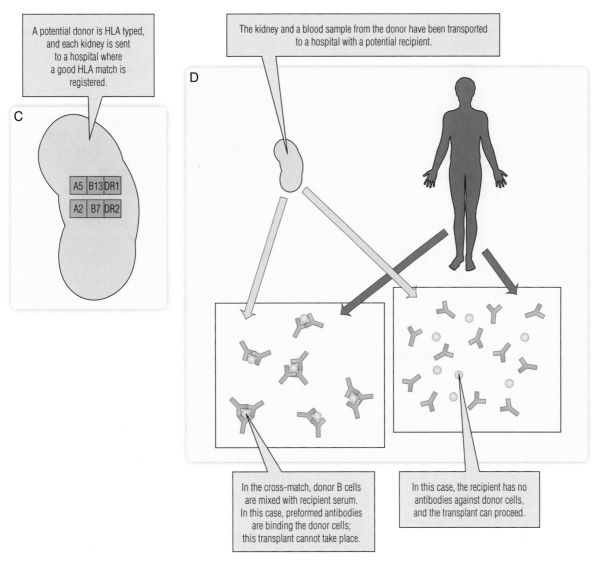

A potential donor is HLA typed, and each kidney is sent to a hospital where a good HLA match is registered.

The kidney and a blood sample from the donor have been transported to a hospital with a potential recipient.

C

| A5 | B13 | DR1 |
| A2 | B7 | DR2 |

D

In the cross-match, donor B cells are mixed with recipient serum. In this case, preformed antibodies are binding the donor cells; this transplant cannot take place.

In this case, the recipient has no antibodies against donor cells, and the transplant can proceed.

Fig 34.4, cont'd The donor is HLA typed (**C**), and the organs are removed. **D,** As a final check, B cells from donor blood (chosen because they express HLA class I and class II) are mixed with recipient serum. This process, the cross match, ensures the donor has not made any antibodies against donor antigens. The kidney is transported on ice, along with a blood sample, to a hospital with a potential recipient with good HLA matches. B cells from the donor blood sample are used in a cross-match to detect antibodies against HLA and potentially other polymorphic alloantigens.

include many millions of donors, it is possible that potential recipients will not find an HLA-identical donor.

Human Leukocyte Antigen Cross-Matching

Cross-matching is performed to rule out preformed antibodies against donor HLA, which could cause hyperacute rejection (see Fig. 34.4D). These antibodies could be produced by exposure to allogeneic HLA during pregnancy, blood transfusion, or a previous attempt at transplantation, as previously mentioned. In the cross-match, donor B cells are incubated with recipient serum. Donor B cells are used in the cross-match because they express HLA class I and II molecules. The presence of antibodies to donor cells rules out the possibility of transplantation.

■ IMMUNOSUPPRESSIVE DRUGS

Immunosuppressive drugs are required to prevent and treat graft rejection and GVHD. The drugs tend to be used in combinations as part of defined regimens. For example, in renal transplantation, combinations such as corticosteroids, cyclosporine, and mycophenolate may be used from the time of transplantation. The exact combination of drugs and timing used varies with the risk for rejection. If the HLA match is known to be incomplete, a combination containing more potent drugs may be used for a longer period. In the event of a rejection episode, stronger drugs may be given. All these drugs carry the risk for infection as a consequence of immunosuppression. In addition, immunosuppressive drugs increase the risk for developing some tumors, as discussed in Chapter 35.

 MCH II

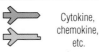 Cytokine, chemokine, etc.

 Complement (C′)

 Signaling molecule

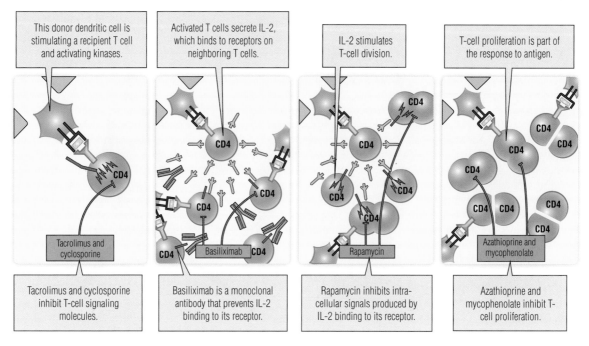

Fig 34.5 Major immunosuppressive drugs (except corticosteroids). *IL,* interleukin. (From Helbert M. *The Flesh and Bones of Immunology.* London: Mosby; 2006.)

Many of these drugs are also used in the treatment of autoimmune disease, and some familiarity with their modes of action is important (Fig. 34.5).

Corticosteroids

Corticosteroids inhibit synthesis of more than 100 proteins, but at low doses they predominantly act on antigen-presenting cells, preventing some of the early stages of graft rejection. Higher doses of corticosteroids have direct effects on T cells and are used to treat episodes of rejection (Chapter 31).

T-Cell Signaling Blockade

Cyclosporine and tacrolimus are discussed in Box 11.3. They work by interacting with proteins in the intracellular T-cell signaling cascade. Cyclosporine was the first to be discovered and improved the outcome of all types of transplant dramatically.

Interleukin-2 Blockade

Monoclonal antibodies against the interleukin 2 (IL-2) receptor can also be given (eg, basiliximab and daclizumab). These antibodies completely block the most important growth factor for all types of lymphocyte and have potent immunosuppressive effects. Because they are so potent, they are only used to *treat* episodes of acute graft rejection. Rapamycin is a drug that can be given orally and interacts with signaling events downstream of the IL-2 receptor. Rapamycin is less potent and easier to take than the monoclonal antibodies, so it is used to *prevent* graft rejection.

Antiproliferatives

Azathioprine, mycophenolate mofetil, and methotrexate inhibit DNA production. These drugs prevent lymphocyte proliferation, but they are not specific for T cells and can cause myelotoxicity.

■ XENOTRANSPLANTATION

Immunosuppressive drugs have dramatically improved outcomes for transplantation. However, waiting lists for solid organ transplants double every 10 years, whereas the number of transplantations carried out remains static. This is because there are too few human organs available to meet the needs of patients. Currently, 10 patients die each day in the United States while on the waiting list to receive life-saving vital organ transplants. Xenotransplants from other species may become an alternative in the future. But before these provide a reliable source of organs, several problems need to be overcome:

• Primates assemble different sugar side chains from other species. Galactose-α1,3-galactose (gal-α1,3-gal) is a sugar present on the cells of most nonprimate species. The immune system can recognize gal-α1,3-gal, and all humans possess antibodies against it following exposure to gut bacteria, for example. Similar natural antibodies were mentioned in Chapter 28. Antibodies against gal-α1,3-gal bind onto xenotransplanted organs, activate complement, and trigger hyperacute rejection.

• Complement inhibitors from other species do *not* inhibit human complement. As a result of this molecular incompatibility, xenotransplanted organs activate complement (Chapter 20).

 T-cell receptor (TCR)   Immunoglobulin (Ig)   Antigen   MCH I

Transgenic pigs are being developed with reduced gal-α1,3-gal expression to prevent natural antibody binding and with human complement inhibitors to bypass molecular incompatibility. Pigs are used because they are a similar size to humans and are easy to rear in captivity. However, two considerable theoretic problems remain:

1. Acute rejection may occur because pig proteins elicit a T-cell response.

2. Even pigs reared in microbe-free conditions are infected with endogenous retroviruses; these have never been known to infect humans, but they could do so after transplantation. Pig viruses are more likely to infect recipients taking immunosuppressive drugs.

BOX 34.1 Acute Graft Rejection

A 43-year-old woman has polycystic kidney disease, a degenerative condition that often leads to irreversible kidney failure. Three years ago her kidney failure became so severe that she started hemodialysis three times a week. She has been referred to the renal transplant team and is a good candidate for a transplant because her renal disease is unlikely to recur in a transplanted kidney. She has been human leukocyte antigen (HLA) typed, and although she has relatively common HLA alleles, she is told that there may be a long wait for a cadaveric kidney. This is because most kidney transplant schemes aim to match the donor and recipient as closely as possible, and only about 1 in 5000 unrelated individuals have identical HLA types.

Living related donors are important in kidney transplantation, provided they are not affected by the same genetic disease. Our patient has three brothers, none of whom is affected by polycystic kidney disease. Because of the long potential wait, the patient's brothers decide to undergo tissue typing, and one of them is found to be an exact HLA and blood group match. The patient's serum did not react with her brother's lymphocytes during cross-match. After transplantation, no evidence of hyperacute rejection was found.

With current technology, it is not possible to match minor histocompatibility antigens, which can trigger graft rejection even in living related donors with HLA-matched organs. For this reason, this patient was given posttransplant rejection prophylaxis with cyclosporine, mycophenolate mofetil, and corticosteroids.

The transplant appeared to be going well, but on day 8 the patient started to feel unwell and feverish. On palpation, the transplanted kidney was swollen, and blood tests showed her renal function had deteriorated.

A renal biopsy showed acute rejection as a result of minor antigen mismatch (Fig. 34.6). Initial treatment with high-dose corticosteroids was ineffective. The patient was treated for 5 days with a monoclonal anti–interleukin 2 (IL-2) receptor antibody, during which time renal function improved, and there were no further episodes of rejection.

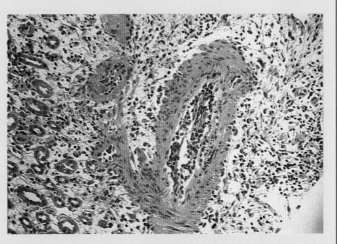

Fig 34.6 Biopsy of a kidney transplant showing lymphocytic infiltration in the graft consistent with acute rejection.

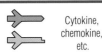 MCH II

 Cytokine, chemokine, etc.

Complement (C′)

 Signaling molecule

BOX 34.2 Infection After Stem Cell Transplant

A 36-year-old woman with lymphoma is at high risk for relapse after initial chemotherapy. Neither of her two siblings is human leukocyte antigen (HLA) identical. After an extensive search on a registry, a donor is found. Although the donor is HLA identical, there is a risk for graft-versus-host disease (GVHD) because of minor antigen incompatibility. Prophylaxis with cyclosporine is used for 6 weeks after stem cell transplant.

Fortunately, her lymphoma does not relapse and she does not develop GVHD. She does, however, have a series of infections.

Conditioning, GVHD prophylaxis, and stem cell transplantation itself cause severe immunosuppression, and infection is the most common cause of death in these patients. Figure 34.7 shows how immune reconstitution takes place and how the specific infections are likely to occur.

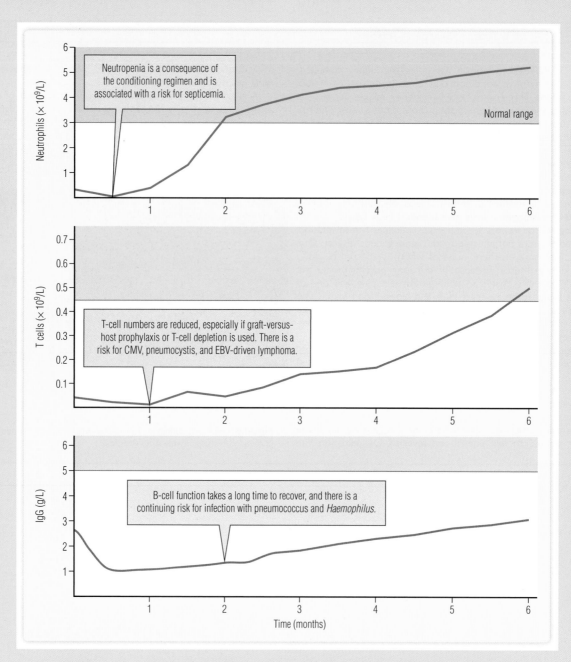

Fig 34.7 Risk of infection after bone marrow transplantation. *CMV,* cytomegalovirus; *EBV,* Epstein-Barr virus.

 T-cell receptor (TCR)

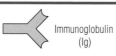 Immunoglobulin (Ig)

 Antigen

 MCH I

LEARNING POINTS   Can You Now ...

1. List the different types of transplants and the organs transplanted?
2. Describe the three phases of rejection of solid organs?
3. Describe the two laboratory procedures designed to reduce the risk for infection?

4. Explain how stem cell transplantation differs from solid organ transplant?
5. List the problems that need to be overcome to make xenotransplantation safe?

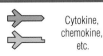 MCH II

 Cytokine, chemokine, etc.

Complement (C')

 Signaling molecule

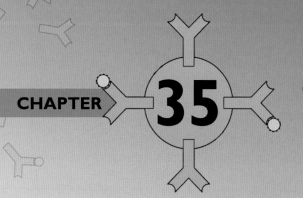

CHAPTER 35

Tumor Immunology

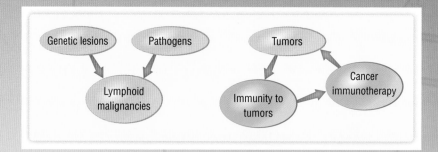

This chapter discusses the two main strands of tumor immunology, including how genetic events and interactions with pathogens lead to tumors of lymphoid cells, how the immune system can respond to tumors, and how this knowledge is being turned into new tumor immunotherapies.

■ LYMPHOID TUMORS

The malignancies that affect the adaptive immune system originate from a single lymphocyte or plasma cell. Each cell of the malignant population has undergone identical immune receptor gene rearrangements and expresses identical immunoglobulin or T-cell receptor (TCR) molecules. The identical nature of the cells is referred to as *monoclonality*.

The cellular origins of lymphoid malignancy are shown in Figure 35.1, and the characteristics of tumor cells are shown in Table 35.1. The characteristics of each type of tumor are dictated by the biology of the originating cell. For example, acute lymphoblastic leukemia (ALL) is derived from rapidly dividing pre–B cells and is extremely aggressive. Untreated ALL can kill within weeks of diagnosis. Myeloma is derived from mature, slow-growing plasma cells, which secrete monoclonal immunoglobulin. Myeloma patients can survive for years without treatment.

Because cells from lymphoid malignancies are easy to remove and grow in vitro, much is known about how they arise. This is usually the result of oncogene activation by chromosomal translocations or the effects of pathogens.

Oncogenesis

Chromosomal Translocations

During immune-receptor gene recombination, chromosomal breaks may not be correctly repaired. In B cells, chromosomal breaks can also occur during class switching. Segments of different chromosomes are occasionally brought together. This often has lethal consequences for the lymphocyte. However, some rare chromosomal translocations have positive effects on cell survival. This may happen because translocation of an oncogene with an immunoglobulin gene promoter or enhancer may result in permanent activation of the oncogene.

In some types of lymphoma, the oncogenes *MYC* (formerly *c-myc*, on chromosome 8) and *BCL2* (formerly *bcl-2*, on chromosome 18) are commonly translocated to the immunoglobulin heavy chain gene on chromosome 14. Activated *MYC* stimulates lymphocyte proliferation. In normal lymphocytes, proliferation is always balanced by apoptosis. Activated Bcl-2 protein protects against apoptosis, which allows unrestrained proliferation of lymphocytes.

Epigenetic changes are also acquired by malignant cells; for example, permanent methylation of tumor suppressor genes leads to decreased transcription of this family of genes.

Oncogene translocations are more likely to occur after exposure to radiation. Myeloma was common in survivors of the Hiroshima atomic bombings.

Pathogens

Herpesvirus family members and retroviruses infect cells without killing them. It is in the interest of viruses to stimulate uncontrolled growth of these infected cells.

Epstein-Barr virus (EBV) causes infectious mononucleosis (Chapter 15), lymphoma, and nasopharyngeal carcinoma. Unlike many other viruses, EBV does not convert the cellular machinery to virus production and destruction of the cell (see Box 15.3). Instead, EBV immortalizes cells by producing proteins that drive B-cell proliferation and inhibit apoptosis. EBV

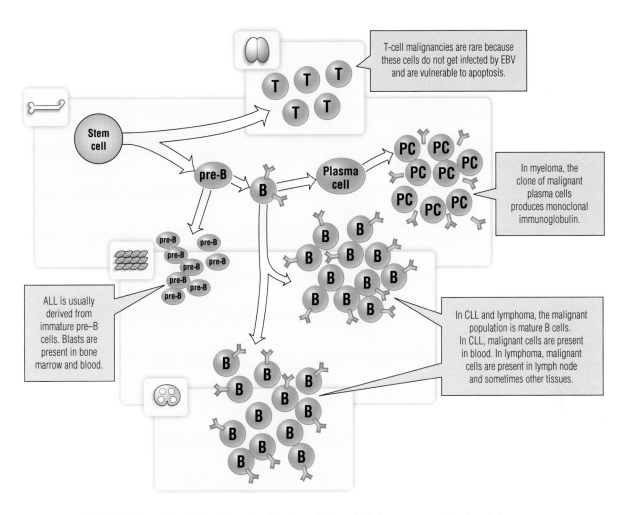

Fig 35.1 Origins of lymphoid malignancies. Clonal populations arise in bone marrow or lymph node but may spill over into blood or other tissues. *ALL,* acute lymphoblastic leukemia; *CLL,* chronic lymphocytic leukemia; *EBV,* Epstein-Barr virus; *PC,* plasma cell.

proteins also help infected cells evade the immune response by blocking antigen presentation.

EBV contributes to the different types of lymphoma (both Hodgkin and non-Hodgkin lymphoma). In regions where malaria is endemic, Burkitt lymphoma occurs in up to 1 in 1000 children and is a consequence of polyclonal activation of B cells by both malaria and EBV. The marked polyclonal B-cell proliferation increases the risk for translocations that involve *MYC,* which leads to the growth of a malignant population.

In immunodeficient patients, the normal response to EBV-infected B cells is lost, and EBV is able to drive B-cell growth. B-cell proliferation is initially polyclonal and presents as a prolonged mononucleosis–like illness with lymphadenopathy. Translocations that involve *MYC* then occur and promote the growth of a malignant monoclonal population. Infection with another herpesvirus, human herpesvirus 8 (HHV8), can cause Kaposi sarcoma in immunodeficient individuals.

Helicobacter pylori is another organism that can contribute to the development of lymphoma. *H. pylori* is a bacterium that triggers chronic inflammation in the stomach. This commonly causes stomach ulcers. More rarely, the inflammation caused by *H. pylori* causes lymphomas to arise in the associated mucosa-associated lymphoid tissue (MALT). Importantly, treatment of the *H. pylori* infection can lead to the lymphoma going into remission.

T-cell malignancy is rare, but when it occurs it is often caused by human T-lymphotrophic virus 1 (HTLV1). This retrovirus encodes Tax protein, which has effects similar to interleukin 2 (IL-2; T-cell growth factor). HTLV1 is rare in the developed world.

Cancers are usually a consequence of at least two events affecting gene expression. Figure 35.2 illustrates this principle.

Diagnosing Lymphoid Malignancy

In some types of lymphoid malignancy, abnormal cells can be recognized by their appearance. For example, in acute leukemia, the presence of high numbers of very immature cells ("blasts") in the blood and marrow is diagnostic. Flow cytometry may then be used to distinguish between acute myeloid leukemia (AML) arising from neutrophil precursors and ALL arising from immature B-cell precursors.

In other situations, the malignant cells look very similar to their normal counterparts. For example, in chronic lymphocytic

 MCH II    Cytokine, chemokine, etc.   Complement (C′)   Signaling molecule

TABLE 35.1   Lymphoid Malignancies and Their Characteristics

Malignancy	Cell Type	Special Characteristics	Diagnosis
Acute lymphoblastic leukemia (ALL)	Immature pre–B cells or B cells	Rare; affects young people; aggressive disease with replacement of bone marrow and invasion of tissues (eg, brain)	Characteristic cells on examination of blood or marrow; flow cytometry may be required to distinguish ALL from acute myeloid leukemia.
Chronic lymphocytic leukemia (CLL)	Mature B cells	Relatively common in the elderly; may be nonaggressive	Lymphocytosis on blood film; CLL lymphocytes express characteristic surface molecules detected by flow cytometry.
Lymphoma	Mature B cells	Frequently associated with EBV or infection and chromosomal translocation; tends to cause solid lesions that often begin in lymph nodes or mucosa-associated lymphoid tissue	Biopsy of affected tissue.
Multiple myeloma	Plasma cells	Relatively common in the elderly	Detection of monoclonal immunoglobulin in blood or light chains in urine. Plasma cells are present in marrow, and osteolytic lesions may be seen on radiography.
T-cell malignancy	T cells	Rare; may be caused by HTLVI infection	This condition can behave either as leukemia (with blood involvement) or as lymphoma (with solid tissue involvement).

EBV, *Epstein-Barr virus*; HTLVI, *human T-lymphotrophic virus I.*

leukemia (CLL), the abnormal cells look very similar to normal, mature lymphocytes. As described Box 35.1, flow cytometry can be used to show the presence of abnormal molecules on the surface of the leukemia cells.

Malignancy of plasma cells, myeloma, is a special case. Box 35.2 describes how the monoclonal immunoglobulin secreted by these cells acts as a marker of malignancy.

■ IMMUNITY TO TUMORS

How cells of the adaptive immune system may give rise to tumors has already been discussed. However, components of the immune system may also recognize and sometimes kill malignancies that arise in other tissues. This is potentially of great importance because it has been surmised that immunotherapy would offer hope to patients with cancer, most types of which remain incurable. To understand this, it is important to know how malignant cells may become antigenic or, in other words, how they express tumor antigens.

Tumor Antigens

Tumor antigens are molecules produced by tumor cells that can potentially be recognized by the immune system. There are a number of different types of tumor antigen:

- *Developmental proteins.* These are normally only transiently expressed during development but may be reexpressed by tumor cells. For example, carcinoembryonic antigen (CEA) is normally expressed on many tissues during fetal life. CEA can be abnormally expressed in gastrointestinal cancer.
- *Lineage-specific proteins.* These proteins are expressed in cancers and in the normal tissues from which they arise. For example, melanoma is a skin cancer of melanocytes. Normal melanocytes and melanoma cells both express the enzyme

tyrosinase, which is not expressed in any other cells, normal or abnormal.
- *Viral proteins.* For example, EBV and human papillomavirus (HPV, in cervical cancer) produce specific proteins.
- *Proteins produced through translocations.* For example, the Bcr-Abl fusion protein is the product of the *BCR/ABL1* translocation.

Developmental and lineage-specific proteins are poorly immunogenic because they are expressed on normal tissues. T cells with receptors capable of recognizing these proteins are deleted through tolerance induction. The same system that protects from autoimmunity thus impairs tumor recognition by the immune system. For example, CEA present in colon cancer does not elicit a strong immune response. Nonetheless, tests to detect CEA are sometimes used to screen for this type of cancer.

Viral and fusion proteins tend to be more immunogenic because they are never present in the normal individual. Each of these has been investigated for its possible clinical role in diagnosing, preventing, and treating cancer.

Vaccination has been used to *prevent* two cancers so far. Hepatitis B virus (HBV) can cause liver cancer, which has been a leading cause of death in some parts of the world. Hepatitis B vaccine has been shown to be nearly 90% effective at preventing liver cancer in Taiwan. Some strains of HPV (the virus that causes warts) cause cervical cancer. HPV vaccine was introduced in the 2000s, and early data suggest that the immunity induced by the vaccines may reduce cervical cancer by approximately 50%. On this basis, HPV vaccines could prevent 50,000 deaths each year in the United States.

After 50 years of research, immunotherapy to treat existing cancer is beginning to show some successes. Knowledge of tumor immunity and how tumors evade the immune system is necessary to understand the problems immunologists face in developing useful therapy for cancer.

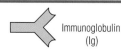 T-cell receptor (TCR)

 Immunoglobulin (Ig)

Antigen

 MCH I

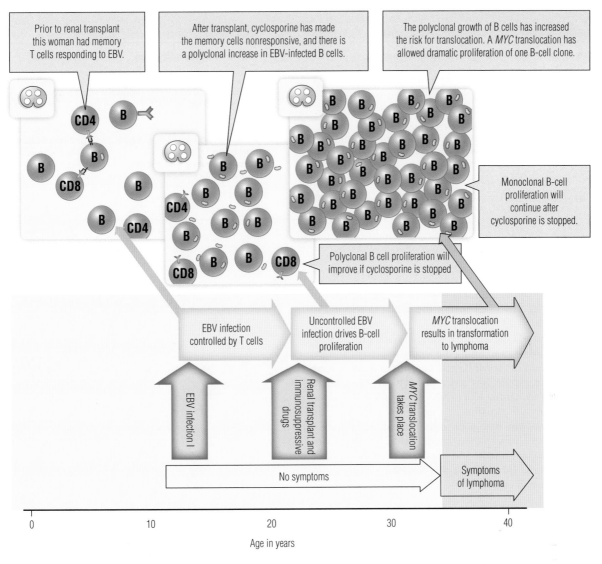

Fig 35.2 A sequence of events is usually required in oncogenesis. In this case, Epstein-Barr virus (EBV) infection, posttransplant immunosuppression, and then a gene translocation led to monoclonal B-cell proliferation.

Evidence for Tumor Immunity

The high frequency of cancers in immunosuppressed patients is often cited as evidence of tumor immunity, such as papillomavirus-driven cervical cancer (100 times more common in immunosuppressed patients). How commonly EBV-driven lymphoma occurs in patients with immunodeficiency has already been discussed. The high prevalence of these tumors in immunodeficient patients is evidence of the more effective role of the immune system in clearing viral infection than in recognizing tumors. Immune surveillance for viruses is much more effective than surveillance for cancers.

However, there is also good evidence that the human immune system attempts to eradicate other types of tumor by recognizing some of the antigens mentioned earlier. Most research has focused on T cells (eg, tumor-infiltrating lymphocytes [TILs]) that are specific for tumor antigens, such as tyrosinase in melanoma. TILs use their TCRs to recognize antigen presented by major histocompatibility complex (MHC).

The immune system occasionally damages the blood supply to tumors and kills them by starving them of oxygen, which leads to necrosis. Very early experiments showed that tumor necrosis factor (TNF) can do this when injected at high doses into mice with cancers. Although this is how the cytokine's full name arose, it is not clear how important these mechanisms are in tumors in humans.

Evasion of the Immune Response by Tumors

Unlike infections, tumors rarely produce danger signals and do not directly activate the innate immune system through Toll-like receptors (TLRs) or other pattern recognition molecules. Apart from natural killer cells (see later), this means that the innate immune system does not usually attempt to kill tumor cells, nor

 MCH II

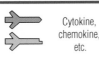 Cytokine, chemokine, etc.

 Complement (C′)

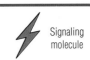 Signaling molecule

TABLE 35.2 Cancer Immunotherapy Approaches

Active or Passive	Type of Immunotherapy	Name of Immunotherapy	Tumor
Passive	Monoclonal antibody	Rituximab stimulates apoptosis	Lymphoma
		Trastuzumab blocks HER2 receptor	Breast
		Bevacizumab blocks VEGF	Colon, lung, breast
Active	Toll-like receptor ligand	BCG	Bladder cancer
		Imiquimod	Basal cell cancer
	Allows costimulatory ligand pair formation T cell	Ipilimumab	Melanoma
		Tumor-infiltrating lymphocyte	
		Engineered T-cell receptor	

BCG, bacille Calmette-Guérin; VEGF, vascular endothelial growth factor.

does it alert the adaptive immune response to the presence of danger. This can lead to T-cell anergy, the failure to respond to antigen.

Some tumors evade the adaptive immune system by decreasing expression of MHC and losing the ability to present antigen to T cells. Mutations in the MHC genes are not unusual in these tumors. Cells that express low levels of MHC make excellent targets for killing by natural killer (NK) cells, which may act as a backup system in this situation.

In most tumors, the malignant cells successfully evade the immune response by using various mechanisms. Rapidly dividing malignant cells may mutate and acquire one or more of these evasion mechanisms. This will give this clone of cells an advantage over nonmutated cells.

Immunotherapy

Attempts at using immunotherapy have been based on the idea that the immune system could eradicate existing tumors. Many approaches at tumor immunotherapy have been attempted, and most have failed. This text mentions only some of the immunotherapy approaches that have been of some success. Immunotherapy can be classified as *passive,* when an existing immune response (usually a monoclonal antibody) is administered, or it may be *active,* when the patient's own immune response is activated to respond to the tumor. Active immunity is considered better because it could provide a lifelong response tailored to the patient's exact tumor antigen. Passive immunity lasts only as long as the infusion and is a generic treatment rather than an exact fit. Table 35.2 shows some cancer immunotherapy approaches.

Passive Cancer Immunotherapy

Monoclonal antibodies (mAbs) can be produced that have a variety of effects against tumors, and they can activate immune system killing mechanisms. For example, they can activate complement (Fig. 35.3). Some mAbs bind to Fc receptors on natural killer cells, which leads to antibody-dependent cellular cytotoxicity (Chapter 22). Alternatively, the mAb may be engineered so that it either delivers radioactivity or a toxin to the tumor cell.

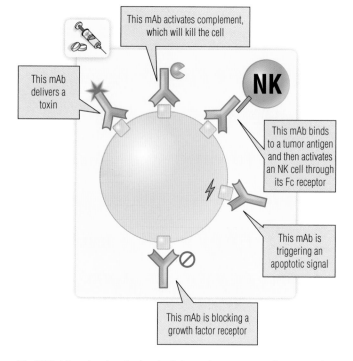

Fig 35.3 Monoclonal antibodies (mAbs) can destroy tumor cells in a number of ways. *NK,* natural killer.

Some tumor antigens are linked to signaling pathways that can be either triggered or blocked by mAbs. For example, rituximab binds to CD20, a signaling molecule present on B cells. When the mAb binds this molecule, it can trigger apoptosis in the malignant B cell.

Trastuzumab (Herceptin) is an antibody against HER2, the epidermal growth factor receptor present on cells from about 30% of breast cancers. Trastuzumab prevents this molecule from signaling and prevents tumor cell growth.

On the other hand, several cancers rely on vascular endothelial growth factor (VEGF) to stimulate an adequate blood supply. VEGF and its receptor can be blocked by mAbs, such as bevacizumab, which are thus of some benefit in some colon,

 T-cell receptor (TCR)   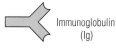 Immunoglobulin (Ig)    Antigen   MCH I

lung, and breast cancers. Chapter 36 discusses mAbs in more detail.

Active Cancer Immunotherapy

Active immunotherapy must overcome tolerance mechanisms to respond to tumor antigen (Fig. 35.4). If TLRs can be stimulated, the innate immune system will be activated, which may help overcome tolerance. A wide range of cells secrete proinflammatory cytokines in response to TLR stimulation. Bladder cancers are sometimes endoscopically injected with the live tuberculosis vaccine, bacille Calmette-Guérin (BCG, Chapter 25). BCG can replicate at the site of injection but will not

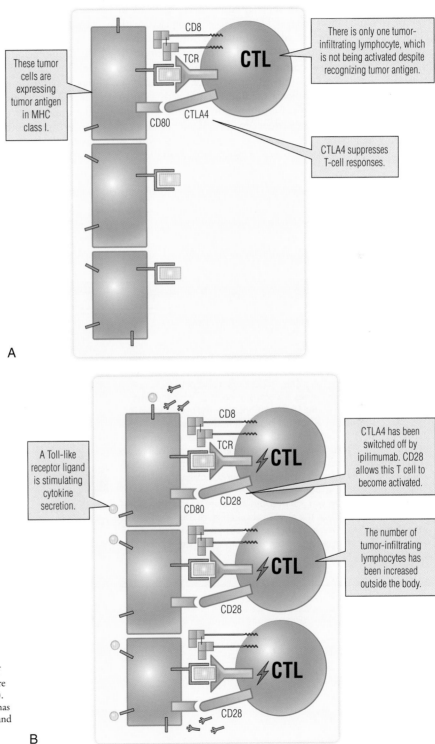

These tumor cells are expressing tumor antigen in MHC class I.

There is only one tumor-infiltrating lymphocyte, which is not being activated despite recognizing tumor antigen.

CTLA4 suppresses T-cell responses.

A

A Toll-like receptor ligand is stimulating cytokine secretion.

CTLA4 has been switched off by ipilimumab. CD28 allows this T cell to become activated.

The number of tumor-infiltrating lymphocytes has been increased outside the body.

Fig 35.4 A, Even though an infiltrating T cell may recognize tumor antigen, it cannot respond because of cytotoxic T-lymphocyte A4 (CTLA4) and because there are no proinflammatory cytokines (no "danger signal"). **B,** After treatment, the number of infiltrating T cells has been increased, there are proinflammatory cytokines, and CTLA4 has been replaced by CD28. *MCH,* major histocompatibility complex; *TCR,* T-cell receptor.

B

 MCH II

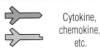 Cytokine, chemokine, etc.

 Complement (C′)

 Signaling molecule

survive long. BCG activates TLRs 2 and 4 and triggers an adaptive immune response. Imiquimod is a synthetic ligand for TLR7 and also indirectly activates the adaptive immune response (Box 21.2). Imiquimod is already in use in some skin cancers, such as basal cell cancer.

Chapter 16 described that one of the costimulatory ligand pairs that forms during successful responses to antigen is CD28 (on T cells) and CD80 (on antigen-presenting cells). This ligand pair provides the second signal to ensure the T cell responds to signals through the TCR. In some circumstances—such as in response to some cancer cells—CD28 on T cells is replaced with CTLA4, which cannot provide costimulation, and the cancer cells are tolerated. Monoclonal antibodies such as ipilimumab bind CTLA4 and allow costimulation to go ahead. This has proven successful in some advanced tumors, such as melanoma.

Another approach is to boost the number and activation of T cells with specific receptors for tumor antigen. Patient T cells must be used because only these express TCRs capable of recognizing self MHC. For example, if a piece of tissue is available, tumor-infiltrating lymphocytes can be extracted and activated, using cytokines, ex vivo. These TILs increase in number and are reinfused into the patient. This approach is reliant on tissue being available and producing sufficient numbers of TILs. Alternatively, T cells can be isolated from the patient's blood and can be genetically altered to express a TCR for the tumor antigen. These cells can then be reinfused after activation with cytokines. This approach requires the patient's tumor antigen to be known.

Many of these approaches are controversial. For example, treatments based on a patient's T cells are expensive and labor intensive and are not guaranteed to be successful. "Off the shelf" monoclonal antibodies can be somewhat cheaper but are only partially effective. For example, when added to conventional cytotoxic chemotherapy, bevacizumab improves median survival in metastatic colon cancer from about 26 to 30 months. The importance of these treatments is that they do show that cancer immunotherapy can work and that further research is justified.

BOX 35.1 Chronic Lymphocytic Leukemia

An elderly man presents with unusually severe shingles (herpes zoster infection), suggestive of a mild secondary immunodeficiency state. On examination, he has generalized lymphadenopathy. These clinical features are consistent with chronic lymphocytic leukemia (CLL) or lymphoma.

The patient undergoes laboratory testing, which shows a raised lymphocyte count (5.6×10^6/mL; the normal range is 1.5 to 3.0×10^6/mL). In a normal blood film, the numbers of neutrophils visible should exceed the number of lymphocytes. In the blood film in Figure 35.5, although six lymphocytes are visible, no neutrophils are present. The lymphocytes have normal morphology without any features that would allow the diagnosis of leukemia or lymphoma to be made.

Flow cytometry was carried out to characterize the molecules on the surface of the abnormal cells. Figure 35.6 shows that the lymphocytes were abnormal B cells expressing the CD5 molecule. The shingles was caused by immunodeficiency secondary to B-cell CLL.

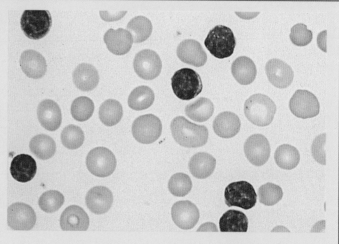

Fig 35.5 A blood sample showing a striking lymphocytosis.

 T-cell receptor (TCR)

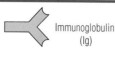 Immunoglobulin (Ig)

 Antigen

 MCH I

BOX 35.1 Chronic Lymphocytic Leukemia—cont'd

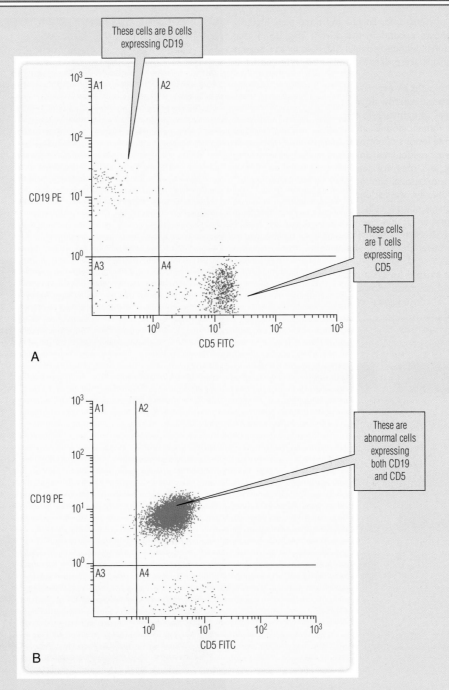

Fig 35.6 A, Flow cytometry from a healthy person. Distinct populations of T and B cells are present. **B,** Flow cytometry in which all the cells express both CD5 and CD19. This is an abnormal combination typical of chronic lymphocytic leukemia (CLL). (Courtesy John Hewitt, Manchester Royal Infirmary, Manchester, United Kingdom.)

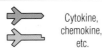 MCH II

 Cytokine, chemokine, etc.

Complement (C')

 Signaling molecule

BOX 35.2 Myeloma

A woman presents with fatigue and bone pain. Electrophoresis shows a band in the serum (Fig. 35.7) that represents monoclonal immunoglobulin (Ig) Gk in the serum. Also, free κ light chains are present in the urine, referred to as *Bence Jones protein*.

A series of radiographs shows multiple lytic bone lesions (Fig. 35.8). In addition, a bone marrow aspirate confirms the presence of excessive numbers of plasma cells (Fig. 35.9). The presence of serum monoclonal immunoglobulin and urinary monoclonal light chains with lytic bone lesions confirms the diagnosis of myeloma.

Monoclonal immunoglobulins can be produced in response to some infections, and they are seen in some healthy elderly people—so-called monoclonal gammopathy of uncertain significance (MGUS). However, monoclonal immunoglobulin is also produced by malignant plasma cells in myeloma, in which case the number of marrow plasma cells is dramatically increased. Bone destruction (osteolytic lesions) is seen in some patients with myeloma but never in MGUS, which helps distinguish the two conditions.

The patient was started on cytotoxic chemotherapy, and she initially made a good response. However, she developed *Haemophilus pneumoniae*, a consequence of her secondary antibody deficiency, and died.

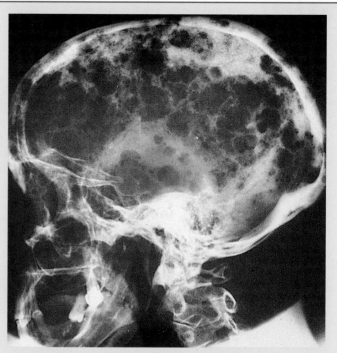

Fig 35.8 A skull survey shows multiple lytic lesions. Hypercalcemia occurs as a result of increased bone resorption and contributes to renal failure. (Courtesy St. Bartholomew's Hospital, London.)

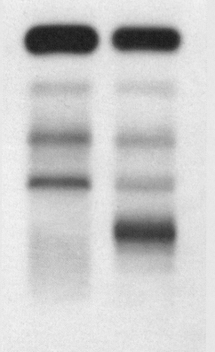

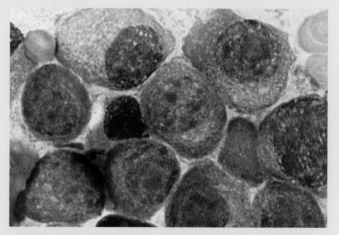

Fig 35.7 The serum electrophoresis strip on the left is from a healthy control. The strip on the right shows a band in the γ region, which reflects a monoclonal immunoglobulin. Compare this image with Figure 4.4. (Courtesy Karen Sneade, Manchester Royal Infirmary, Manchester, United Kingdom.)

Fig 35.9 This figure shows bone marrow aspirate from the patient. All the cells in this field are plasma cells, which secrete the monoclonal immunoglobulin seen in Figure 35.7.

 T-cell receptor (TCR)   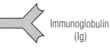 Immunoglobulin (Ig)   Antigen   MCH I

LEARNING POINTS   Can You Now...

1. Describe the different lymphoid malignancies?
2. List the techniques used to diagnose lymphoid malignancies?
3. Explain how host and viral oncogenes interact to cause cancer?
4. Describe the different types of tumor antigen and explain how tumors evade the immune response?

5. List several approaches to cancer immunotherapy?
6. Describe two different examples of therapeutic monoclonal antibodies used to treat malignancies?

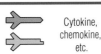 Cytokine, chemokine, etc.

MCH II

 Complement (C′)

 Signaling molecule

CHAPTER 36 Biopharmaceuticals

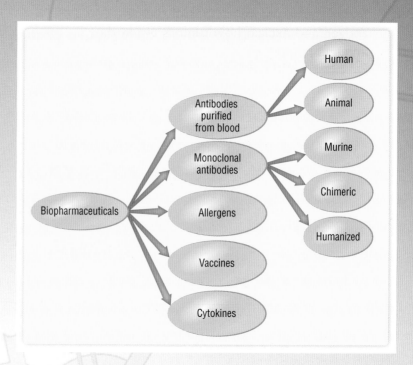

Biopharmaceuticals are also known as *biologic medicinal products* and *biologics*. They can be defined as medications that can only be produced by living cells. The oldest biopharmaceuticals included antibodies purified from humans (eg, immunoglobulin replacement; Chapter 32) or from animals (eg, digoxin fab fragments; Chapter 4). Vaccines (Chapter 25) and allergens used for allergy immunotherapy (Chapter 27) are also biopharmaceuticals. These may be produced by purifying extracts or organisms or using molecular biology. Biopharmaceuticals include therapeutic monoclonal antibodies (mAbs) and recombinant cytokines, which are the topic of this chapter. These are produced using molecular biology and cellular technologies. Remember that the specialized tests described in Chapter 5— such as lateral flow tests (eg, pregnancy tests), enzyme-linked immunosorbent assay (ELISA), and flow cytometry—would not be possible without mAbs. Recombinant cytokines and mAbs are the newest biopharmaceuticals, and their use is doubling every 4 years.

Biopharmaceuticals are proteins, and all have the potential to elicit an immune response. In the case of vaccines and allergens, this is a desirable characteristic. In the case of mAbs and cytokines, an immune response is not desired, and these protein molecules are usually altered to reduce immunogenicity.

This chapter describes some of the ways that biotechnology is being used to improve mAbs and cytokines for use in clinical medicine (see figure above). An enhanced understanding of biotechnology has been used to improve mAbs, for example, by reducing the amount of murine genetic sequence and increasing the amount of human genetic sequence while preserving the original specificity of the mAb ("humanized" mAbs). Genetic approaches have also been used to alter the oligosaccharide side chains of mAbs to make them less "murinelike" and less likely to react with anti-carbohydrate antibodies that recognize species-specific differences (Chapter 34).

Recombinant cytokines have also been altered by derivation with polyethylene glycol (PEG) to make them less likely to induce anti-cytokine antibodies and to increase their half-life in serum. This chapter reviews some material presented in Chapters 4 and 5, and it illustrates some practical uses of biotechnology applied to immunology for clinical medicine.

■ MONOCLONAL ANTIBODIES

Two key regions of antibodies have made them attractive molecules for biotechnologists to develop as drugs (Fig. 36.1):

- The Fab region (Chapter 4) of any given antibody confers specificity for antigen and could act as a "magic bullet," directing its effects against pathogens or tumor cells. This specificity results in predictable therapeutic effects and reduced side effects compared with other drugs that cannot be directed to specific target cells.
- The Fc region of antibody is the effector region. For immunoglobulin G (IgG), the physiologic effects of the Fc region include activation of the complement cascade and of macrophages, natural killer (NK) cells, and mast cells. The Fc region can also be altered to deliver drugs and toxins to specific cells.

Historical Approaches to Antibody Therapy

During the past 100 years, various biotechnologic approaches to antibody treatments have been tried. Animal polyclonal immunoglobulin, given as injections of serum, was previously used to treat infections and to neutralize snake venom (antivenin). Horse serum was frequently used but often induced antihorse antibodies, which formed immune complexes with the horse proteins. These circulating immune complexes triggered a type III hypersensitivity reaction, leading to serum sickness (Chapter 30). How Fab fragments against digoxin can be used to "mop up" excess digoxin after an overdose has already been discussed (Chapter 4).

Polyclonal human immunoglobulin is sometimes given as a form of passive immunity. Immunoglobulin replacement therapy is given to patients with antibody deficiency (Chapter 32). Anti-D immunoglobulin is given to rhesus-negative women

pregnant with rhesus-positive fetuses to prevent hemolytic disease of the newborn (Chapter 29). However, obtaining large quantities of human immunoglobulin from donors is expensive and always carries a risk for transmitting blood-borne infection. In addition, because human volunteers cannot be deliberately immunized with infectious agents or with tumor cells, the scope of therapeutic antibodies available from human sources is limited.

Monoclonal Antibody Technologies

Mouse monoclonal antibodies (murine mAbs) were invented in 1975 with the specific aim of developing large quantities of very specific antibody that could be given cheaply and safely. Murine mAbs also have the advantage that they can be raised against antigens that could not be used to deliberately immunize humans, such as dangerous pathogens or tumor cells.

The conventional approach to making murine mAbs has been to fuse B cells from immunized mice with mouse myeloma cells (see Box 36.2). This leads to production of high levels of murine mAb.

Murine mAbs were widely used but have some significant problems. Murine mAbs have mouse Fc regions and do not always interact well in vivo with human complement molecules or Fc receptors on human macrophages and NK cells. In addition, therapeutic murine mAbs invoke the production of antimouse antibodies. These antimouse antibodies can recognize either the unique oligosaccharide side chains expressed on mouse proteins or the amino acid sequence of the constant regions of the mouse immunoglobulin chains. Antimouse antibodies can cause immune complex disease (IgG antimouse antibodies) or anaphylaxis (IgE) (Chapter 30). Antimouse IgG antibodies also neutralize the effects of the murine mAb and are produced in about 40% of patients. Neutralizing antibodies block the beneficial effects of the mAbs. For example, a patient with rheumatoid arthritis may notice that a drug that has previously worked may stop working. For these reasons, murine mAbs are no longer used. To overcome these problems, several approaches have been used to increase the proportion of human genetic sequences used in manufacturing mAbs (Fig. 36.2).

1. Chimeric mAbs use mouse immunoglobulin variable region gene sequences derived from immunized mice and human constant region gene sequences, both cloned into mammalian cells, which then express a chimeric immunoglobulin molecule. Chimeric mAbs contain only about 30% mouse amino acid sequence but still tend to elicit antibodies when used therapeutically. Chimeric mAbs contain the letters "xi" in their name, for example, rituximab (Chapter 35), infliximab, and basiliximab (transplantation; Chapter 34).

2. Humanized mAbs use a technique similar to chimeric antibodies, but only the mouse hypervariable region gene sequence is used. Only about 10% of the amino acids are derived from mouse sequences. Humanized mAbs contain the letter "u," for example, rituximab, trastuzumab, bevacizumab, and ipilimumab; all of these are used in cancer treatment (Chapter 35).

These technologies have been used to develop mAbs with humanlike amino acid sequences, and they reduce the risk of evoking antimouse responses. A further complication is provided by the differences in glycosylation of immunoglobulin

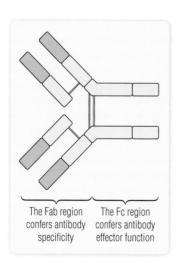

The Fab region confers antibody specificity   The Fc region confers antibody effector function

Fig 36.1 Immunoglobulin structure (covered in Chapter 4).

 MCH II

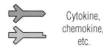 Cytokine, chemokine, etc.

 Complement (C')

 Signaling molecule

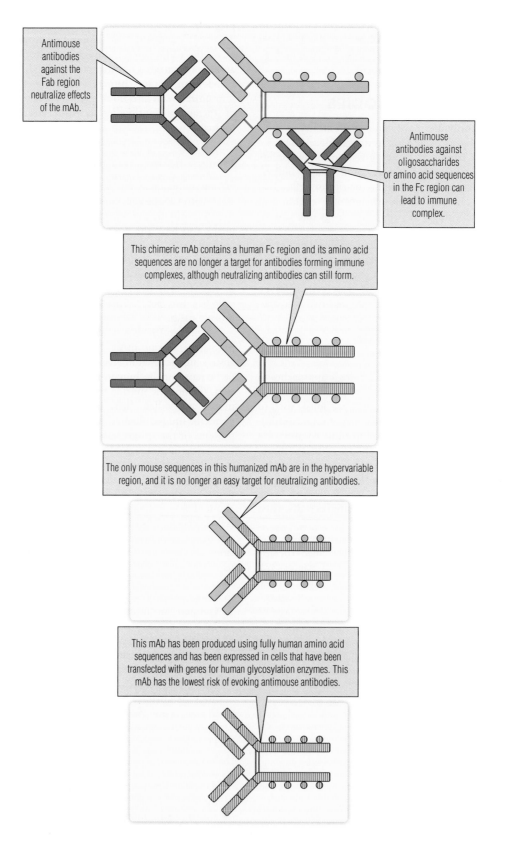

Antimouse antibodies against the Fab region neutralize effects of the mAb.

Antimouse antibodies against oligosaccharides or amino acid sequences in the Fc region can lead to immune complex.

This chimeric mAb contains a human Fc region and its amino acid sequences are no longer a target for antibodies forming immune complexes, although neutralizing antibodies can still form.

The only mouse sequences in this humanized mAb are in the hypervariable region, and it is no longer an easy target for neutralizing antibodies.

This mAb has been produced using fully human amino acid sequences and has been expressed in cells that have been transfected with genes for human glycosylation enzymes. This mAb has the lowest risk of evoking antimouse antibodies.

Fig 36.2 Modifications aimed at reducing the risk of antimouse antibodies being produced against monoclonal antibodies (mAbs). The small circles represent oligosaccharide molecules on the surface of the immunoglobulin.

 T-cell receptor (TCR)

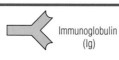 Immunoglobulin (Ig)

 Antigen

 MCH I

produced in human and nonhuman cells. *Glycosylation* refers to the addition of oligosaccharide side chains to proteins. The structure of these side chains has species specificity due to species-specific enzymes involved in their synthesis. Chapter 34 discussed how different mammals have different glycosylation patterns, and antibodies can recognize these. When mAbs are expressed in nonhuman cells, there is a tendency for them to be recognized by anticarbohydrate antibodies. Molecular biology techniques can also be used to alter the glycosylation of humanized antibodies (see Fig. 36.2).

With conventional small molecule drugs, such as penicillin or aspirin, it is possible to switch between different manufacturers without any clinical problems. With biopharmaceuticals, because they are produced in living cells, switching between different drugs must be done much more carefully because different mAbs may have different benefits and side effects. So, for example, switching between two different anti–tumor necrosis factor (TNF) mAbs, infliximab and adalimumab, in rheumatoid arthritis must be done carefully (see Box 36.2). Even when two manufacturers use the same hybridoma to produce a biopharmaceutical, these two drugs should not be considered identical. The two mAbs are described as "biosimilar" and may subtly differ as a result of differences in the manufacturing technique.

Increasing the Effects of Monoclonal Antibodies

The technology described so far has been used to produce mAbs that elicit fewer problematic immune responses in humans. In many cases, these simple antibodies are quite effective. For example, mAbs that block the effects of cytokines have already been widely used. These include anti-TNF mAbs used in rheumatoid arthritis (Chapter 31; see Box 36.2) and anti–interleukin 2 (IL-2) receptor mAbs used to treat transplant rejection (Chapter 34).

However, in cancer immunotherapy, only a minority of mAbs tested so far have been effective at killing target cells through complement activation and antibody-dependent cell-mediated cytotoxicity (ADCC). These include the anti-CD20 and anti-HER2 mAbs mentioned in Chapter 35. In most other cancers, simple mAbs do *not* deliver potent enough effects. Various approaches have been used to increase the effects of mAbs, which are illustrated with cancer immunotherapy in Fig. 36.3.

Biospecific Antibodies

Biospecific antibodies combine the specificities of two different antibodies. In the case of cancer immunotherapy, these have been manufactured against the T-cell receptor (TCR) on cytotoxic T lymphocytes (CTLs) and target antigens on tumor cells. The biospecific antibody brings the CTL and target cell together and activates the CTL to initiate cell killing.

Conjugates

Monoclonal antibodies can be combined with substances that would otherwise be too toxic when administered at higher concentration alone. For example, mAbs can be conjugated to toxins or radioactive isotopes to deliver them to the target cells. Conjugation thus increases the specificity of the toxin or isotope for the target cells.

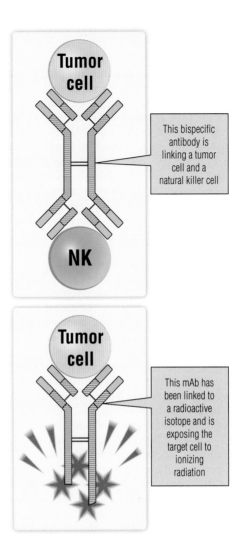

Fig 36.3 Modifications to the Fc region of monoclonal antibodies (mAbs) can enhance effector function. *NK,* natural killer.

Some Successes and Failures in Monoclonal Antibody Therapy

Monoclonal antibodies have gained an important place in the treatment of many common diseases. It is interesting that mAbs are beginning to provide useful therapy in cancer, when there is little evidence that antibodies are part of the normal human immune response to cancer. On the other hand, although antibody has a very clear role in the physiologic defense against infection, mAbs have so far proved to be rather unsuccessful. Much research has been carried out using passive immunotherapy with mAbs to combat infection. For example, mAbs have been raised against lipopolysaccharide (LPS), the substance released from organisms that trigger cytokine release in septic shock (Chapter 21). It is possible to produce mAbs against LPS, but the diversity of antigens in wild-type organisms means that these mAbs are not always effective in a strain that causes infection and symptoms. Similar to other types of pathogens, the very high specificity of mAbs limits their use in treating infections. On the other hand, active immunity using vaccines induces

 MCH II   Cytokine, chemokine, etc.   Complement (C′)   Signaling molecule

polyclonal responses that have been very successful at preventing infection (Chapter 25).

Monoclonal antibodies have been successful in one final arena in which humans do not normally produce helpful antibodies: the treatment of drug overdose and substance abuse. Some drugs—for example, digoxin—are dangerous in overdose and cannot easily be removed from the body by conventional means. Treatment with antidigoxin mAbs leads to rapid clearance of the offending drug (Chapter 4). In addition, mAbs have been used in drug-dependent patients who wish to reduce or eliminate their dependence. The drug and mAb form an immune complex, preventing the drug from reaching specific receptors in the brain and instead directing the drug to the spleen. Patients do not receive the normal "reward" from drug consumption, and hence dependency can be broken.

■ RECOMBINANT CYTOKINES

Most research on recombinant immunologic cytokines has been on the potential role of stimulatory or growth factor cytokines on improving immunity. The major immunologic cytokine in relatively frequent use is interferon-α (IFN-α).

IFN-α is used to treat some forms of viral hepatitis (Chapter 20). Treatment needs to be continued for up to 1 year to be successful. IFN-α induces a mild acute-phase response, which makes most patients feel unwell during treatment (Chapter 24). Some patients produce anti–IFN-α, which neutralizes the effects of the treatment. The major problem has been the cost of treatment—up to $15,000 per year. This cost is at least in part attributable to the very short, 4-hour half-life of IFN-α, which means that infusions have to be given on a daily basis.

Some of these problems can be overcome by adding polyethylene glycol (PEG) molecules to the IFN-α structure. During so-called PEGylation, PEG molecules are covalently joined onto the IFN-α molecule. This increases the half-life of the molecule by increasing its molecular weight so that it is not filtered at the kidney. PEGylation also effectively surrounds the IFN-α molecule so that it is not digested by proteases (Fig. 36.4). Together, these effects increase the half-life to 40 hours, meaning treatment can be given weekly instead of daily. PEGylation also protects the IFN-α molecule from the patient's immune system and reduces the risk for inducing anti–IFN-α antibodies. When PEGylation is carried out appropriately, it does not affect binding to the IFN-α receptor.

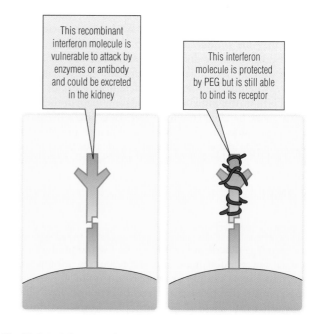

Fig 36.4 PEGylation can be used to increase the biologic half-life of some recombinant molecules. *PEG,* polyethylene glycol.

BOX 36.1 Production of Monoclonal Antibodies

Monoclonal antibodies (mAbs) are homogeneous immunoglobulins. They can be prepared with almost any desired specificity. The basic production technique produces a hybridoma, a combination of a B cell that produces a specific antibody and a myeloma cell. Hybridoma production is illustrated in Figure 36.5. The aim is to produce immortalized cells that secrete only immunoglobulin directed against the antigen used in immunization. It is important to be sure that myeloma cells that have not fused with immunized B cells do not survive. To do this, the myeloma cells that are used have a mutation that results in lack of a specific metabolic enzyme, without which they die in some culture media. After fusion, the cells are grown in these media, and both nonimmortalized B cells and nonfused myeloma cells die. Only myeloma cells that have fused with B cells and that received the correct metabolic enzyme survive. Colonies of hybrid cells are grown and screened for the production of antibody of the desired specificity. Screening for antibody-positive colonies usually involves an enzyme-linked immunosorbent assay (ELISA), described in Chapter 5.

This basic process produces murine mAbs, which are modified using molecular biology techniques to produce chimeric or humanized monoclonal antibodies.

An alternative method is to avoid immunizing an animal altogether and to use phage libraries (not illustrated). These are libraries of random and slightly differing light and heavy chain variable domain genes expressed in bacteriophages. Many different phages can be produced, each of which expresses different variable region molecules. These can be screened for binding to the antigen of interest and then cloned into a mammalian cell (along with constant-region genes) for expression.

The conventional way of producing mAbs derived from hybridomas or phage display libraries has been to grow the cells secreting the mAb in large vats, which can be expensive. Newer technologies allow the mAbs to be produced in farm animals or even plants; vaccines and other proteins can be produced in the same way. It is hoped that these "pharming" technologies will reduce the price of biopharmaceuticals considerably.

 T-cell receptor (TCR)   Immunoglobulin (Ig)   Antigen   MCH I

BOX 36.1 Production of Monoclonal Antibodies—cont'd

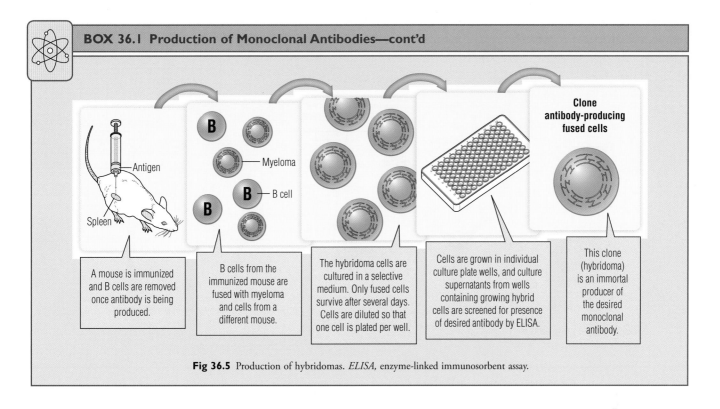

A mouse is immunized and B cells are removed once antibody is being produced.

B cells from the immunized mouse are fused with myeloma and cells from a different mouse.

The hybridoma cells are cultured in a selective medium. Only fused cells survive after several days. Cells are diluted so that one cell is plated per well.

Cells are grown in individual culture plate wells, and culture supernatants from wells containing growing hybrid cells are screened for presence of desired antibody by ELISA.

Clone antibody-producing fused cells

This clone (hybridoma) is an immortal producer of the desired monoclonal antibody.

Fig 36.5 Production of hybridomas. *ELISA*, enzyme-linked immunosorbent assay.

BOX 36.2 Tumor Necrosis Factor Blockade in Rheumatoid Arthritis

Tumor necrosis factor (TNF) is a key cytokine in delayed hypersensitivity reactions, such as rheumatoid arthritis (RA). Three strategies have been developed to prevent TNF binding to receptors on cells involved in the inflammatory response (Fig. 36.6).

- Mouse monoclonal antibodies can prevent TNF binding to its receptor. However, patients produce antibodies against the mouse-specific epitopes on the immunoglobulin. These neutralizing antibodies prevent the anti-TNF from working, which can cause serum sickness–like reactions (Chapter 30).
- Chimeric antibodies such as infliximab are engineered to combine mouse and human fragments; chimeric anti-TNF antibodies are highly effective—up to 80% of patients with RA have clinical improvements. Humanized monoclonal antibodies such as adalimumab are not produced in humans but contain no molecules of mouse or other nonhuman origin.
- Another strategy has been to make recombinant TNF receptor/Fc molecules to "mop up" TNF (eg, etanercept).

These are constructed using human protein sequences to overcome problems with neutralizing antibodies. These molecules are also effective in RA.

Each of these approaches has been successful in RA, but none of the anti-TNF drugs completely switches off RA. This is because of the redundancy of cytokines; in other words, the fact that in most situations, several cytokines are involved in immunologic processes. An anti–interleukin 1 (IL-1) drug, anakinra, has been developed and is also successful in some patients with RA. It may be that combinations of anticytokine drugs will ultimately be used in these situations.

TNF has a physiologic role in combating infections. One concern over drugs that block the effects of TNF is that they may predispose to infections such as tuberculosis, *Listeria* (Chapter 24), or hepatitis B. Another problem with these drugs has been the high cost. It is hoped that the careful use of biosimilars will lead to the introduction of more cost-effective treatments.

Continued

 MCH II   Cytokine, chemokine, etc.   Complement (C′)   Signaling molecule

BOX 36.2 Tumor Necrosis Factor Blockade in Rheumatoid Arthritis—cont'd

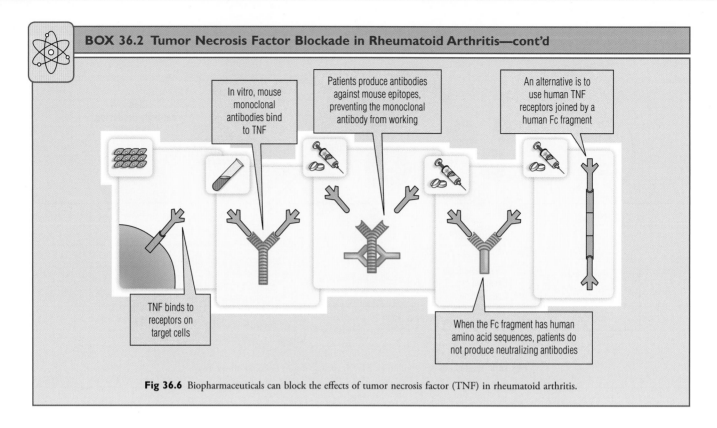

In vitro, mouse monoclonal antibodies bind to TNF

Patients produce antibodies against mouse epitopes, preventing the monoclonal antibody from working

An alternative is to use human TNF receptors joined by a human Fc fragment

TNF binds to receptors on target cells

When the Fc fragment has human amino acid sequences, patients do not produce neutralizing antibodies

Fig 36.6 Biopharmaceuticals can block the effects of tumor necrosis factor (TNF) in rheumatoid arthritis.

LEARNING POINTS Can You Now…

1. List the problems encountered with early therapeutic antibodies derived from horse or human plasma?
2. List several strategies to reduce the antigenicity of murine mAbs?
3. Describe with diagrams two ways in which the Fc region of mAbs can be modified to enhance effector function?

4. Explain the terms *hybridoma*, *humanized*, *chimeric*, and *biosimilar*?
5. List several examples of mAbs proving successful and where they have been so far disappointing in clinical medicine?
6. Explain how PEGylation makes some cytokine therapies more feasible?

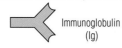 T-cell receptor (TCR)   Immunoglobulin (Ig)    Antigen   MCH I

GLOSSARY

Activation phase. Phase of the immune response when a lymphocyte divides to give many more of the same cell (clonal expansion).

Active immunity. Protective immunity that develops after exposure to infection or vaccination.

Acute-phase response. A systemic reaction to infection or inflammation, mediated by cytokine production and characterized by fever and production of acute-phase proteins.

Adaptive (acquired) immune system response. Part of the immune system in which genetic recombination is used to recognize specific molecules. Slow to respond, but produces lasting memory.

Adjuvant. Substance that increases the immunogenicity of a vaccine, usually by activating the innate immune system.

Affinity. Strength of binding between antigen and antibody or T- or B-cell receptor.

Affinity maturation. Process by which B cells undergo somatic hypermutation and increase the affinity of the B-cell receptor.

Allele. Normal genetic variants that occur in more than 1% of the population. For example, eye color or different human leukocyte antigen types.

Allelic exclusion. Any one B cell expresses only immunoglobulin of one allotype in a heterozygous individual.

Allergen. An environmental substance capable of eliciting an immediate hypersensitivity reaction.

Allergy. Immediate hypersensitivity reaction to an otherwise harmless environmental substance, mediated by immunoglobulin E.

Allogeneic. Immune reactions to a genetically different member of the same species.

Allogeneic transplant. Transplant between genetically different members of the same species.

Allotype. Genetic polymorphisms (different alleles) of both heavy and light chain immunoglobulin genes that can be detected by antibodies.

Alternative pathway. Activation of the complement cascade by exposure to a solid surface lacking complement inhibitors.

Anaphylatoxin. Low-molecular-weight product of complement activation that increases capillary permeability and attracts leukocytes.

Anergy. State of dormancy induced by exposure to antigen in certain circumstances.

Antibody. Protein produced in response to and capable of binding specifically with an antigen. Antibodies have an immunoglobulin structure.

Antigen. Molecules specifically recognized by receptors of the adaptive immune system.

Antigen recognition molecules (ARMs). The ARMs are the B- and T-cell receptor molecules and the proteins encoded by the major histocompatibility complex.

Antigen-binding site. The portion of the antibody that makes contact with antigen.

Antigenemia. High levels of antigen circulating in the bloodstream.

Antigenic drift. Gradual change in an organism's antigens consequent to acquisition of mutations.

Antigen-presenting cells (APCs). Cells that can process antigen and present antigen to T cells.

Apoptosis. Deliberate, programmed cell death.

Asthma. Transient airflow limitation due to bronchial smooth muscle constriction and mucus secretion.

Atopy. Genetic predisposition to allergy.

Attenuated vaccine. Vaccine produced by genetically modifying a pathogenic organism.

Autoantibody. Antibody produced against self antigen.

Autoimmune disease. Disease caused by hypersensitivity reactions that occur as exaggerated autoimmunity.

Autoimmunity. Recognition of normal components of the body by the adaptive immune system. Occurs in healthy individuals but can also cause autoimmune disease.

Autologous transplant. Tissue returning to the same individual after a period outside the body, usually in a frozen state.

B-cell receptor (BCR). The cell surface–located receptor for antigen on B cells.

B lymphocytes. Subset of white blood cells that can secrete antibody molecules.

Bence Jones protein. Monoclonal light chain present in the urine in myeloma.

Biopharmaceutical (biologic). Medication, usually proteins, produced by living cells.

Biosimilar. Two biopharmaceuticals with identical amino acid sequences but produced by different manufacturers. Cannot be assumed to be identical.

Blasts. Immature, rapidly proliferating cells.

Bone marrow. The major hematopoietic organ in humans. Particularly important in B-cell generation, but all the blood cell types—except mature T cells—are generated in the bone marrow.

Caspase. Proteolytic enzymes involved in triggering apoptosis.

CD. Cluster of differentiation nomenclature system for cell surface molecules (and thus for cell subsets).

CD4 count. Number of circulating CD4$^+$ T cells; used to monitor HIV infection.

Cell-mediated immunity. Refers to the function of T cells as opposed to humoral or antibody-mediated immunity.

Central tolerance. Tolerance induced in immature T or B cells in the thymus and bone marrow, respectively.

Chemokines. Chemotactic cytokines; these attract cells to the site of infection.

Chemotaxis. Directed movement of cells, often to the site of infection.

Chimeric monoclonal antibody. Monoclonal antibody using mouse immunoglobulin variable regions and human immunoglobulin constant regions.

Class switching. The process by which an individual B cell can, during maturation, switch immunoglobulin heavy chain usage while retaining the same variable genes and antigen specificity.

Classical pathway. Activation of the complement cascade by exposure to aggregated immunoglobulin.

Clonal selection theory. The idea that each lymphocyte expresses a unique antigen receptor and that this preexisting cell divides on exposure to antigen and gives rise to many daughter cells (clones).

Clone. In immunology, a series of genetically identical lymphocytes, all derived from one B cell or T cell after receptor recombination.

Cognate antigen. The precise antigen that a given antigen receptor has specificity for.

Cognitive phase. Phase of an active immune response during which antigen is recognized by a cell bearing a receptor specific for the antigen.

Collectin. Molecules forming part of the innate immune system, containing lectin (carbohydrate-binding) domains and collagen-like domains.

Colony-stimulating factor (CSF). Growth factors that induce differentiation of specific cell lineages during hematopoiesis.

Combinatorial diversity. Refers to immunoglobulin or T-cell receptor variable region gene segments recombining in multiple combinations (eg, 30 Vκ × 5 Jκ = 150 different variable regions).

Complement. Cascade of serum enzymes activated by the presence of pathogens.

C-reactive protein (CRP). Acute-phase protein produced at high levels during inflammation.

Cross-reactivity. Occasionally, an antigen recognition molecule is specific for a particular antigen, but a different antigen fits well enough for stable binding to occur.

Cytokine. Soluble molecules used to transmit messages from cell to cell. Interferons and chemokines are types of cytokines.

Cytokine network. System of cytokines used to regulate interactions between cells of the innate and adaptive immune systems.

Danger signals. Molecular signals produced by the body's cells indicating damage, usually because of infections.

Defensin. Low-molecular-weight peptide capable of damaging bacteria.

Degranulating cell. Innate immune system cell that releases toxic granules on activation.

Delayed hypersensitivity. Reaction that takes several days to develop and involves antigen-presenting cells and T cells.

Dendritic cell. Irregularly shaped cell with many branchlike processes that is critical in antigen capture and presentation to T cells.

Desensitization. Type of treatment for allergy involving increasing doses of antigen.

Diapedesis. Term used to describe lymphocyte passage through the tight junction between adjacent endothelial cells into the tissues.

Effector cell. Effector B cells are the plasma cells that secrete antibody molecules, and effector T cells are the T-helper and cytotoxic T-lymphocyte populations.

ELISA. Enzyme-linked immunosorbent assay.

Eosinophil. Short-lived degranulating cell.

Eotaxin. Chemokine that attracts eosinophils to the site of inflammation.

Epithelioid cell. Type of mature macrophage.

Epitope. Area of an antigen with which an antibody reacts/binds specifically.

False positive. Erroneous positive test result, for example, produced by a cross-reacting antibody.

Fas. Cell surface molecule that, when bound, can trigger apoptosis.

Flow cytometry. The process of enumerating live cells that express an antigen that can be recognized with an antibody, usually a monoclonal antibody.

Follicular dendritic cell. Antigen-presenting cell found only in lymphoid follicles that may have a different origin from bone marrow–derived dendritic cells. Antigen-antibody complexes are retained on their surface attached to Fc and complement receptors.

Germinal center. Area of lymphoid follicles that contains chiefly activated B cells.

Germline diversity. Term that refers to the multiple copies of V, D, and J gene segments.

Giant cell. Type of mature macrophage.

Glial cell. Type of mature macrophage.

Glomerulonephritis. Inflammation of the glomerulus.

Graft-versus-leukemia effect. Beneficial effects of stem cell transplant against malignancy in the recipient.

Granuloma. A localized area of chronic inflammation, usually produced in response to a pathogen that is hard to clear.

Granzyme. Protein in granules found in cytotoxic T cells and natural killer cells.

Haplotype. A block of alleles that are inherited together, such as in the major histocompatibility complex.

Hapten. Small molecule capable of acting as antigen only after combining with host proteins.

Heaf test. Skin test for exposure to *Mycobacterium tuberculosis*.

Heat shock protein (HSP). Stress-induced protein found in a wide range of organisms.

Hematopoietic stem cells. Pluripotent, self-renewing stem cells that give rise to all blood cell types.

Hemolysis. Damage to red cells.

Herd immunity. High levels of immunity sufficient to prevent epidemics in a given community.

Histamine. Mediator produced by activated mast cells.

Histiocyte. Type of mature macrophage.

HLA. Human leukocyte antigen, also referred to as *major histocompatibility complex*; genetically polymorphic proteins whose function is to bind and present antigen to T cells.

HLA cross matching. Laboratory procedure to rule out reactions between patient and donor cells prior to transplantation.

HLA typing. Laboratory procedure to determine patient or donor human leukocyte antigen type prior to transplantation.

Homing. Migration of lymphocytes to specific tissues.

Human immunodeficiency virus (HIV). Virus capable of infecting cells and damaging the immune system.

Humanized monoclonal antibody. Monoclonal antibody in which only the mouse hypervariable region is used. The rest of the molecule uses human amino acid sequences.

Humoral (antibody-mediated) immunity. Antibody-mediated immunity.

Hygiene hypothesis. Hypothesis that exposure to organisms, particularly mycobacteria, early in life prevents allergies from developing.

Hypermutation. A process of rapid mutation of sequences that encode the binding site for antigen in antibody molecules.

Hypersensitivity. Inflammation caused by an exaggerated response to an antigen. The immune response, rather than the antigen, causes disease.

Hypervariable region (hv). Amino acids that are part of the binding site for antigen and are also contact residues for the antigen.

Idiosyncratic adverse drug reactions. Unpredictable reactions to drugs, often with an immunologic basis.

IL (generic). *Interleukin* (IL) is an old name for *cytokine*. The IL abbreviation is used as a naming system for cytokines.

Immediate hypersensitivity. Reaction that occurs within a few minutes after a response to a trigger, usually mediated by immunoglobulin E.

Immune complex. Lattices of antibody and antigen formed in the body.

Immunofluorescence. Laboratory techniques used to show the presence of a substance in a tissue (*direct immunofluorescence*) or antibody in the blood (*indirect immunofluorescence*).

Immunogen. A substance that by itself causes an immune response (eg, antibody production).

Immunoglobulin. A soluble molecule composed of variable and nonvariable domains with antibody function.

Immunoglobulin domain. Parallel β-sheet structure folded into globular domains that are held together by disulfide bonds.

Immunoglobulin superfamily. A family of molecules with a domain structure similar to that of immunoglobulin. Each has a different role in the immune system (eg, immunoglobulin, T-cell receptor, and major histocompatibility complex molecules).

Immunologic synapse. The area of close binding between an antigen-presenting cell and a T cell that involves multiple receptor-ligand interactions and facilitates cell activation.

Immunotherapy. The treatment of disease by inducing, enhancing, or suppressing an immune response. Most frequently applies to allergen immunotherapy.

Inflammation. Defined clinically as the presence of redness, swelling, and pain. Histologically, *inflammation* is defined as the presence of edema and white cells in a tissue.

Innate (nonadaptive) immune system response. The older part of the immune system, which responds rapidly to infection but with exactly the same response each time.

Insertional mutagenesis. Mutations caused in the genome, for example, after random insertion of a therapeutic gene.

Interferon. A cytokine with antiviral effects.

Invariant chain. A nonpolymorphic protein that facilitates "loading" of major histocompatibility complex class II molecules with antigen.

Junctional diversity. Different sequences created by random addition of nucleotides during formation of junctions between gene segments (eg, V and J, leads to greater antibody diversity).

  T-cell receptor (TCR)

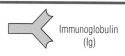 Immunoglobulin (Ig)

 Antigen

 MCH I

Killer immunoglobulin-like receptors (KIRs). Receptor on the surface of natural killer cells.

Kupffer cells. Type of mature macrophage.

Lactoferrin. Bactericidal protein produced by neutrophils and macrophages.

Late-phase response. Follows immediate hypersensitivity in some allergic reactions and is mediated by T cells and eosinophils.

Lectin pathway. Activation of the complement cascade by mannan-binding lectin.

Lymph nodes. Structures that function to concentrate and survey lymph-borne antigens for presentation to T and B cells.

Lymphocyte homing. When effector and memory T lymphocytes migrate and lodge in selected tissue sites, such as peripheral tissues, where they may remain for some time. The process is controlled by interactions between several adhesion molecules.

Lymphocyte recirculation (trafficking). Constant circulation (trafficking) of mature lymphocytes that occurs from one tissue to another. A lymphocyte may make a complete circuit of the body once or twice a day.

Lymphoid tumors. Tumors derived from cells of the adaptive immune system.

Macrophage. Large phagocytic cells with many granules that function as a critical link between the innate and adaptive systems because these cells are active in antigen processing and presentation.

Major histocompatibility complex (MHC). Gene cluster that contains genes for cell surface proteins that present antigens to T cells. The human version of MHC is referred to as *human leukocyte antigen* (HLA).

Mantoux test. Skin test for exposure to *Mycobacterium tuberculosis*.

Mast cell. Cells resident in tissues that are able to release granules during some types of infections.

Membrane attack complex (MAC). Final part of the complement cascade, capable of damaging cells or pathogens.

MHC polymorphism. Polymorphism refers to the existence of allelic alternatives, and the major histocompatibility complex (MHC) with a large number of allelic determinants is the most polymorphic locus known.

MHC restricted. T lymphocytes recognize antigen in association with major histocompatibility complex (MHC) class I or II molecules, and their antigen recognition is therefore said to be MHC restricted.

Molecular mimicry. Idea that infections may trigger autoimmunity when pathogen antigens cross-react with autoantigens.

Monoclonal. A population of B cells or T cells with identical immunoglobulin molecules or receptors. Monoclonal populations are often neoplastic.

Monoclonal antibody. A homogeneous immunoglobulin of defined specificity generally prepared using hybridoma technology for biomedical research, diagnostic use, or therapy.

Monocyte. Immature circulating macrophage.

Mucociliary escalator. Innate defense of the airways.

Mucosa-associated lymphoid tissue (MALT). Lymphoid tissue in the respiratory and gastrointestinal tracts that is enriched in immunoglobulin A–producing plasma cells and specialized epithelial cells, M cells, that take up antigen by pinocytosis.

Naïve lymphocyte. A lymphocyte that is mature but has not yet encountered the nonself antigen that it has specificity for.

Natural antibody. Immunoglobulin M antibody produced without previous exposure to antigen.

Natural killer (NK) cell. These large granular lymphocytes have two major roles: (1) to kill some virally infected cells, such as herpesvirus-infected cells, and (2) to help activate the adaptive immune response.

Negative selection. The deletion of lymphocytes capable of recognizing self antigen.

Nephritis. Kidney inflammation.

Neutralizing antibody. An antibody that impairs antigen function—for example, as a toxin or as a docking mechanism—without destroying the antigen.

Neutrophil. Short-lived phagocytic cell.

NKG2/CD94. Receptor on the surface of natural killer (NK) cells.

Opsonization. Particles that have been opsonized with either immunoglobulin or complement become targets for phagocytosis.

Oral tolerance. Suppression of an immune response to antigens that have previously been administered orally.

Osteoclast. Type of mature macrophage.

Oxidative burst. Production of toxic molecules by activated phagocytes.

Passive immunity. Transfer of effector components (eg, immunoglobulin, T cells) from one individual to another.

Pathogen. Disease-causing organism.

Pathogen-associated molecular patterns (PAMPs). Molecules associated with groups of organisms recognized by the innate immune system.

Pattern recognition molecules. Molecules of the innate immune system capable of recognizing molecules characteristic of infection, for example, double-stranded RNA and some sugars.

Perforin. A protein found in the granules of natural killer and cytotoxic T cells that can polymerize and form a pore in the membrane of target cells.

Periarteriolar lymphoid sheath (PALS). Concentric cuffs of lymphocytes (chiefly T cells) found around central arterioles in the spleen.

Peripheral tolerance. Tolerance induced in mature T or B cells in the nonlymphoid tissues.

Phage libraries. Collections of genetic sequences expressed in bacteriophages.

Phagocyte. Cells capable of engulfing and destroying particulate matter.

Plasma cell. Terminally differentiated B cell capable of secreting large quantities of immunoglobulin.

Polyclonal. A population of B cells or T cells that produces a complex mixture of immunoglobulin molecules or T-cell receptors.

Polygenic disorder. Disorder caused by a combination of several genetic and environmental factors.

Polymorphism. Slight genetic differences between members of a population. See Allele.

Positive selection. The ability of T cells to recognize self major histocompatibility complex with moderate affinity, and so they survive in the thymus.

Pre–B cell receptor (Pre-BCR). A light chain–like structure expressed transiently during B cell development.

Primary immunodeficiency. Immune deficiency caused by genetic defects.

Primary lymphoid organs. The organs in which lymphocytes are produced (the bone marrow and thymus in adult humans).

Prion. Infectious particle that contains no genetic sequences.

Prostaglandin. Mediator released from mast cells and eosinophils.

Proteosome. A cytoplasmically located complex of proteases involved in creating peptides that may bind to major histocompatibility complex class I molecules.

Pyogenic. Pus forming.

Receptor editing. The process in certain immature B cells of reinitiating V(D)/J rearrangement to attempt to alter the B-cell receptor specificity and create a receptor with no self-reactivity.

Rejection. Ability of the host immune response to destroy transplanted tissue.

Replicative senescence. Loss of ability to proliferate by aged lymphocytes.

Retrovirus. Virus that transcribes a DNA genomic sequence from an RNA template.

Reverse transcriptase. Enzyme capable of translating RNA to DNA.

Rhinitis. Nasal inflammation.

Secondary immunodeficiency. Immune deficiency caused by disease after birth.

Secondary lymphoid organs. The organs in which lymphocytes come into contact with antigen, clonally expand, and mature into effector cells (ie the spleen and lymph nodes).

Selectins. Family of adhesion proteins that bind sugars on the surface of cells, for example, to selectively attract the cells to specific tissues.

Self-restriction. Refers to T cells capable of recognizing antigen only if presented on self major histocompatibility complex molecules.

Septic (endotoxic) shock. Hypotension caused by exposure to substances released from bacteria.

Serum sickness. Disease caused by circulating immune complexes.

Skin prick testing. Test for allergy.

Somatic recombination. The process of gene segment rearrangement that occurs to create a repertoire of antigen receptors.

 MCH II

  Cytokine, chemokine, etc.

 Complement (C′)

 Signaling molecule

Spleen. A secondary lymphoid organ that functions as a filter for the blood and as the main site of immune responses to blood-borne antigens.

Subcapsular zone. An area of the thymus that contains the earliest progenitor thymocytes.

Subunit vaccine. Vaccine that uses parts of a pathogen.

Syngeneic transplant. Transplant between genetically identical individuals.

T-cell receptor (TCR). The receptor for antigen on T lymphocytes.

T-cell tolerance. Tolerance is the process of preventing the immune response to autoantigens. T cells are initially made tolerant to self antigens in the thymus, and only those T-cell receptors with appropriate specificity for self major histocompatibility complex and nonself peptides are selected.

TH1 cell. T-helper 1 cell; provides help for cytotoxic T cells, macrophages, and immunoglobulin G production.

TH2 cell. T-helper 2 cell; provides help for immunoglobulin E secretion and eosinophil activation.

Thymocytes. Progenitor T cells.

Thymus. A organ found in the anterior mediastinum that is responsible for T-cell development.

Thymus-dependent antigen. Antigen that requires B- and T-cell cooperation to produce an immune response.

Thymus-independent antigen. Antigens that can activate.

Tolerance. A state of unresponsiveness to molecules the immune system has the capacity to recognize and attack B cells without T-cell help (eg, certain common bacterial cell wall components such as lipopolysaccharide).

Transgenic mice. Genetically altered mice.

Tumor antigen. Antigen expressed on a tumor that is either absent or present at only very low levels on healthy cells.

Vasculitis. Inflammation of the blood vessels.

Viral latency. Part of a viral life cycle when there is no active replication or host cell damage.

Western blotting. An immunoblotting technique used to characterize complex mixtures of antigens biochemically.

Wild-type organism. Unaltered (native) organism used to manufacture vaccines.

Xenogeneic transplant. Transplant between members of different species.

 T-cell receptor (TCR)

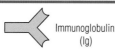 Immunoglobulin (Ig)

 Antigen

 MCH I

INDEX

Page numbers followed by "*f*" indicate figures, "*t*" indicate tables, and "*b*" indicate boxes.